W9-CJY-784

The Partnership Model in Human Services

Sociological Foundations and Practices

CLINICAL SOCIOLOGY
Research and Practice

SERIES EDITOR:

John G. Bruhn, *New Mexico State University*
Las Cruces, New Mexico

CLINICAL SOCIOLOGY: An Agenda for Action
John G. Bruhn and Howard M. Rebach

THE LIMITS OF IDEALISM: When Good Intentions Go Bad
Melvyn L. Fein

THE PARTNERSHIP MODEL IN HUMAN SERVICES: Sociological Foundations and Practices
Rosalyn Benjamin Darling

The Partnership Model in Human Services

Sociological Foundations and Practices

Rosalyn Benjamin Darling
Indiana University of Pennsylvania
Indiana, Pennsylvania

Kluwer Academic / Plenum Publishers
New York, Boston, Dordrecht, London, Moscow

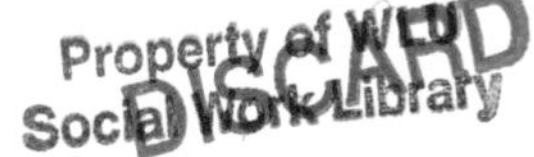

Library of Congress Cataloging-in-Publication Data

Darling, Rosalyn Benjamin.
The partnership model in human services: sociological foundations and practices/ Rosalyn Benjamin Darling.
p. cm.—(Clinical sociology)
Includes bibliographical references and index.
ISBN 0-306-46274-5 (alk. paper)
1. Social case work. 2. Clinical sociology. 3. Interviewing in social work. 4. Social work education. I. Title. II. Series.

HV43 .D2 2000
361.3—dc21

00-038632

ISBN 0-306-46274-5

233 Spring Street, New York, N.Y. 10013

http://www.wkap.nl/

10 9 8 7 6 5 4 3 2 1

A C.I.P. record for this book is available from the Library of Congress

Printed in the United States of America

For the newest Darlings:
my granddaughter Evelyn and
daughter-in-law Karen

Preface

Academic disciplines tend to develop separately. As a result, interdisciplinary work is not common and points of convergence between disciplines often are not recognized. This volume represents a synthesis of human service practice and the academic field of sociology. Although I was trained as an academic sociologist, I spent 15 years as the director of a human service agency. Frequently in my work at the agency, I saw parallels between sociological theory and methods and the helping process that I supervised.

As I began to read the journals of various helping professions and to participate in national associations of practitioners in these fields, I realized that the human service system was moving toward what I considered to be a sociological approach. When these professionals talked about becoming more client and family centered, the rhetoric they used sounded like the *Verstehen* tradition in sociology. They seemed to have independently discovered what sociologists had known all along: that individuals cannot be considered apart from their social contexts.

Because most of these practitioners had not been trained in sociology, they often "reinvented the wheel" and coined new terms for the concepts they thought they were inventing. In some cases, they did this very well. In others, their lack of sociological training resulted in versions that were not as well structured as their sociological counterparts. I began to realize that the systematic infusion of sociological knowledge into the helping professions would be valuable in guiding them in the new directions they were taking. Several years ago, I coauthored a volume for early childhood special educators on applications of sociology to their discipline. This volume has a broader focus in applying sociological theory and methods to the entire spectrum of human service work.

The volume developed out of a course I have been teaching for the past 6 years entitled Clinical Sociological Theory. The sociology majors at the university where I teach can select a clinical track, which requires a series of four courses—beginning in the junior year—in addition to other requirements. Clinical Sociological Theory is the first course in the clinical track sequence and is followed in order by Clinical Sociological Practice, an internship, and Social Change. The first two courses are taught primarily from a microperspective, with a focus on individuals and families. In the social change course, the focus shifts to the macrolevel. I designed this volume to serve as a text for both the clinical theory and clinical practice courses. In particular, the first five chapters are covered in the theory course, and the remaining chapters are covered in the practice course.

Although the primary audience for the book is upper-level undergraduate sociology students, I also have used the material successfully in a graduate course on sociological practice. In addition, I believe that it would be useful to professionals practicing in the human service field, especially those without backgrounds in sociology who are trying to align their practices with the newer client- and family-centered partnership models.

The volume is organized into three parts. Part I, entitled Background and Theoretical Foundations, includes four chapters. The first, "The Partnership Approach: A Sociological Model of Practice," indicates the parallels between sociological theory and methods and the new partnership approach in human services. The second chapter documents the shift to a partnership approach in a variety of fields, including education, social work, mental health and mental retardation services, medicine, and police work. The last two chapters in Part I provide the theoretical foundations for the practice model described in the rest of the volume. The first of these chapters presents some concepts from sociological theories of social structure that are especially relevant to human service work. The second theoretical chapter discusses social process and shows how client–professional interaction reflects the tenets of symbolic interaction theory.

Part II is entitled The Client's Social World and Methods for Discovering It. The first chapter in this part shows how clients' worldviews are shaped by their locations in society in relation to their gender, social class, race, and ethnicity. The remaining chapters in this part present methods for identifying clients' resources, concerns, and priorities. Identification is the first step in the partnership model of human service practice.

The final part of the volume, Models of Intervention and Evaluation, includes two chapters on intervention, which is the second step in the practice model. The first of these chapters discusses microlevel interventions with individuals and families, and the second describes mesolevel interventions to change service systems. The last chapter presents the final step in the model, service evaluation.

A number of people assisted in the development of the ideas in this book. I would like to thank John Bruhn and an unknown reviewer for many helpful suggestions relating to the organization of the material and the clarity of the writing. In addition, Harry Perlstadt provided valuable comments that resulted in a more focused discussion of levels of intervention and a much improved chapter on service evaluation. I also would like to thank Christine Baxter, my coauthor of the previously mentioned textbook for early childhood special educators; her contributions to that volume provided the basis for many of the ideas in the techniques chapters. Mike Fleischer suggested the parallel between the partnership model and grounded theory. I also want to acknowledge the assistance of Eliot Werner,

Executive Editor at Kluwer Academic/Plenum Publishers, whose patience during a lengthy writing and review process I greatly appreciated. Anne Meagher, Production Editor at Kluwer Academic/Plenum, was extremely conscientious in helping me bring the publication process to a successful conclusion. I am grateful to Jeff Himes and Larry Metts, who prepared the Index. The students I have taught at Indiana University of Pennsylvania during the past 6 years also have played a role in the volume's development by reacting to, and thus helping me to refine, the ideas it contains. Finally, I want to thank my husband, Jon. A major book project always takes time and energy away from family life and cannot be accomplished without patience, understanding, and support.

I hope that this volume will reward the efforts of the people who helped make it possible by contributing significantly to the education of students who plan to work in the human service field. I hope, too, that the partnership model that the volume espouses will result in a more humane and effective human service delivery system for the many clients who, like most people, need some help in confronting a society in which opportunities are inequitably distributed.

Contents

I. BACKGROUND AND THEORETICAL FOUNDATIONS

II. THE CLIENT'S SOCIAL WORLD AND METHODS FOR DISCOVERING IT

I

Background and Theoretical Foundations

1

The Partnership Approach
A Sociological Model of Practice

The human services have been undergoing some significant changes. In the past, the helping professions were based on a *status inequality model*, which tended to value the practitioner's perspective more than the client's; as a result, recommended interventions did not always appropriately address client concerns. More recently, a *partnership* model has become the norm in a variety of human service fields. In this model, the client's point of view is valued and serves as the basis for service delivery. This volume will suggest that the partnership model has much in common with a sociological perspective, especially one based on the principle of *Verstehen*. This principle, which derives from the work of Max Weber and emphasizes the importance of *understanding* the people being studied, has guided much sociological inquiry during the last 100 years. The remainder of this chapter will suggest some connections between partnership-based practice in human services and sociological theory and methods.

The infusion of the sociological perspective into the helping professions has important implications for the theory and practice of human service delivery. One model that has long driven the human services has focused on defining the individual in need of help as the source of the problem. The practitioner's task, in this model, is to change the individual, to adjust the individual to society, or to bring the individual into line with more normative standards. The sociological perspective, on the other hand, links individuals with social structures and recognizes that individuals and their behaviors are expressions of their social worlds, that is, their cultural and family backgrounds and the settings within which they regularly interact. This perspective suggests that practitioners must look more closely at the social worlds of service users in planning interventions. Ultimately, practitioners may need to make efforts to restructure society itself in order to address their clients' concerns.

The sociological perspective refers to the application of the theories and methods of sociology. The key sociological concepts that will be used in this book are *definition of the situation* and *opportunity structure*. For human service delivery, the application of the sociological perspective asserts that before they can help their clients service providers need to understand clients' definitions of the situation, or the clients' understanding of the problem, their priorities and resources, and their understanding of their encounters with the helping professional. The perspective also means recognition that interactions between service providers and service users create a new social system based on a client–professional partnership in which both parties make significant contributions to service outcomes. This model rejects the idea of professional as expert who dictates to the client and requires compliance.

Further, the sociological perspective emphasizes the need for practitioners to understand their clients' social worlds and to make social change the goal of service provision. Consequently, professionals work to change their clients' situations by adding resources to their opportunity structures in order to help clients gain access to the means to achieve the outcomes they define. Finally, this practice model includes the application of the methods of sociologists, including observation, interviewing, questionnaire development and administration, and social systems analysis. These principles and methods will be explained further, applied, and illustrated throughout this volume.

The *Verstehen* Approach in Sociology

A partnership model of practice, which is firmly rooted in sociological tradition, and especially in the *Verstehen* tradition, centers on an understanding of actors' meanings. In the early 1900s, Weber wrote:

> Sociology . . . is a science which attempts the interpretive understanding [*Verstehen*] of social action in order thereby to arrive at a causal explanation of its course and effects. In "action" is included all human behaviour when and in so far as the acting individual attaches a subjective meaning to it. . . .
>
> . . . In no case does [meaning] refer to an objectively "correct" meaning or one which is "true" in some metaphysical sense. It is this which distinguishes the empirical sciences of action, such as sociology and history, from the dogmatic disciplines in that area, . . . which seek to ascertain the "true" and "valid" meanings associated with the objects of their investigation. . . .
>
> . . . For the verifiable accuracy of interpretation of the meaning of a phenomenon, it is a great help to be able to put one's self imaginatively in the place of the actor and thus sympathetically to participate in his experiences . . .
>
> . . . Empathetic or appreciative accuracy is attained when, through sympathetic participation, we can adequately grasp the emotional context in which the action took place. (Parsons, 1947, pp. 88–91)

Weber goes on to suggest that people who share similar values will be better able to understand each other's meanings.

Meanings are learned through a process of *socialization* in a social context. Both the client and the professional emerge from social contexts. The client has a gender and is a member of a social class and of racial and ethnic groups, which shape his or her view of the world. Similarly, professionals operate within a social context that includes agency structure, educational background, and other determinants of their perspectives in addition to their own gender, social class, and racial and ethnic backgrounds. Professionals who understand both their clients' social contexts and their own can help develop more realistic solutions to their clients' problems. Moreover, a *Verstehen* approach implies that, because meaning is relative to one's social situation, the views of the professional are different from but not better or more correct than those of the client. This implication supports a partnership approach in which client and professional are viewed as equally important members of a problem-solving team.

In sociology, the *Verstehen* approach has traditionally been applied to research. Researchers using this approach work to understand their subjects' subjective meanings in a nonjudgmental way. I will suggest in this volume that the approach is equally appropriate for human service practice and is especially supportive of a partnership model.

The following sections will present an overview of the partnership model that will serve as the basis for the remaining chapters of this volume. In addition, they will suggest the similarities between this model and other currents in sociological thinking, including clinical sociological approaches and the philosophy of grounded theory. The final section will discuss a related approach in social work and suggest that sociology can provide it with a theoretical and methodological basis.

The Parntership Approach

Figure 1.1 presents the partnership approach to human service practice as a process that begins with the client's opportunity structure and ends with service evaluation. A review of this process will introduce the material to be presented in later chapters.

Before the client and professional meet for the first time, each has had experiences determined by the social structure within which each resides. The professional's background includes educational and work experience, along with the experiences that result from being a member of certain racial, ethnic, socioeconomic, gender, age, religious, and other groups. Similarly, the client belongs to a variety of groups and may have had previous experience in the human service system.

Because the partnership approach is based on an understanding of the *client's* structural constraints and resources, the starting point in the helping process is the client's opportunity structure. This concept, which is based in structural–functional theory in sociology, will be explained in detail in Chapter 3. Certain principles are inherent in an opportunity–structure based model:

- *Opportunities are not equally distributed in society*. Large amounts of data support the knowledge that some groups in society have more power and advantages than others. Some of the bases for social inequality include gender, social class, race, and ethnicity. Weber, Marx, and other sociologists have developed theories to explain social inequality.

- *Understanding the client's location in the social structure is more useful than trying to attribute blame for the client's problem.* Although the motivations of individuals affect their social situations, all behavior occurs within a social context that places limits on available alternatives. Karuza,

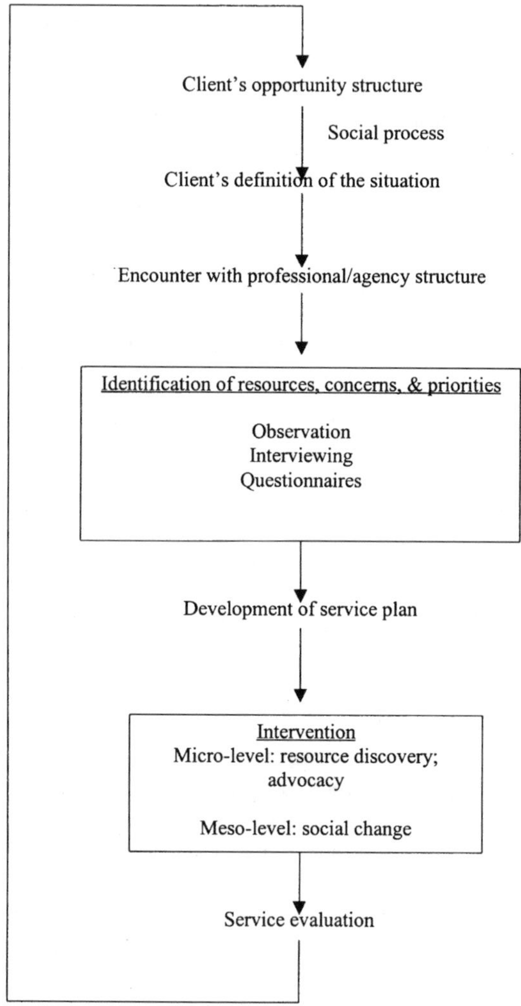

Figure 1.1. The process of partnership-based practice.

Zevon, Rabinowitz, and Brickman (1982) and others suggest that most (status inequality) models of helping attribute responsibility to the client. The helping process then involves an attempt to convince the client of the correctness of the model. The inappropriateness and often futility of such an approach will be explained in Chapter 2.

- *An understanding of the organizational context is essential in helping relationships.* As will be discussed in Chapter 3, the outcome of the client–professional encounter will be determined at least in part by both the structural conditions in the client's life and the organization of the helping agency. Organizational forms such as bureaucracy may limit the possibility of helpful interactions with professionals. Crandall and Allen (1982) note other organizational variables, such as role definition, role conflict, and organizational demands, that can influence the outcome of helping relationships.

The concept of definition of the situation is based in symbolic interactionist theory in sociology, which will be discussed in Chapter 4. A client's definition of the situation will derive in large measure from his or her opportunity structure. Clients with limited opportunities resulting from poverty or other structural conditions generally are aware of these limitations and are interested in improving their life situations. In a partnership approach, the professional accepts the client's definition as valid for the purpose of providing help. This acceptance is based on the assumption that:

- *Most clients are acting in their own best interest.* Although the client's definition of the situation might not match the professional's, it is the appropriate starting point for interaction. In most instances, professionals who try to impose a different definition on their clients are not likely to meet with success. Although some clients are ordered to receive services by the courts or are coerced into receiving services by family members or authority figures, most human service clients seek help voluntarily. At the outset, then, their definitions of the situation include an acceptance of the efficacy of the help-seeking process.
- *Client empowerment is necessary for eliciting the client's definition of the situation.* As DePaulo (1982) and others have noted, client definitions may include notions of inadequacy because our society values independence and the ability to help oneself. The result is a potential power imbalance, in which the professional is likely to control the interaction that ensues. In a partnership approach, professionals need to convince their clients that their experiences and resulting perspectives are valid and important, in an attempt to equalize the power in the relationship. Otherwise, clients may be reluctant to reveal their true definitions.

After an empowerment-based rapport has been established between the client and professional, the professional can proceed to learn as much as possible about the client's opportunity structure, which, as Chapter 5 will suggest, is related to the client's socioeconomic and cultural background. This learning process involves the identification of the client's resources, concerns, and priorities.

In Chapters 6, 7, and 8, three identification methods will be presented: observation, interviewing, and questionnaires. The purpose of these methods is to help the professional understand the client's social world, including his or her resources and concerns in the areas of information, material support, informal support, and formal support. In order to be effective, the professional must come to know as much as possible about the opportunities (resources) available to the client, as well as the client's perception of a lack of or limitations in opportunities (concerns). In addition, the professional needs to understand which concerns are priorities for the client.

The result of the identification process is a service plan. This plan, which serves as a contract between the professional and the client, lists a series of actions that will produce desired outcomes. The ultimate goal of the service plan is to expand the client's opportunity structure.

Intervention strategies for expanding opportunities may occur at the micro- or mesolevel. Most human service programs operate on a microlevel. Partnership-based practitioners engage in activities to aid their clients in resource discovery when opportunities already exist and in advocacy to expand opportunities in the client's family or community when existing opportunities are inadequate. Sometimes, though, client concerns are just the individualized expression of communitywide social problems. In these cases, human service professionals may need to engage in mesolevel activities to bring about social change. Some social problems, though, are societal in scope. As Chapter 10 will suggest, human services are not designed to create macrolevel change.

Finally, professionals need to evaluate their efforts. In a partnership approach, evaluation is based on client perceptions regarding expanded opportunities. Chapter 11 will present methods for eliciting those perceptions. Because evaluation results are used to increase opportunities, the process is circular, ending where it began—with the client's opportunity structure.

The Partnership Model and Sociological Practice

The sociological tradition includes approaches that stress theory and related empirical research, as well as an approach that has come to be called sociological practice. In sociological practice, theory and research are used in the solution of social problems. The idea that sociology could be used for the betterment of society can be traced to Auguste Comte, the 19th-century French sociologist who argued that sociological research would lead to the discovery of universal social laws, the application of which would produce social progress.

In the United States, Comte's thesis was refined by Lester Frank Ward, who distinguished between "pure," or theoretical, sociology and "applied" sociology. Applied sociology would involve "social telesis," or the use of sociological knowledge for the improvement of society (Barnes, 1948). Because of the work of Ward and others, one of the principles of early American sociology was "melioristic intervention" (Hinkle & Hinkle, 1954). This principle suggested that sociologists had an obligation to use their knowledge to bring about social reform. Not all American sociologists accepted this approach (a notable early exception was William Graham Sumner), and some suggested that sociology should be simply an academic discipline and that sociologists should not impose their views on government. However, the applied tradition has continued to exist as an important thread in sociological thinking throughout the history of American sociology.

Over time, the term "applied" has come to characterize the work of sociologists who engage in research to improve society. At the same time, another group of sociologists has worked to use theory and research to intervene in people's lives on the individual, group, and societal levels. This latter practice is generally called "clinical sociology." The American Sociological Association includes both applied and clinical sociology within the category of sociological practice.

The subject matter of this volume could be characterized as clinical sociology, and the partnership model outlined above is entirely compatible with the principles of clinical sociology presented by Bruhn and Rebach (1996). In their text, which is the most comprehensive recent treatment in this field, these authors define clinical sociology as "active intervention that is rooted in the perspectives, theory, and methods of sociology" (Bruhn & Rebach, 1996, p. 2). They note further that "clinical sociology is active, humanistic, and change oriented" (p. 2). These statements clearly describe the partnership model of practice.

Bruhn and Rebach (1996) use the concept of "the sociological spectrum" to describe the range of interventions that can occur through clinical intervention. This spectrum involves a "macro–micro continuum" (Bruhn & Rebach, 1996, p. 6). Macrolevel interventions attempt to change world and national systems and large corporate structures. Mesolevel interventions focus on smaller corporate structures and secondary and primary groups. Finally, microlevel interventions attempt to change individuals. In this volume, microlevel interventions will be addressed in Chapter 9 and will describe efforts to change the immediate social structures of individuals, that is, their families, neighborhoods, schools, and work environments. This usage is a little broader than Bruhn and Rebach's. Mesolevel approaches, which will be discussed in Chapter 10, will address activities such as grant writing and political action that are designed to change community-, state-, and occasionally, national-level service systems. I have adopted Bruhn and

Rebach's usage of macrolevel and use it to refer to interventions at the societal level that are usually beyond the purview of traditional human service approaches.

Bruhn and Rebach note that human behavior is influenced by biological, psychological, and social factors. They offer the example of substance use during pregnancy, in which health (biological) is affected, along with the ability to cope with the responsibilities of motherhood (psychological) and the individual's relationship with family members, employers, and others (social). No single perspective can address all the issues involved. However, the sociological perspective adds a necessary element that is not present in other explanatory approaches: the importance of social interaction in shaping an actor's (client's) perceptions and actions. While recognizing the validity of other perspectives for explaining some aspects of human behavior, this volume focuses exclusively on the contribution of the sociological perspective.

The model of the client–professional relationship suggested by Bruhn and Rebach (1996) also is consistent with the partnership approach being advocated here. They write,

> A model of status inequality—professionals (high status) dictating to clients (low status)—in most instances will fail. To be effective, working relationships must be democratic in character, and clients' autonomy, ability to problem-solve, and to make choices must be respected. (p. 22)

This statement supports the principle stated earlier that clients are assumed to be acting in their own best interest.

Bruhn and Rebach (1996) state that "intervention proceeds through four functional stages: assessment, program planning, program implementation, and program evaluation" (p. 22). These stages mirror the processes of identification, plan development, intervention, and service evaluation described in this volume. They suggest that assessment begins with recognizing the client's "presenting problem" or "the client's statement of the problem as they see it, and is framed in their own words" (p. 22). This client-centered view is entirely consistent with the approach to be taken throughout this volume.

Bruhn and Rebach (1996, pp. 24–25) also suggest a series of ethical guidelines for clinical practice, which are completely consistent with the partnership approach:

- Do no harm. This guideline includes the principles of not going beyond the scope of one's professional expertise and being accountable for the outcomes of intervention.
- Respect people's autonomy and their right of self-determination. This guideline implies a professional–client relationship that is a partnership between equals.

- Respect people's right to confidentiality. [This guideline is sometimes waived in cases of potential danger to a client or others (e.g., a client who threatens violence). Such exception will be discussed further in Chapter 6.]

Respecting clients' rights to autonomy and self-determination is the cornerstone of the partnership approach. Bruhn and Rebach trace this approach to the psychotherapist, Carl Rogers, who used the term "client centered" as early as 1951. Their description of this approach provides a good summary of the perspective:

> Though you will eventually focus on a problem, you must see the client as someone who has strengths and resources that must be acknowledged and learned about. The person also has a history, is a member of various social systems, and has roles and interacts within them. The person is striving to be effective and solve problems, is striving for positive social relationships within social contexts, and is striving to maintain dignity, a positive definition of self, and to have some control over life. The person also has a range of feelings, values, expectations, and goals. (Bruhn & Rebach, 1996, pp. 75–76)

In the field of social work today, the term "client centered" is commonly used to describe a partnership model similar to the one being presented in this volume.

Sociological intervention, according to Bruhn and Rebach, can be separated into four phases: selection, process, outcome, and follow-up. Selection involves a determination of value compatibility between professional and client. However, compatibility does not imply congruence. Although professionals should not work with clients whose values they cannot accept, training in a partnership approach should include skill development in the areas of accepting diversity and being nonjudgmental. Narrow-minded people do not make good partners.

The process phase concerns the development of rapport. Bruhn and Rebach discuss techniques such as reflection, legitimation, support, and respect. These techniques are similar to methods for establishing rapport to be discussed in the technique chapters of this volume.

The outcome phase involves the actions taken by the professional to bring about change. Bruhn and Rebach note that helping relationships extend along a continuum from information giving to counseling and psychotherapy. The intervention methods suggested in this volume clearly fall along the information giving end of the continuum. Sociological expertise tends to produce cognitive rather than affective kinds of assistance. Psychological interventions, on the other hand, sometimes tend more toward affective change.

Bruhn and Rebach suggest that follow-up is perhaps the most neglected aspect of intervention. As Chapter 11 will note, assuring the efficacy of service delivery is essential. Evaluation can be incorporated into the process of intervention itself or can be conducted after services have been terminated to determine whether desired outcomes have been achieved.

Finally, Bruhn and Rebach note that sociologists have not always been successful in marketing their intervention skills. For most of the 20th century, the helping professions have been dominated by the fields of medicine, social work, and psychology. As this volume will show, sociological knowledge includes a wealth of relevant information for the helping professions.

The Partnership Model and Grounded Theory

The partnership model to be presented in this volume also converges in some ways with the grounded theory approach promoted by Glaser and Strauss (1967). Although this approach was intended to guide research, its basic principles are similar to those of intervention based on partnership. Glaser and Strauss argue that some research needs to precede rather than follow theory, because theory must be grounded in actual social life.

Grounded theory must be credible, plausible, and trustworthy (Glaser & Strauss, 1967, p. 223). In other words, it must fit the facts. Glaser and Strauss suggest that a theory should be understandable to the people who work in the substantive area it purports to explain. They advocate qualitative research as the best means of coming to understand an area of social life in order to extrapolate explanatory principles and concepts. Further, they suggest that the resulting theory can be applied in the improvement of social relationships. To illustrate this application process, they argue that a knowledge of the theory of awareness contexts (see Chapter 4) by medical professionals can result in improvements in the quality of their interactions with dying patients.

Glaser and Strauss contend that insights into social life develop from experience, either one's own or that of others. In partnership-based practice, the professional's insights must come from the client's experience. Often, professionals can build on insights developed over the course of their careers, as a result of their interactions with many clients. Yet, each new client presents a unique set of circumstances. Thus, the identification techniques presented in this volume are essential to the development of a more complete understanding of the client's situation.

In a sense, human service practitioners are like grounded theorists. They continually revise and refine their theories as they encounter new clients whose experiences do not exactly fit the facts of past experience. Interventions are applications of the professional's current understanding of the client's situation. For example, the identification process may reveal that a client's greatest concern is obtaining health care for an aging family member. The professional may provide information about a clinic in a neighboring city that has provided satisfactory services to previous clients. However, the family member in question may refuse to leave the house. The professional will then have to revise his or her thinking and consider home-based alternatives. The resulting "theory of intervention" to be used with future clients in similar situations might include the corollary that "treatment settings need to be individualized to the client," which, in turn, might result in the more general principle that the client's definition of the situation must be taken into account.

The primary basis for convergence between grounded theory and partnership-based practice is that experience matters. Just as theory that is not empirically grounded is not very useful in explaining social life, human service practice that derives from unrealistic theoretical approaches is not very helpful to clients. This lack of grounding can explain some of the failure of status inequality approaches that have been popular in the human service field. The starting point of the helping process must be the client's social situation and experience.

The Structural Approach in Social Work

Chapter 2 will illustrate how human services, including social work, education, health care, law enforcement, and other fields, have experienced a shift during the past decades from a status inequality service model to a more partnership-based approach. Practitioners in a variety of helping professions have recognized that client–professional relationships based on partnership rather than professional dominance are generally more productive. What has been lacking in this shift is a comprehensive theoretical and methodological basis.

The structural approach in social work (Wood & Middleman, 1989) is a good example of a practice model based on partnership that does not acknowledge a debt to sociological theory. Wood and Middleman write:

> In contrast to other orientations to practice that may aim to help individuals adjust to their situations, to understand their motivations, to gain insight, or to change their ways of thinking and acting, the structural approach aims to modify the environment to the needs of the individuals. (1989, pp. 12–13)

They go on to state that environmental causes need to be explored first, before making assumptions about individual pathology. Based on this perspective, they argue that the social worker's role is "to help people connect with needed resources" and "to change social structures where existing ones limit human functioning and it is feasible to change them" (p. 28).

Wood and Middleman (1989) argue further that a primary guiding principle in social work should be accountability to the client. They write:

> The client, with the help of the worker, describes the pressures on him . . . , and these pressures, in turn, define the task to be accomplished. . . . When a task acceptable to both client and worker has been determined, the worker defines the way in which she will help the client accomplish it. (p. 36)

This approach clearly reflects a partnership orientation to service planning.

The structural approach relates further to the process in Fig. 1.1 in its treatment of situations in which microlevel interventions are not sufficient:

> The demand that the worker consistently look beyond the client to see if others are suffering in relation to the same phenomenon translates the essence of a structural approach to social work—meeting social needs through social change—into actual practice behavior. (Wood & Middleman, 1989, p. 41)

Although their approach is clearly compatible with a sociological perspective, the authors do not use sociological theory as the basis for their arguments. Rather, they cite ideological and practice precedents in the field of social work itself. Although these suggest the historical roots of their work, they do not help to explain *why* their approach is better than others in the field.

The methodological sections of their book also would benefit from a systematic exploration of various methods for identifying client concerns. Although they state that "clients tend to be the best consultants about their own pains and needs" (Wood & Middleman, 1989, p. 70), they rely primarily on interviewing as the means for learning what clients want and need. Their discussion of social change on a larger scale would similarly be improved by an exploration of methods such as needs assessment. In general, the systematic application of sociological methods would strengthen the practice aspects of their approach.

The Contribution of Sociological Theory and Methods

This volume will provide a theoretical and methodological framework for the newer partnership approaches in human services, including the structural approach in social work described above. As noted earlier, the *Verstehen* strand in sociology provides a philosophical basis for understanding clients on their own terms. In Chapter 3, structural theory in sociology will be used as a basis for understanding the constraints that both clients and professionals face. Chapter 4 will use symbolic interaction theory to explain how clients' and professionals' understandings develop in the course of their interactions with each other and with others in their social worlds. Together, these theoretical strands can help professionals understand their clients' lives and make sense of their clients' views of the world.

Sociological methods also provide an important contribution to a partnership approach, in which practitioners need to understand their clients' points of view. The methods of observation, interviewing, and questionnaire development and administration, which were originally developed for research purposes, can be applied equally well to human service practice. These methods were designed to get as much information as possible from research subjects, but within a context of respect for diversity. As Chapters 6, 7, and 8 will show, these methods are ideally suited for partnership practice in the human services.

Although all human service practitioners need not be trained as sociologists, two principles for professional socialization in the human services are suggested by the discussion above:

1. The incorporation of sociological content into the training programs of other professions is important.
2. Because of their special expertise, sociologists should be employed as human service practitioners in greater numbers than they have in the past.

The first of these principles may be easier to implement than the second. The recognition of the value of sociological knowledge is, at least in part, a matter of marketing. In the past, sociologists have not done a very good job of promoting their knowledge and skills. Although many medical schools today include sociologists on their faculties and require sociology courses of their students, sociologists are still rare in schools of education and social work.

Both the scarcity of sociologists in preprofessional programs and the absence of sociologists from some areas of human service practice are related to the issue of credentialing. Many states have restricted human service practice to individuals with licenses in fields such as social work or psychology. In part, these restrictions are the result of organized lobbying by those disciplines. The advent of managed care and other forms of service control also has contributed to practice restrictions. Although sociologists have been developing their own credentials (e.g., a certification in clinical sociology), these have not been widely recognized.

Sometimes credentials of any kind can interfere with the provision of partnership-based services. In the early intervention agency I directed, for example, a licensed social worker was employed to assist families of children with disabilities in identifying their resources, concerns, and priorities. She was very competent and caring and related well to the families in the program. However, her personal experience did not include parenting a child with a disability. This social worker, who believed firmly in the value of partnership, suggested that we employ a parent whose child had been in the program to assist with the identification process. She thought that parents would be able to relate better to someone who had shared their experience.

I subsequently hired a parent who was a former client to make home visits to current program clients. This parent, whose own child with autism was progressing nicely in a preschool program, was able to offer support to parents of younger children. In addition, clients felt comfortable sharing their concerns with someone who could "really understand." On the annual client satisfaction survey, many parents commented about the helpfulness of this employee.

However, when our agency attempted to bill for the services provided by this nonprofessional "family service worker," the public funding agency refused to pay. "Social work" services, we were told, could only be provided by a licensed social worker. Interestingly, this state also endorsed the principles of "family-centered" early intervention, based on a partnership model. In this case, the managed care environment created a conflict between acknowledged best practice and bureaucratic requirements.

Partnership-based practice requires flexibility. Services that are valuable and meaningful to one client may not be valuable or meaningful to another. Client advocates should oppose strict credentialism and other practices based on status inequality when those practices are not in the best interest of the people they serve.

Client advocacy is not a new idea. However, typically it has not been promulgated in the context of a complete model of practice theory and methods. This volume provides such a context. By situating partnership-based practice within a sociological framework, this volume attempts to ground such practice in a knowledge base that offers it a logical home.

Chapter Summary

This chapter has introduced the concept of partnership-based practice in human services and suggested its congruence with a sociological perspective. The partnership approach shares a philosophical basis with the *Verstehen*, clinical, and grounded theory strands in sociology, and students of this approach would benefit from an understanding of the sociological concepts of opportunity structure and definition of the situation. In addition, sociological methods, including observation, interviewing, and questionnaire development and administration, are useful in helping practitioners identify their clients' resources, concerns, and priorities. The chapter concludes by suggesting that sociological theory and methods be incorporated into training programs for human service practitioners.

Suggestions for Further Reading

Bruhn, J.G., & Rebach, H.M. (1996). *Clinical sociology: An agenda for action.* New York: Plenum Press.

Wood, G.G., & Middleman, R.R. (1989). *The structural approach to direct practice in social work: A textbook for students and front-line practitioners.* New York: Columbia University Press.

2

Changing Practices in Human Services

The previous chapter suggested that sociology is relevant to practice in human services. This relevance has increased as services have moved from a status inequality model to a partnership model in recent years. This chapter will explain and document this shift and show how it applies to a variety of human service fields.

During the period from the 1940s through the 1970s, practitioners of the helping professions focused primarily on changing individuals in order to aid them in adjusting to society. During the 1980s, a shift in emphasis occurred. Practitioners in fields as diverse as social work, psychology, medicine, and education began to look more closely at the perspective of service users and at restructuring some aspects of society to address their concerns. These emphases on understanding diverse perspectives and on social change to accommodate those perspectives have long been principles guiding research and theory in the field of sociology. Thus, in some ways, the helping professions are becoming more sociological. At the present time, then, sociological practitioners are positioned to make important contributions to thinking and practice in the human services.

An Illustrative Study: Parents of Children with Mild Mental Retardation

The sociological perspective to be used in this volume can be illustrated by a study done by Jane Mercer in the early 1960s (Mercer, 1965). Mercer was interested in why some parents of children with mild mental retardation insisted on removing their children from an institutional treatment setting, while other parents found the same placement to be appropriate for their children. After interviewing these parents, she concluded that the major difference between the two groups of parents was socioeconomic. Parents of higher status seemed to approve of the placement, while lower-status parents disapproved.

Her interviews suggested a reason for this difference. Among families of lower socioeconomic status (SES), mild mental retardation was not defined as a form of deviance. Because many individuals in this population group did not achieve educational and occupational success, the achievement levels of individuals limited by slightly lower IQ scores were not significantly different from the community norm. On the other hand, in the upper classes, where educational and occupational achievement were more common, and thus more highly valued, children who were not able to succeed in college and career were more likely to be labeled as deviant and to be an embarrassment to their families. Consequently, upper-SES parents found institutional placement to be appropriate for their children who could not play a valued role in the community. Parental attitudes, then, were determined more by their social situation than by their children's mental status, as measured by an IQ test.

In this case, the parents' attitudes sometimes came into conflict with those of the professionals working in the institution. These professionals had what Mercer calls a clinical perspective; that is, they believed that their tests provided an appropriate measure of deviant behavior. To them, a score below a certain level indicated that a child would benefit from institutional treatment. Thus, upper-SES parents tended to support the professionals' perspective, while lower-status parents tended to reject it. This conflict in perspectives is illustrative of many similar conflicts that have occurred in other areas of the human services when professionals have not understood their clients' views of the world. Thus, Mercer's model is useful in understanding the shift in thinking that has been taking place in fields as diverse as health care, education, social work, and mental health services.

The Status Inequality Perspective

The status inequality perspective (what Mercer calls the "clinical" perspective) characterized most human service practice in the decades preceding the 1980s. Mercer suggests that this perspective is defined by the following components (all terms used are hers):

- *The development of a diagnostic nomenclature.* Professionals typically determine appropriate treatments on the basis of a set of diagnostic categories. These categories vary by discipline. For example, physicians and other health care providers use the International Classification of Diseases (ICD), which includes labels such as "unspecified anomaly of the respiratory system," "congenital hydrocephalus," and "blindness, unspecified"; mental health professionals use the Diagnostic and Statistical Manual (DSM), which lists conditions such as, "organic delusional syndrome," "separation anxiety disorder," and "paranoid schizophrenia"; professionals in special education have used a series of categories, including "trainable mentally retarded," "socially/emotionally disturbed," and "visually impaired," among others; legal professionals have used the criminal code; and so forth.

Although these categories are treated as though they are objective and empirically based, they appear to be somewhat arbitrary and subject to change. For example, "borderline mental retardation" has been eliminated as a category from the DSM, as has homosexuality [see Kirk and Kutchins (1992, pp. 81–90) for a discussion of the political context of the elimination of the homosexuality category]. Changes in professional views of homosexuality seem to reflect changes in lay conceptions, and what was once regarded as a disease is now seen as a lifestyle difference. On the other hand, alcohol-related behaviors that might have been regarded as crimes during Prohibition are now more likely to be viewed as diseases, and drug addiction, which was once socially acceptable in certain circles, is now seen as a disease as well. Many cases of label change appear to be related to a trend toward the "medicalization" of society. As Conrad and Schneider (1980) and others have suggested, illness is more socially acceptable than badness: Parents who are embarrassed by a child who is a "school failure" are likely to encounter sympathy after their child has been relabeled as "learning disabled." Kirk and Kutchins (1992) further note that deliberate misdiagnosis commonly occurs to help clients avoid a stigmatizing label or to help them obtain needed services. Similarly, Daniels (1978) shows how in the military psychiatrists use their diagnostic power to assist either their patients or the system in achieving certain ends. She concludes, "The categories that the psychiatrist uses do not exist in a vacuum. . . . the construction of psychiatric reality may be almost entirely social" (p. 391). Thus, although such labels may be useful in certain contexts, their basis in empirical reality is questionable.

- *The creation of diagnostic instruments.* Service users are placed in diagnostic categories on the basis of their performance on standardized tests, such as IQ tests, or through generally accepted assessment techniques. The use of these techniques is generally part of the preprofessional curriculum in medical schools, graduate programs in psychology, and other training milieus.
- *The professionalization of the diagnostic function.* Professionals such as physicians and psychologists, then, become the gatekeepers of the human service system. They are believed to be the only ones who are qualified to determine whether or not a client is in need of services. Related to this principle is the concept of professional dominance (Freidson, 1970b). Freidson argues that, in the field of medicine in particular, the patient or client is expected to defer to the authority of the physician or professional. To some degree in all human service fields, professionals maintain control over their clients because of their perceived expertise, based on their training and experience.
- *The assumption that the professional is right.* Mercer (1965) argues, "if persons in other social systems . . . do not concur with official findings . . . , the

clinical perspective assumes they are either unenlightened or are evidencing psychological denial" (pp. 19–20).

- *Services are designed to change the individual or the individual's family.* As a result of the diagnostic process, individuals or families acquire labels, as noted above. These labels then determine the treatment methods that will be employed. The medical model of acute illness is the most familiar one: An individual acquires a disease; the doctor prescribes medication; the individual takes the prescribed medicine and becomes well. The assumption in this model is that the pathology rests in the individual. Thus, the cure involves "doing something" to the individual to eliminate the pathological condition. This model also provides the basis for much of the counseling that occurs in the mental health field and the teaching that is done in the field of education.

  In a discussion similar to Mercer's, Batson, O'Quin, and Pych (1982) describe the dispositional bias that causes some professionals to "infer that a client's problem lies with the client as a person even when it is really due to some aspect of the client's situation" (p. 60). They cite studies by Goffman, Rosenhan, and others in which mental illness is *assumed* to be present in those being presented for admission to mental hospitals. Some of the sources of this bias include (1) information from third-party sources, (2) assessments done in clinical rather than natural settings, (3) training in the medical model, (4) concern with protecting society, and (5) the ready availability of clinical treatment modalities.

This status inequality perspective served as the basis for service provision in most human service areas during a large portion of the 20th century. Sometimes, it led to successful treatments and cures. Certainly, the health status of people around the world has improved dramatically as a result of various medical and surgical interventions based on this model. Diagnostic categories are useful when they point the way toward effective intervention. On the other hand, the status inequality model has failed miserably in treating some problems. Social workers have been counseling poor people for years but have not succeeded in eliminating poverty by this method. Similarly, programs for the rehabilitation of drug addicts, juvenile delinquents, and adult criminals have experienced frustratingly high rates of recidivism. Even in the field of medicine, established treatment regimens do not always work.

Failed attempts at intervention are often the result of a poor understanding of the nature of a problem. Although some pathologies do rest within individuals, often the source of a problem is external to the individual and the family. With respect to early education programs for poor children, Bowman (1992) has written,

> [M]any of us who work in poverty communities believe that we can and should be able to change the developmental outcomes of children in these profoundly depriving envi-

> ronments. But success is limited and burnout is rampant. . . . The truth of the matter is that trying to cure sociological problems with treatments aimed at the intrapsychic organizations of individuals is counterproductive at best. It may be immoral. (pp. 104–105)

The importance of recognizing the difference between individual and social problems will be discussed in greater depth in Chapter 9.

Mercer argues that the source of the problem often lies within the social system, rather than within the individual. In the case of the families that she studied, a child's label was contingent on the situation in which the child was placed. In the institutional setting, lower-SES children might be regarded as mentally deficient; however, when these same children are removed from the institution and returned to their home communities, they are likely to be regarded as normal. Thus, Mercer suggests that the solution to some problems might involve changing the norms of the social system or, alternatively, relocating, the individual to a system that does not regard his or her behavior or condition as pathological.

The Partnership Approach

Mercer (1965) proposed an alternative perspective, which she calls the social systems approach, that "attempts to see the definition of an individual's behavior as a function of the values of the social system within which he is being evaluated" (p. 20). What Mercer calls the social system perspective is the approach that most sociologists have used to help them understand patterns of human behavior. Individuals are viewed as products of their interactions with others in their families, communities, and societies. Thus, human behavior is regarded as situational: what is deemed to be appropriate in one social context may be seen as deviant in another. This social system perspective is in many ways identical to the partnership approach described in Chapter 1. In the partnership approach, the professional's definition of the situation is not necessarily seen as "right." Rather, the definitions of all parties are accepted as meaningful for the purpose of designing effective interventions. In this approach, the client and professional become partners in the problem-solving endeavor. The professional contributes expertise based on his or her training and past experience and the client contributes the expertise that comes from being intimately familiar with his or her social world.

One of the major difficulties in human service work in the past resulted from the failure of human service professionals to take the situational nature of human behavior into account. Juvenile delinquents who appear to be "cured" in a treatment setting are very likely to revert to their former delinquent behaviors when they return to the situations that prompted those behaviors in the first place. Most human service programs, at least until fairly recently, have addressed only a small sector of their clients' social lives. If we are serious about helping people, we must try to understand their social worlds; the contexts within which they interact on a daily basis. A number of human service fields already have recognized the importance of this principle. The independent movement of a variety of disciplines toward a partnership approach will be explored in the next section.

The Shift toward a Partnership Perspective

Education

In the field of education, the shift toward a partnership perspective has been most notable in the area of early intervention, in the movement toward "full-service schools," and in the recognition of cultural diversity. These approaches are explored below.

Early Intervention

This aspect of the field involves special education for young children with disabilities. Much of the early literature in this field tended to take a victim-blaming stance toward the families of these children. When families had difficulty coping with their children's disabilities, professionals typically assumed that the family was at fault, and even when families were coping well, they were sometimes thought to be "in denial" (see, for example, Mandelbaum & Wheeler, 1960; Solnit & Stark, 1961). However, studies (see, for example, Schonell & Rorke, 1960) began to reveal that most families' difficulties were attributable to a lack of appropriate services in the community rather than to parental shortcomings. Still, diagnostic instruments continued to be developed to measure levels of family functioning (see, for example, Crnic, Friedrich, & Greenberg, 1983; Abidin, 1983). Service plans generally focused on the child and did not take family concerns into account. When families were included at all, they were typically treated as clients themselves, and treatment centered around improving their ability to cope with and adjust to their children's disabilities [cf Darling and Darling (1992) and Gliedman and Roth (1980) for a further discussion of families as clients].

As recently as 1986, a major journal in the early intervention field published a thematic issue entitled "Assessment of Handicapped Children and Their Families: New Directions" (*Topics in Early Childhood Special Education*, 1986). The assessment of families was based on a status inequality model that suggested that professionals knew better than parents what was best for their children. However, just 4 years later, the same journal published an issue entitled, "Gathering Family Information: Procedures, Products, and Precautions" (*Topics in Early Childhood Special Education*, 1990). The change in terminology marked a shift in thinking about families. In a relatively short period of time, the field had moved from talking about assessing families to viewing families as equal partners who could provide valuable information.

This newer perspective is reflected especially in the writing of Carl Dunst and his colleagues, who suggest an "enablement and empowerment" perspective:

> A fuller understanding of empowerment requires that we take a broader-based view of the conditions that influence the behavior of people during help-seeker and help-giver exchanges. . . . Empowerment implies that what you see as poor functioning is a result of social structure and lack of resources which make it impossible for the existing competencies to operate. (Dunst, Trivette, & Deal, 1988, p. 3)

They go on to describe how a social system perspective views a family as a social unit embedded within other formal and informal social units and networks. Dunst et al. (1988) propose a "social systems definition of intervention": . . . the provision of support (i.e., resources provided by others) by members of a family's informal and formal social network that either directly or indirectly influences child, parent, and family functioning."

In a similar vein, Donald Bailey and his colleagues have developed a curriculum and materials for early intervention professionals based on a "family-focused" perspective (see, for example, Bailey et al., 1986; Winton & Bailey, 1988). They discuss the need for intervention to fit the individualized needs of families. Among intervention goals they list the following: "To preserve and reinforce the dignity of families by respecting and responding to their desire for services and incorporating them in the assessment, planning, and evaluation process" (Bailey et al., 1986, p. 158). Thus, the family's definition of the situation rather than the professional's becomes the focus for service provision.

Why has this shift occurred? Several factors seem to have played a role: (1) Probably most important is the role played by families themselves. Increasingly, parents of children with disabilities began to speak out against practices based on status inequality and to demand a larger part in determining the services their children received (for a further discussion of the parent movement of the 1970s–1980s, see Pizzo, 1983; Darling, 1988). (2) Professionals also began to realize the inefficacy of status inequality approaches in their day-to-day work with families. Especially as home visiting became a more popular method in the field, professionals began to acquire a new respect for the family's perspective. One professional, who herself became the parent of a child with a disability, noted, "Before I had Peter I gave out [physical therapy] programs that would have taken all day. I don't know when I expected mothers to change diapers, sort laundry, or buy groceries" (Featherstone, 1980, p. 57). (3) Research with families also led increasingly to an appreciation of their point of view. For example, one early study of parents of children with disabilities in an Australian city with few services available (Schonell & Watts, 1956) concluded that the parents' concerns were pathological. When the same population was studied following the establishment of new services in the city (Schonell & Rorke, 1960), their "neurotic" symptoms had disappeared. Their "pathology," then, seemed to be an artifact of the lack of resources—their limited structure of opportunities—rather than the manifestation of some inherent, psychological disorder.

Newer, system-based perspectives in the field of early intervention have been reflected in practice. The "Individualized Family Service Plans" mandated by law now tend to be products of a partnership between families and professionals, and services are based on the family's resources, concerns, and priorities. Guidelines for practice usually reflect the new approaches, as illustrated by the following "underlying principles" from a seminal document in the field:

- Each family has its own structure, roles, values, beliefs, and coping styles. Respect for and acceptance of this diversity is a cornerstone of family-centered early intervention.
- Respect for family autonomy, independence, and decision making means that families must be able to choose the level and nature of an early intervention program's involvement in their life.
- An enabling approach to working with families requires that professionals re-examine their traditional roles and practices and develop new practices when necessary (Johnson, McGonigel, & Kaufmann, 1989, p. 3).

This newer perspective does not deny the existence of clinical, diagnosable developmental disabilities in children. However, it asserts that the existence of diagnosable disabilities in children does not require that their parents be diagnosed and categorized as well. Rather, parents have become respected members of the treatment team.

Full-Service Schools

As Hendrickson and Omer (1995) and others have noted, educators have been realizing that children do not always learn well when they are taught in isolation from their families and communities. Further, they have become increasingly aware of the lack of integration between in-school services and out-of-school services, such as probation, family counseling, and foster care. Families also have tended to be fragmented, with some family members receiving services from one or more agencies, while other members receive services from different agencies. These problems seem to be magnified in communities marked by high levels of poverty.

As part of the school reform movement of the 1980s, educators became interested in using the schools to address these problems. Two types of solutions have been proposed: school-based services and school-linked services (Hendrickson & Omer, 1995). In school-based services, the school serves as a site for the provision of services such as child care, probation, family counseling, adult literacy, and other programs. In school-linked services, the school plays a role in coordinating services provided elsewhere. Schools thus are becoming partners with other community members in providing for a variety of family needs.

A popular model for integrating education with other services has been "full service schools." When this approach is used, schools become community centers, and the goal is to provide many services under one roof, in a manner similar to that of the settlement houses that were popular in American cities during the period of large-scale European immigration during the early 20th century. In Pennsylvania, for example, the state has been providing funding to school districts since 1991 to establish "family centers" that provide programs as diverse as teen parenting, adult education, home visiting to "at-risk" infants and preschool children, domestic abuse support groups, and job training (Moffett, 1997). Similarly, the Beacons Initiative in New York increased the number of hours that certain school buildings were open and provided a variety of school-based programs in those buildings, including GED classes, recreation programs, parent support groups, youth leadership groups, family dinners, educational enrichment, and business partnerships that located part-time jobs for students (Schorr, 1997).

The goal of these programs has been prevention. Educators have come to believe that students cannot perform well in school if they are experiencing hardships outside of school. By providing for their students' extracurricular needs, they are hoping to reduce some of the risks for school failure that exist in these children's daily lives. Thus, older, status inequality models that focused exclusively on changing the child through education are giving way to newer approaches that take the social system into account. Interestingly, at the other end of the socioeconomic spectrum, middle- and upper-class parents also are becoming increasingly involved in their children's education (Wells, 1998).

Cultural Diversity

Another way in which the field of education has undergone a shift from a status inequality to a partnership perspective is the increasing recognition and incorporation of principles of cultural diversity. In the past, many models of education took a "one size fits all" approach. In this approach, when children did not learn, victim blaming was the rule. Either the children were seen as lazy or slow learners or their parents were seen as poor facilitators of the educational process. Typically, such blaming was applied most commonly to the poor and to members of ethnic and racial minority groups.

More recently, a shift in thinking has taken place. A number of recent books and articles have stressed the importance of taking a child's and family's social and cultural background into account. Swadener and Lubeck (1995), for example, argue that older approaches tended to negatively label children and to prevent them from achieving to their fullest potential. They suggest an alternative "at promise" perspective that restructures the educational process to build on children's strengths rather than expecting children from diverse backgrounds to learn within a single framework.

Similarly, a number of recent books have attempted to increase practitioners' understanding of the lifestyles of diverse groups of parents and children and to suggest educational approaches that take these differences into account. For example, in the field of special education, Harry (1992a) has written a textbook in which she shows how the beliefs about education vary in the African American, Latino, and other communities. Similarly, in the field of early intervention, Wayman, Lynch, and Hanson (1991) suggest that professionals working with culturally diverse families need to take the following areas of difference into account in their practice: family structure, childbearing practices, family's response to a crying infant, family's perception of child's disability, family's perception of health and healing, family's perception of help seeking and intervention, language, and interaction styles. Two of these authors have also edited a textbook in this area (Lynch & Hanson, 1992).

Social Work

A strand that values the strengths and perspectives of service users has always existed in the field of social work (Simon, 1994). However, for a number of years, that strand seemed to be overshadowed by approaches based more on status inequality. Specht and Courtney (1994) note, for example, a trend toward the private practice of psychotherapy among social workers during the past 60 years. Recently, however, social system approaches have experienced a resurgence.

Adams and Nelson (1995) suggest that the new movement toward community- and family-centered practice was stimulated by concerns about the "fragmented, bureaucratic, rule-driven, ineffective way" (p. 3) that human service agencies had been operating. They pose a series of questions suggesting their vision of a more effective, social system model:

> What would it be like if services were designed to strengthen rather than substitute for the caring capacity of families and communities? What if services were shaped by and available to all citizens in their communities, so people could get a little help when they needed it, without always having to fit into a narrow category or be formally processed as "clients"? What if services were geared to recognizing and building on the strengths and resources of families and communities, rather than focusing on their deficits? (p. 2)

A major component of newer, social system approaches in social work has been the concept of empowerment. Lee (1994) argues that an empowerment approach is based on a number of underlying principles, including the following:

- People empower themselves: social workers should assist.
- Social workers should establish an "I and I" [partnership] relationship with clients.
- Social workers should encourage the client to say her own word [and not use the language of the oppressor].

- The worker should maintain a focus on the person as victor and not victim.
- Social workers should maintain a social change focus. (pp. 27–28)

She argues further that social workers need to develop “fifocal vision,” based on historical, ecological, “ethclass,” feminist, and critical perspectives.

One model of community- and family-centered practice in social work has been the “patch” approach developed in Great Britain (Adams & Krauth, 1995). This approach is neighborhood-based and proactive: “Families receive a little help when they need it, instead of having to wait for a crisis. There is no need to be categorized, diagnosed, or ‘clientized’ to get help” (p. 87). Rather, professionals work in teams that come to know a community well and to understand the strengths of its residents.

The “family support movement” also has been growing rapidly in the United States. As Zigler and Black (1989) have noted, a number of recent social trends have increased stresses on families, creating a need for support. The goal of family support programs is “not to provide families with direct services, but to enhance parent empowerment—to enable families to help themselves and their children” (Zigler & Black, 1989, p. 7). The need for agency services often can be avoided when support is provided to families even before problems occur. Such models also suggest that all families could use some help from time to time; yet being labeled as a client can be demeaning and may discourage people from seeking the help they need.

In the child welfare field, family-centered practice has resulted in the creation of “family preservation programs” (Cameron & Vanderwoerd, 1997; Fraser, Pecora, & Haapala, 1991; Nelson & Allen, 1995; Wells & Biegel, 1991; Whittaker, Kenney, Tracy, & Booth, 1990). Rather than removing “at-risk” children from their homes and placing them in foster care, these programs build on family strengths and work to keep families together. The family support and preservation philosophy has guided funding for child protective services in recent years and has given rise to new programs throughout the United States, many of which are based on home visiting or family center models. The following testimony from a service user extols the value of one such program:

> At the time, I had my sister and her two children who were burned out of their home; I had my niece’s three children who were 2, 3, and 7; and my granddaughter who was about 12 . . . and we were all living in five rooms. You name it. I needed food, clothes, beds—we were in trouble. . . . I didn’t know where to go, who to contact for any of the stuff I needed and I didn’t have money to buy it. . . .
>
> [After learning about the family support center,] all I had to do was pick up the phone and make a phone call—to anyone there. . . . It helped me a lot because I really don’t have family members to go to, nobody I could call and just talk, cry on their shoulder. . . . I learned so much. . . . I love it [in the new housing the center helped me find]. . . . We’re doing fine now. We have a house. In fact, we’re doing pretty good. We’re doing just about great. (Ellis, 1995, p. 6)

Such family support centers are similar to those discussed in the section on education above. In some cases, the centers are school based; in others, they are located in shopping malls, housing projects, and other community buildings. Much of their funding comes from federal, state, and local government sources, suggesting the institutionalization of this newer model in the administrative bureaucracy. In Pennsylvania, for example, the Family Center Initiative is part of a larger Department of Public Welfare initiative called, Family Service System Reform, which is designed to be community planned and to provide a coordinated format for service provision based on a philosophy of family empowerment and support. Like the patch and other programs discussed above, services provided through this initiative are intended to be preventive and supportive rather than corrective. The popularity of the approach is suggested by the fact that in one Pennsylvania county alone, 22 family support centers are currently operating. (Certainly, not all families are able to use community resources to help themselves. Those addicted to drugs, for example, may have difficulty providing for their children's needs even with help. A critique of the family support/preservation approach is presented in Chapter 3.)

Psychology/Mental Health

The field of psychology has been moving toward a partnership model in a number of areas. Social system principles underlie the theoretical literature in the ecological and family systems approaches that have been popular in recent years. These principles can also be seen in several practice models, including behavioral healthcare delivery and children's mental health care, among others.

Theory

Social ecology theory in the field of psychology derives primarily from the work of Bronfenbrenner (1979). This theoretical perspective suggests that the behavior of individuals is a function of their interaction within systems operating at four levels: micro, meso, exo, and macro. The microsystem generally consists of the individual's family; the mesosystem involves those with whom the family interacts, including neighbors and co-workers; the exosystem consists of external agencies that can affect the family, such as health care and social welfare; and finally, the macrosystem includes societal and cultural features, such as religion and the economy, that have an impact on individuals and families. The ecological model is sociological in that it takes into account the interaction of the individual with larger social systems and recognizes the importance of family, community, and society in shaping individual outcomes.

The social ecology model has been used in interventions with individuals and families. One application (Hartman, 1978) uses a diagrammatic assessment tool called an Eco-Map, which graphically depicts the relationships between clients and others in their social systems, such as friends and family, and institutions such as school, work, and social service agencies. A key tenet in the social ecology model is that if one wishes to change behavior, one must change the environment.

Family systems theory in psychology owes its greatest debt to the work of Minuchin (1974), who argued that individuals could not be understood apart from their families. He suggested that, because families are systems, the actions of any family member will have repercussions for all other members of the same family. Elman (1991) suggests that families are like objects hanging from a baby's crib mobile. When one object is touched, all the objects move. Family systems theory serves as the basis for much of the family therapy that occurs in the United States today.

Family systems theorists have looked at various family interaction styles and the nature of the bonds between the members of different family subsystems. Although this perspective relies on professionally defined levels of family functioning, it also takes the social system into account. In more recent writings, family systems theorists seem to be moving closer and closer to a partnership perspective, as illustrated by the following statement by the father of family systems theory:

> At first the helpers used the words that everyone used. But as they helped, they began to notice peculiarities among the poor, and they gave them names. The world of the helped was transformed. Some of the helped began to resemble their labels (such is the power of naming). And the helpers made more and more labels. As more words and signifiers appeared, organizations were developed to carry on the task of assigning the labels and writing formulas that explained the meaning of behaviors they had labeled. And as the behavior of the poor was categorized, and the meaning of their behavior, thinking, and feeling was elucidated, the helping professionals, in their zeal, proliferated and differentiated. . . .
>
> As history evolved, a number of the helpers began to notice that the poor did not always improve with help, and sometimes they got worse. . . .
>
> A way of working evolved in which the helpers and the poor people together determined the goals of their joint tasks. Words like teamwork, coconstruction, community, systems, neighborhood, ecology, family, and empowerment began to replace the tired old words like deficit, concern, problems. (Minuchin, 1995, pp. vii–viii)

Practice

In a recent publication (National Community Mental Healthcare Council, 1997), the National Community Mental Healthcare Council proposes a new model for services that is consumer centered and based on an understanding of the importance of the social system. A series of "principles for consumer-centered care" include, among others:

- The provision of services and support should take place in the consumer's environment and be directed by his or her needs and desires, wherever possible.
- Consumer needs, strengths, and choices should be considered, and the involvement of the individual should be demonstrated, in service planning and implementation, in order to help consumers take charge of their lives through informed decision-making.

- Services should be culturally and linguistically appropriate. Providers should demonstrate responsiveness, understanding, and respect for the consumer's culture and language and should make every effort to provide services in the person's preferred language. (pp. 15–16)

A shift in perspectives in the mental health field is also apparent in professional support for self-help groups. As Wasow (1997) has noted, in the past consumer organizations were seen by professionals as suspect. Today, many professionals recommend such groups to their clients, and the consumer advocacy movement is growing.

One area of mental health practice that seems to have moved almost completely toward a partnership model is services to children. In the past, when children were diagnosed with behavioral and emotional disorders, their families were typically seen as the cause of their problem. In characteristic victim-blaming fashion, parents were labeled as "overprotective" or "too permissive," or by some other term suggesting their ineptness as parents. Although some parents certainly do contribute to their children's difficulties, blaming models have not been productive in creating positive outcomes for children and families. More recent models have regarded families as allies and have looked beyond the family for system-based causes of children's behavior.

The federally sponsored Child and Adolescent Service System Program (CASSP) approach is based on a partnership between service providers and families (Cohen & Lavach, 1995). In this model, parents are acknowledged to be experts about and advocates for their children. Parent involvement has been encouraged through mutual support or self-help groups, joint service planning, and increased recognition by professionals of the constraints on families imposed by their social and cultural environments. Greater flexibility in service delivery is also an important feature of the model.

Today, mental health services are delivered in a variety of settings, including schools, child care centers, and family homes, in addition to the offices and clinics that are the "natural habitats" of professionals. Although older, status inequality models still determine eligibility for services in many cases, (especially in some of the newer, managed care plans), professionals seem to be more aware of the importance of the service user's usual environment and definition of the situation. Thus, like the other helping professions, psychological practice has been moving toward a more partnership-based approach.

Health Care

Family-centered health care has been tried in various forms throughout much of the 20th century (Doherty, 1985). Projects such as the Peckham Experiment, the Cornell Project, and the Montefiore Medical Group attempted to apply a holistic perspective, rather than treating patients in isolation from their familial and social milieus. However, the area in the health care field that has moved the closest to a partnership perspective is probably maternal and child health. Perhaps the role of the family was most obvious in the case of infant and child patients.

During the past 20 years, the family-centered care movement has been gaining momentum in maternal and child health. This movement recognizes that "families are the primary caregivers and advocates for their children" and encourages parent–professional collaboration rather than professional dominance (Hostler, 1991). "Within this philosophy is the idea that families should be supported in their natural care-giving and decision-making roles by building on their unique strengths as people and families" (Brewer, McPherson, Magrab, & Hutchins, 1989). Family-centered care has also been incorporated into the 1989 amendments to Title V of the Social Security Act.

The US Bureau of Maternal and Child Health has been providing funding for various initiatives, including the Center for Family-Centered Care at the Association for the Care of Children's Health and various Special projects of Regional and National Significance (SPRANS), including physician training projects in several states. The Healthy Tomorrows Partnership between the Maternal and Child Health Bureau and the American Academy of Pediatrics requires that all funded projects be community-based, family-centered, comprehensive, and culturally relevant. Further, Ireys and Nelson (1992) have suggested that pediatric training programs at all levels will need to incorporate the principles of community-based, family-centered care into their curricula.

The Institute for Family-Centered Care lists the following core principles:

- In family-centered health care, people are treated with dignity and respect.
- In family-centered health care, health care providers communicate and share complete and unbiased information with patients and families in ways that are affirming and useful.
- In family-centered health care, individuals and family members build on their strengths by participating in experiences that enhance control and independence.
- In family-centered health care, collaboration among patients, families, and providers occurs in policy and program development and professional education, as well as in the delivery of care. ("Core Principles of Family-Centered Health Care," 1998, pp. 2–3)

Physician training programs based on a partnership model have been especially prevalent in the area of children with special health care needs. Parents of such children are being used as faculty in these programs throughout the country, at both the medical school and residency levels, as well as in continuing education programs for practicing physicians. Usually, pediatricians and family physicians are targeted.

One model program at the medical school level (Lewis & Greenstein, 1994) requires first-year medical students to make six to eight home visits to a family of a child with special health needs over the course of one semester. These students clearly come away with a new appreciation of the family's definition of the situation:

> Above all, no one can really see what this family experiences. I think I see a window into their life: their daily routines, their minor setbacks offset by victories. One of their most fervent desires is to make me understand that I cannot feel their painful experience, but that I should recognize and acknowledge it and incorporate this into my fiber as a professional. Another lesson: chronic illness does not stop when the patient leaves the office; it is a way of life. . . . There is some sort of lesson here, although I don't think I fully understand it yet. It is something about the value of having a relationship that is close enough to be painful. (Lewis & Greenstein, p. 89)

Similar programs also exist at the residency level (Cooley, 1994). Many of these programs bring families into the classroom. Others require pediatric residents to spend time with families, either as observers or as respite care providers.

Physicians practicing in the community also have been targeted by newer training programs. For example, a major SPRANS grant project in Hawaii developed a curriculum for practicing physicians based on the American Pediatric Association's concept of "medical home" (Peter & Sia, 1994). This concept designates physicians as service coordinators for their patients and suggests the integration of medical services with those provided by school and community agencies. The Hawaii curriculum has been adopted in many states. [For a further discussion of this and other projects designed to train physicians in a partnership perspective, see Darling and Peter (1994.)]

Thus, the professional dominance of physicians seems to be declining in favor of a newer perspective that takes the patient's (and/or patient's family's) views into account. Newer training programs in the health care field are acknowledging that patients seen in medical offices, clinics, or hospitals are impacted by their lives in nonmedical settings and that medical professionals cannot gain a complete understanding of their patients' needs unless they come to recognize the totality of their patients' social worlds.

Other Services

Although the fields discussed above seem to have taken the lead in the shift away from a status inequality perspective and toward a partnership approach, other human services also seem to be moving in the same direction. For example, in many communities, police officers are moving away from their traditional role as authority figures toward more service-based activities, under a "community policing" model (Thurman, 1995). In this model, police officers become involved in the communities they serve in a proactive, preventive way. As a result, community members come to perceive them as partners in community-building, rather than as feared enemies.

Similarly, the field of mental retardation services has changed considerably since Mercer's (1965) studies were published in the 1960s. The guiding principle for many years has been that of "normalization" (Wolfensberger, 1972) or "social role valorization." This principle suggests that people with mental retardation have the right to be recognized as having value and to make important life decisions themselves. Much of the deinstitutionalization of the past decades has been justified by this principle. Thus, as in other human service fields, professionals in the field of mental retardation have seen their role change from that of dominant expert to that of partner as service users have been recognized to have expertise of their own.

The field of drug abuse treatment also seems to have developed a new respect for clients. At the Parkdale Center in Toronto, for example, the concerns expressed by clients serve as the basis for research, which has led to the establishment of a nonjudgmental harm reduction program (Cavalieri, Clarke, & Polych, 1997). A number of other human service fields also are involving clients in "participatory action research."

After a review of 130 published sources in a variety of disciplines, a group of researchers ("Family-Centered Service Delivery," 1997, p. 1) found a number of key components of these newer models of practice, including the following:

- Organizing assistance collaboratively (e.g., ensuring mutual respect and teamwork between team workers and clients).
- Organizing assistance in accordance with each individual family's wishes so that the family ultimately directs decision making.
- Considering family strengths (versus dwelling on family deficiencies).
- Addressing family needs holistically (rather than focusing on a member with a "problem").
- Normalizing perspectives (i.e., recognizing that much of what those receiving services are experiencing is typical).
- Structuring service delivery to ensure accessibility, minimal disruption of family integrity and routine.

In addition, newer models focus on prevention rather than social control (providing a safety net) or assistance (resuscitation) (Heckman, 1996).

Some of the creators of these changes in the human services have acknowledged a debt to sociological theory and research; in other cases, theorists and practitioners have been "reinventing the wheel." In this volume, I argue that the sociological literature already provides concepts and practices that are useful in the provision of human services. The following chapters provide an overview of this literature as it can be applied in the helping professions. Such applications seem especially relevant at this time, given the recent independent movement of so many human service fields toward a recognition of the value of a sociological perspective.

When Is Sociological Intervention Appropriate?

Although the remainder of this volume will explore the applicability of the sociological perspective to the human services, an important caveat needs to be acknowledged. Although many human service fields have been moving away from a status inequality model, no single perspective is appropriate in all human service situations. The sociological perspective is especially useful in situations in which social change is possible. On the other hand, some situations are relatively inflexible, requiring adjustments by affected individuals. For example, an individual may have difficulty accepting the fact that he or she has an incurable illness. When such lack of acceptance is problematic for the individual or the family, a partnership model may not be appropriate. Interventions based on status inequality may be needed to facilitate adjustment and coping. Professional-centered interventions are also appropriate when problems are caused by biological, psychological, and other nonsocial factors. Clearly, antibiotics are a more appropriate treatment for a bacterial infection than any sociological intervention might be.

On the other hand, interventions based on status inequality too often have been inappropriately applied to socially caused problems, resulting in the kind of victim-blaming discussed above. A social problem such as poverty cannot be solved by counseling poor people to change their thinking. Motivating people to want to work is not a pragmatic intervention when jobs that pay a living wage are not available.

Practitioners, then, need to be able to assess situations to determine the nature of their antecedents. They should have a good understanding of social problems and their causes in order to recognize the difference between personal and social problems (Mills, 1959). Social problems can affect people at various levels. Sometimes the effect is limited to a few individuals or families; other times, the effect is community- or societywide. In all cases, though, the cause rests either in social structure, that is, the organization of social relationships, or in social process, that is, the dynamics of those relationships.

Sociological intervention, then, is action that changes either social structure or social process. These changes can assist individuals and families by creating new resources for them and expanding their opportunity structures. When system-changing intervention occurs at the societal level, it is usually called social change; when it occurs at the individual or family level, it is sometimes called advocacy. The human services have traditionally regarded the individual or family as the unit of intervention. For this reason, this volume will focus more on advocacy techniques than on changing society as a whole, although advocacy is sometimes contingent on broader social change.

Human services cannot solve all social problems. Practitioners need to recognize the limits of their field. Probably a large part of the "burnout" that occurs so commonly among human service professionals can be attributed to the frustration of trying to affect societal problems by changing individuals. After years of receiving services, most poor clients are still living in poverty, and the conditions that produce domestic violence and drug abuse persist for treated batterers and abusers. The importance of understanding the difference between individual and social problems will be considered further as part of the discussion of intervention techniques in Chapter 10.

Chapter Summary

This chapter has highlighted the differences between traditional status inequality models of human service practice and newer partnership approaches. An overview of recent developments in education, social work, mental health, medical care, and other fields provides strong evidence of a paradigm shift. In the past, practitioners tended to impose their perspective on their clients; today, many professionals are listening more closely to their clients and working in partnership with them. Sociological theory and methods can provide a framework for practitioners interested in understanding the foundations of these newer partnership approaches, as well as techniques for applying them.

Exercise

The cases below are based on real clients encountered by human service professionals. In each case, the reader should consider the nature of the causes: are they based in the client's psyche, or in the client's social system, or both?

Case #1

You are a counselor at a mental health treatment center. Your client is Mary, age 42. She has been diagnosed with depression.

In your first session with Mary, you learn that she is trained as a secretary. However, she quit her job a year ago to take care of her 75-year-old mother, who has Alzheimer's disease. She says that her mother cannot be left alone in the house for more than a few minutes. Mary is divorced and has a 10-year-old son. Her father is deceased. Mary says she will have to ask for public assistance, because her ex-husband has not been making his child support payments and her mother's social security payments are not enough to support the family. She is afraid she will lose her house and car.

Which do you think should be tried *first* in treating Mary's depression: a status inequality or a partnership approach?

Case #2

You are a juvenile probation officer. Your client, John, age 15, has a history of truancy from school and petty theft. He has been found to be "incorrigible" by the court, because his mother says she cannot control him or make him go to school. John is reported to be a member of a gang.

You learn from the family history that John lives with his mother and younger brother. His mother is a drug addict and has been arrested several times for prostitution. A grandmother lives nearby. All John's friends have been adjudicated delinquent; they all have records of truancy from school.

What interventions might you use with John? Would you try to change his social system?

Case #3

You are a school social worker. Maria, age 14, has been referred to you because she is often absent from school and is failing most of her classes. She has been tested by the school psychologist and has an IQ of 79. The school has recommended to her parents that she be placed in special education classes, but they have refused. The guidance counselor has referred the family to you with the hope that you can convince them that Maria is mildly retarded and needs special education.

In your first meeting with the family, you learn that they came to the United States from Puerto Rico 2 years ago and do not speak English very well. They say that they do not think Maria is retarded, because she has no trouble learning and understanding things at home and because she did well in school in Puerto Rico.

Would you follow up on the guidance counselor's referral and try to convince the family that Maria should be placed in a special education program, or would you explore other, social-system-based interventions? Why?

Case #4

You are a medical social worker. Your client is 2-year-old Jimmy and his family. Jimmy has cerebral palsy and is seen at a clinic at the hospital where you work. The family is referred to you because they are not following through with Jimmy's therapy at home. The physical and speech therapists say that he is not making progress. They are concerned, because his mother does not seem interested in working on the exercises they suggest. They think she is "in denial" and unable to accept Jimmy's cerebral palsy.

In your first meeting with the family, you learn that Jimmy lives with his 21-year-old, single mother, two brothers, aged 4 and 3, and a 3-month-old sister. The family has recently moved to the city; they have no friends or relatives nearby. They receive public assistance, and the mother says she has trouble providing what her family needs. They have just been evicted from their apartment for not paying rent and have not yet found another place to live.

What intervention would you consider *first:* counseling Jimmy's mother to help her "accept" Jimmy's disability and his need for therapy, or trying to change the family's social situation? Why?

Case #5

You are a case manager in a child abuse prevention program. Your client is Susan, age 19. She has been referred to your program by Child Protective Services. Susan was reported to that agency by neighbors, because her 18-month-old son, Bobby, was found alone in the house on several occasions. The case-worker from Child Protective Services believes that Susan is irresponsible and that Bobby should be removed from her home and placed in foster care. However, she has made the referral to you, because her agency is required to try newer methods of family preservation before removing a child.

When you meet with Susan in her home, you get the impression that she is intellectually limited. She has difficulty responding to your questions and is unable to fill out the forms you give her. You notice that the house is dirty. Bobby is crying and holding his bottle, which is empty. However, Susan seems concerned about Bobby. She shows affection toward him and expresses her fear that he might be taken away from her. When you ask her why she has left Bobby alone in the house, she says that she has no one to leave him with and cannot afford to pay a babysitter.

How might you try to change Susan's social situation to try to keep the family together?

Suggestions for Further Reading

Adams, P., & Nelson, K. (Eds.). (1995). *Reinventing human services: Community- and family-centered practice.* New York: Aldine deGruyter.

Bowman, B. (1992). Who is at risk for what and why? *Journal of Early Intervention, 16(2),* 101–200.

Darling, R.B., & Peter, M.I. (Eds.). (1994). *Families, physicians, and children with special health needs: Collaborative medical education models.* Westport, CT: Greenwood.

Mercer, J.R. (1965). Social system perspective and clinical perspective: Frames of reference for understanding career patterns of persons labelled as mentally retarded. *Social Problems, 13,* 18–34.

3

Theoretical Foundations I

Social Structure

Sociological theory can be useful in understanding the nature of professional–client interaction. In this volume, the strands of theory that will provide a foundation for the partnership model introduced in the last chapter are structural–functionalism and symbolic interactionism. The former is useful in explaining the context within which professionals and clients interact, and the latter provides a basis for understanding how the viewpoints of clients and professionals develop. This chapter will focus on context. The professional milieu will be examined in terms of the organization of human service agencies, with an emphasis on bureaucracy and its consequences and the roles that practitioners are expected to play. The client's situation will then be explored in terms of role expectations and opportunity structures. An understanding of the opportunity structure concept is important, because the practice model being advocated in this volume is based on intervention that increases clients' opportunities.

Two theoretical concepts will be explored in some depth: social structure and social process. The theoretical underpinnings of the social structure concept to be discussed in this chapter can be found in structural–functional theory in sociology. The discussion of the social process concept in the next chapter will be based on symbolic interactionist theory. These sociological theories are separate and distinct, and each has strengths and weaknesses in terms of explaining different aspects of social life. Structural–functional theory helps us to understand social organization in terms of the expectations that people in a society share. Symbolic interaction theory, on the other hand, helps to explain how these expectations come to exist and how they change. An understanding of both aspects of social life is important in human service practice. Because understanding can lead to respect, professionals in a partnership relationship with their clients will want to understand the bases for their clients' thinking and behavior. In addition, an understanding of social structure and social process is required for intervention to bring about change.

The relationship between structure and process, with respect to the interaction between service users and service providers, is illustrated in Fig. 3.1. The structural elements included in the boxes on either side of the figure will be discussed in this chapter, and the concepts listed in the "Process" box in the middle will be explained in Chapter 4. The relationship between structure and process is addressed below.

Social structure refers to the way a society is organized, which in turn relates to generally accepted cultural practices. Prior to meeting for the first time both the client and the professional have certain beliefs, values, and expectations based on their prior life experiences. These experiences derive from their respective locations in society. The thinking and behavior of clients are based on such structural conditions as their socioeconomic status, their family status, and their ethnic group membership. Professionals, in turn, have expectations based on their family backgrounds, education, occupational experience, and other aspects of their position in society. Such structural conditions provide a baseline for the interaction that will occur between client and professional.

Once the client and professional meet, their preexisting worldviews will be shaped by the interaction that takes place. If both professional and client are listening to each other, both will have somewhat different worldviews when their relationship ends than they did when it started. Through a process of symbolic interaction, each learns from the other. The conditions that give rise to preexisting worldviews will be considered in this chapter, and the changes that occur during the course of interaction will be considered in Chapter 4.

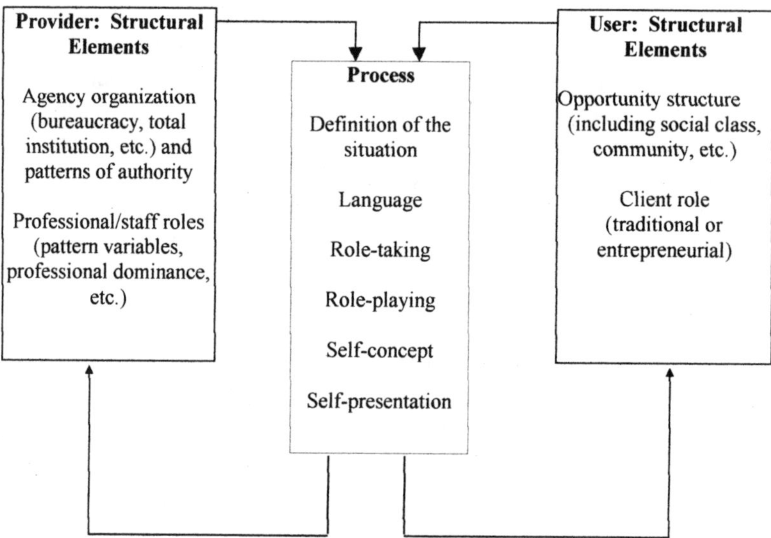

Figure 3.1. The relationship between elements of social structure and social process in the service provider–service user relationship.

The conditions that affect service users and service providers derive from the society within which they live and are based on the culture of that society. The role of cultural diversity in shaping social structure and the worldviews of individuals in different parts of society will be discussed further in Chapter 5. The present chapter will suggest that the way a society (or a human service agency) is organized will have an impact on service users. Further, the organization of a society involves certain expectations about how people occupying various positions in society will act. The chapter will show how these expectations affect the way that professionals and clients interact with one another.

The Organization of Human Service Agencies: Bureaucracy and Its Consequences

Like many other large organizations in society today, most human service agencies are bureaucracies. Our sociological understanding of bureaucracy owes a large debt to the work of Max Weber, who became concerned with the changes he saw occurring in society in the late 1800s. Weber (1949) argued that older forms of authority in society were giving way to newer forms with a rational–legal basis. In the past, much authority was based on tradition and personal relationships. In large, modern societies, on the other hand, people's personal networks are usually limited to their families, neighbors, friends, and co-workers, and other relationships are generally impersonal.

When people do not know one another well, their relationships are best governed by rules, so that everyone is treated equally and fairly. This principle provides the basis for bureaucratic organization. According to Weber, the staff in a bureaucratic organization are appointed and function according to the following criteria:

1. They are personally free and subject to authority only with respect to their impersonal official obligations.
2. They are organized in a clearly defined hierarchy of offices.
3. Each office has a clearly defined sphere of competence in the legal sense.
4. The office is filled by a free contractual relationship. . . .
5. Candidates are selected on the basis of technical qualifications. . . .
6. They are remunerated by fixed salaries in money. . . .
7. The office is treated as the sole, or at least the primary, occupation of the incumbent.
8. It constitutes a career. There is a system of "promotion" according to seniority or to achievement, or both. . . .

9. The official works entirely separated from ownership of the means of administration. . . .
10. He is subject to strict and systematic discipline and control in the conduct of the office. (Weber, 1949, pp. 333–334)

Thus, obedience is to an impersonal order, rather than to a particular individual, and positions are determined by competence and specialized training, rather than by personal characteristics.

The sociologist, Talcott Parsons suggests that cultures can be characterized by a series of opposing "pattern variables" (Parsons, 1951). Although he does not discuss these variables in connection with bureaucratic or personal forms of organization, they are helpful in explaining the conflict that sometimes arises between structural conditions and the expectations of individuals and between human service agencies and their clients. Figure 3.2 lists the variables associated with these two organizational forms, which are explained in the following paragraphs.

Bureaucratic organizations are designed to be *universalistic*. In other words, they treat people in similar situations in similar ways. Ideally, democratic societies are universalistic, with all members having equal representation in government. The opposite of universalism is *particularism*. In particularistic organizations, some people may receive better treatment than others. Nepotism is a form of appointment based on particularism. When nepotism occurs, a person may be appointed to a job because he is the boss's son, regardless of whether or not he is qualified for the position. Another term that is sometimes used for particularism is favoritism.

Bureaucracies also are *functionally specific*, that is, they define tasks in terms of clearly delimited activities, avoiding overlap. The field of medicine, for example, is becoming increasingly functionally specific. In the past, physicians were "general practitioners," who were expected to treat a variety of ailments. Today, physicians are divided among many specialties, including gastroenterology, neurology,

Bureaucracy	**Personal Organization**
Universalism	Particularism
Functional specificity	Functional diffuseness
Achievement	Ascription
Affective neutrality	Affectivity

Figure 3.2. Pattern variables associated with bureaucracy and with personal organizational forms.

ophthalmology, and obstetrics, among others. Thus, patients may have to consult a variety of specialists for their medical needs. The opposite of functional specificity is *functional diffuseness*. In the past, physicians were functionally diffuse, and patients could have all their medical needs met with "one-stop shopping."

Positions in a bureaucratic organization are determined by *achievement*. In other words, hiring and promotion are based on performance. Jobs in the government bureaucracy, for example, are filled on the basis of scores on civil service examinations. Promotion is usually determined by such factors as further examination, job performance, and seniority. The opposite of achievement is *ascription*. In ascription, who you are is more important than what you do. Thus, in some societies, the oldest son of the king will become the next king, regardless of his abilities or experiential qualifications.

Finally, bureaucracies are based on *affective neutrality*. Bureaucratic staff are not expected to become emotionally involved with their clients. The bureaucratic culture suggests that universalism may be compromised when staff develop personal relationships with the people they serve. Other relationships in society, on the other hand, are *affective*. Families in particular are expected to be based on the emotional bonds that exist among their members.

As a form of organization, bureaucracy characterizes institutions as diverse as the Catholic Church, the government of the United States, the Boy Scouts, and most universities. Although some small, neighborhood-based, grassroots, human service organizations have avoided bureaucracy, most human service agencies today are organized bureaucratically. Wilensky and Lebeaux (1965) note that in one typical human service agency, 51% of all expenditures were for record keeping, case consultation, and other aspects of bureaucratic communication, while less than half the agency's expenditures were for direct contact with clients. Agencies in the public sector are part of the larger government bureaucracy, and large nonprofit and for-profit agencies typically constitute bureaucracies in their own right. Thus, most clients of these agencies are treated according to universally applied written rules and must work with a variety of qualified human service specialists, according to the number and type of their needs. They can also expect to be treated impersonally and rationally, without appeal to emotion.

Advantages for the Service User

The bureaucratic organization of human service agencies can have both positive and negative consequences for service users. Potential positive consequences will be discussed in this section and potential negative ones in the next. Probably the major advantages of bureaucratic organization for clients of human service agencies are efficiency, fairness, and effectiveness. These will be discussed below.

Ideally, because of their clearly defined functions and well-established chains of command, bureaucratic agencies can operate very efficiently. Rather than making determinations on a case-by-case basis, these agencies can act swiftly and decisively when faced with client situations that meet predetermined criteria. Thus, when clients apply for medical assistance or some other form of service, trained workers know the procedure to follow. They ask the clients to complete a series of forms, and the information from those forms is matched with established criteria, such as income levels, to determine whether the clients are eligible for the service. The forms are then processed in a timely fashion by staff who are qualified and specially trained to do this work. Clients then receive their medical assistance cards or other services as quickly as possible. Of course, in the "real world," bureaucratic staff are not always as well trained as they should be, and forms sometimes get lost. However, as an ideal form of social organization, bureaucracy is designed to be the most efficient way to handle large numbers of service users in the shortest amount of time.

The second advantage of bureaucratic organization derives from the principle of universalism. In an ideal bureaucracy, all service users in any given category can expect to be treated equally. Thus, clients with particular attributes, such as wealth, charismatic personality, good looks, or relationship with the agency administrator, would not be given preference over those without those attributes. One method that human service agencies typically use to ensure fairness is a waiting list based on a "first-come, first-served" principle. When such a list is used, potential clients can expect to receive services in the order in which they apply for them, regardless of the identity of the other potential clients on the list.

The final, major advantage of bureaucracy is effectiveness. This advantage is based on the principles of achievement, functional specificity, and affective neutrality. In the ideal bureaucracy, clients can expect the human service workers assigned to them to be well qualified and competent. Moreover, staff whose functions are very specific can be expected to be experts in their area. A person desiring counseling to cope with a difficult marriage would probably feel more comfortable with a professional who specializes in marriage counseling than with one whose specialty is drug addiction. Further, if the counselor becomes emotionally involved with the client, his or her professional judgment may be impaired, resulting in ineffective treatment. Thus, the bureaucratic principles that govern the hiring, assignment, and conduct of staff can help to ensure the quality of the services that the client receives.

Disadvantages for the Service User

Principles, such as universalism, that can produce advantages for service users can also create disadvantages. Some of the potentially negative consequences of bureaucratic organization for the client include depersonalization, ritualism–inflexibility, and compartmentalization. These will be discussed below.

Depersonalization

Although affective neutrality, functional specificity, and universalism can produce services that are fair and effective, they also can contribute to feelings of depersonalization on the part of clients. This quote from the parent of a child with a disability suggests these feelings:

> We went to a clinic at . . . Children's Hospital. . . . We saw a different doctor every time and we always had to wait a long time. One time, Kathy was so fussy by the time they got around to examining her, they couldn't even examine her. . . . The doctors treated her like a "thing." (Darling, 1979, p. 152)

Actual employees of bureaucratic agencies may only approximate the stereotypic bureaucrat in the brown suit who never smiles and rarely looks up from his paperwork, but clients commonly tell stories about staff who do not seem to care about them and about being treated like a "number" (usually a case number or social security number used for identification purposes). A commonly cited example of the most extreme case of depersonalization is that of Nazi Germany, where bureaucrats who sent Jews and others to their deaths ceased seeing their victims as human beings.

Depersonalization also occurs for reasons other than bureaucratic organization, with perhaps the primary one being the power imbalance between service users and service providers. Clients of human service agencies tend to be of lower socioeconomic status than the professionals who serve them; further, they are likely to come from the least powerful segments of society. As a result, their personal identities may be lost in blanket condemnation or labeling:

> Staff came with many different attitudes. Some, both volunteers and paid staff, actively resented homeless people. To them, homeless persons had chosen to be where they were, and were too weak-minded, too lazy or crazy to better themselves. Freeloaders. Undeserving poor....
>
> Others believed that homeless people are generally undeserving freeloaders except for the real-life women they had come to know personally. (Liebow, 1993, pp. 126–127)

This form of depersonalization will be discussed further in Chapter 5.

Ritualism–Inflexibility

Although the written rules that govern a bureaucratic organization can ensure fair and efficient treatment, they can have the opposite effect as well. Sometimes, the rules take on a life of their own rather than being seen as they were intended—as the means to an end—resulting in ritualism. Ritualism occurs most commonly when universalism is practiced regardless of the exceptional needs of individuals. For example, when I was a student, one of my summer jobs involved scheduling appointments for the written test required to receive a driver's license at an office of the Department of Motor Vehicles in a large city. Because many people wanted to take the test and only a fixed number of time slots were available, the waiting period between the date of scheduling and the date of the test was approximately 2 weeks. I was instructed to follow the "first-come, first-served" principle and schedule appointments in the order in which I received requests. Sometimes, someone who already had a driver's license from another state would try to schedule an appointment. Occasionally, one of these people would say to me, "I have been offered a job driving trucks. I need to start working right away; my employer will not wait 2 weeks, and I really need this job. Can't you squeeze me in this week?" As a good bureaucrat, I would refuse to violate the rules. I would say, "I'm sorry. I can only give you the next available appointment."

Thus, bureaucratic rules designed for the benefit of most people can disadvantage individuals with particularistic needs. This problem is especially acute in human services, because potential clients are often people in serious need of help. Because of funding limitations, most agencies that provide nonentitlement services have waiting lists. Sometimes an effort is made to use a triage process or to serve people with the greatest need first. However, determining degree of need is not always easy, and more reticent clients with great needs may wait longer than those with lesser needs who are more outspoken. Clients who are poor or who are members of racial or ethnic minority groups may be too intimidated to demand special treatment. Group differences in empowerment will be discussed further in Chapter 5.

Rules that take on a life of their own produce "red tape." Clients are likely to see them as impediments to service even when their needs are not unusual. They may question why they must fill out so many different forms or see so many different people before they can receive the help they need. Sometimes cumbersome procedures are required to satisfy the requirements of different, uncoordinated funding sources. In such an instance, the bureaucratic effects are compounded by the fact that more than one bureaucracy is involved (both state and local government, for example).

The following discussion, by the mother of a child with severe disabilities, humorously illustrates the perils of red tape and inflexibility:

> If you were to ask me the most difficult aspect of rearing this unique little girl, the answer would not be the countless hospitalizations, the equipment demands, the sleepless nights or the too-long stares when we're in public. It would be the government bureaucracies we face to provide for her, protect her and help her tap her potential. . . .
>
> I . . . begin by introducing . . . the five or so caseworkers assigned to our Claire. One is from Arizona's Department of Developmental Disability. Another is with Arizona Long Term Care. Another is with the Arizona Health Care Cost Containment System. Another is with APIPA, and I don't know what that stands for. I lost track of acronyms, agencies and caseworkers long ago.
>
> These caseworkers, assigned as advocates for my daughter's needs, come to our house, one by one, once each year to conduct two-hour interviews and verify in person

> that Claire, a child who is now six and has never spoken, has not been the recipient of a miracle cure.
>
> I don't know what the caseworkers do beyond this interview, but two things have occurred to me. First, burglars could just arrive at our door with a lot of forms and an acronym and anyone in the household would let them in. Second, there must be yet another contrived constitutional privacy right or some insider trading rule that prohibits state and federal employees who work with the same family from using one file, comparing notes, sharing information or even carpooling for interviews. . . .
>
> Title XIX qualifies children on the basis of need (i.e., income) or degree of disability. Claire qualified on the basis of disability, but we are still required once each year to submit to an in-office interview (with yet another caseworker) in which I must give copies of our car titles, house deed, bank account statements, W-2s, and the like. A sample caseworker comment from one year's interview: "I see you have a new piano in your home. Claire doesn't play this, does she?" I had to wonder why someone looking at a child who can't sit, hold her head up or make any discernible voluntary movements felt compelled to ask such a question.
>
> One year, we made the monumental mistake of adding Claire to our car title. Claire must be on the car title in Arizona for us to have a handicapped license plate. . . . But I had to face the glare of a Title XIXer who said, "Is Claire driving this car?" I was required to sign a witnessed statement that said our cortically blind kindergartner did not take the Chevrolet Suburban out for spins. . . .
>
> I began using our newly discovered Title XIX medical benefits in August. In just six weeks, I received authorization for a new wheelchair and a scoliosis jacket. In October, I got a call from a caseworker who informed me that Claire's Title XIX benefits were being terminated as of that day. He had discovered on the forms that I fill out for the financial interview a $1,600 bank account for Claire. It was a burial account within the $1,500 limit allowed by statute, but it had earned interest. Claire had too much income. I offered to close the account. "Too late," he said. Then he added, "But you can always come down and reapply for Title XIX." It took me six months to get qualified the first time. I should have us reinstated just in time for summer school this year.
>
> I am a lawyer who teaches and writes about administrative process. Yet this system is beyond my expertise. How do parents with language barriers, little or no knowledge of due process and noncompulsive personalities cope? (Jennings, 1994)

Compartmentalization

Functional specificity tends to compartmentalize people and to prevent professionals from seeing them in a holistic way. In lay settings, people tend to think of one another as individuals with many statuses. For example, a man might be seen as a carpenter, a father, a husband, a son, an uncle, a churchgoer, and a golf enthusiast. However, when he is at the hospital for surgery, he may simply be thought of as "the knee" by the doctors and nurses who are treating him. The following quotes are from parents of children with disabilities who came to resent physicians who did not treat their children as diffuse individuals:

> (Our pediatrician) treated her as an article in a medical journal.
>
> The pediatrician didn't seem interested in anyone with a problem. . . . He would keep him alive but he wasn't interested in Brian as a person.

> It's like when you take your dog to the vet. . . . Not many doctors pick him up and try to communicate with him as a child. (Darling, 1979, pp. 151–152)

The Effect of Automation and Funding Changes

All the disadvantages discussed above seem to be made worse by recent trends in human services toward increasing automation. Garson (1988) looked at a public assistance office that had recently moved from a system that relied on personal contact between caseworkers and their clients to one in which computers were used to make eligibility determinations. At the same time, caseworkers began to be evaluated on the basis of their productivity, that is, the number of computer-related operations they performed in a month. One of the caseworkers she interviewed explained the system:

> "Just talking isn't an action," Eddy explained. "Opal earned over 150 percent of her budget the week before last as a Kelly Girl, and the downtown computer automatically threw her off. I spent half an hour this morning telling her how to get back on. I won't get credit for that. . . . But when I make up a T.D. [Turnaround Document] and an MRW [Monthly Report Worksheet] and send it to EDP then I'll get .3."
>
> "What we run here is a garage," he explained as we walked upstairs. "They come in for air, a valve job, oil. It's a service station, that's all. (Garson, 1988, p. 80–81)

Garson suggests that the automation of the eligibility determination process serves to distance caseworkers from their clients' life situations. Although workers were happy to be relieved of the tedious calculations involved, "newer workers who'd never done the calculation themselves couldn't estimate for a client that cutting her rent from \$200 to \$150 a month might in fact make the family poorer" (Garson, 1988, p. 89).

An even more damaging consequence of the new system was related to the emphasis on productivity, as measured by specific, instrumental actions, rather than on the more qualitative ways in which caseworkers had helped their clients in the past. Garson quotes a caseworker:

> The way it is now you're not a social worker, you're an FAW [Financial Assistance Worker]. If you take ten minutes out to help one kid in a family you're gonna' fall behind. . . . If they say, "I think my baby is sick. I don't know where to take him," I don't say, "What's the matter?" I say, "I can recommend you to Project Good Health." And I don't even look. (Garson, 1988, p. 93)

The consequences for the service user are similar to those of bureaucracy—depersonalization, ritualism–inflexibility, and compartmentalization.

The changes Garson discusses are becoming ever more common in human services today, as a result of both automation and funding imperatives. Newer managed care models are designed to increase efficiency, sometimes at the expense of service quality. The trend toward such models seems to be having the effect of increasing bureaucracy, with its attendant disadvantages for the client. Changes in the early intervention system in Pennsylvania provide an example from the author's experience as the director of an agency in that state during the 1980s and early 1990s.

In the past, families interested in receiving early intervention services generally contacted various government-funded, nonprofit agencies directly. Many of these agencies were organized bureaucratically and required a certain amount of paperwork to initiate services. Under the new system, instituted during the 1990s, case managers, who were Civil Service employees, were designated as "single point of contact" service coordinators. The intention of this designation was ostensibly to make it easier for families to access services but would also have the effect of controlling costs by monitoring the number and type of services received. The immediate effect of the change was to confuse families. Now, instead of simply completing the service agency's paperwork, they had to submit to an additional intake process, involving interviews and form completion with the case manager. Most of the families entering the early intervention service system are under a considerable amount of stress, because they have recently learned that their child has or might have a disability. Undergoing a complex intake process at that time is likely to add to rather than to alleviate their stress.

At the same time that the early intervention system added an extra service layer by expanding the role of its case managers, it also restructured the way it provided funding to agencies. In the past, agencies generally received their funding by billing the government for the number of children served each month. Reimbursement rates varied from one county to the next, because of differences in transportation and personnel costs in urban and rural areas, among other factors. The system involved some record keeping, but paperwork was kept to a minimum. During the early 1990s, the state did a study to determine average service costs across counties. The impetus for the study was the need to standardize rates in order to institute Medical Assistance billing (a way to draw down additional federal funds for these services), although some in state government also thought that more accountability was needed in the system. The consequences for service users were twofold.

First, when rates were standardized throughout the state, those agencies that had had higher rates in the past had to find ways to make up the shortfall in their budgets. Thus, like the agency studied by Garson (1988), they had to find ways to increase their productivity. Service providers who had previously spent 1 ½ or 2 hours on home visits with families had to limit their visits to 1 hour or less in order to complete more visits during a day. As a result, some families began to complain about depersonalization and other consequences of bureaucracy discussed above.

Second, paperwork increased. Under the new system, providers had to submit service plans for each client twice a year, along with a variety of new "authorization" forms. These forms had to be approved by several people before services could begin, generally resulting in a delay in the onset of needed services. Further, all services had to correspond exactly to those listed on the service plan, otherwise the government would not pay for them. Thus, rather than a working document that could be readily adjusted to take a family's developing needs into account, the plan became the inflexible basis for the ritualized provision of certain designated services. Plan changes were still possible but required a cumbersome approval process. Agencies intent on providing appropriate and necessary services to families were forced to find creative ways to circumvent the system in order to continue to receive sufficient funding to operate their programs.

Providers in a bureaucratic system are frequently faced with conflicts involving the goals of compliance and service quality. Although bureaucratic rules are intended to make the service system more effective and efficient, they are typically made by bureaucrats who have little direct contact with clients. Conversely, workers involved in the direct provision of services are usually not in a position in the bureaucratic hierarchy to make the rules that govern them. As a result, established procedures may not be "best practice" in the field and, in the worst cases, may actually interfere with service quality. Although change is possible, it tends to come slowly, because bureaucrats are trained to enforce the rules, not to change them. Bureaucratic careers are commonly built on enforcement ability, and those who "rock the boat" are not often rewarded in a bureaucratic system. Further, as Hagedorn (1995) suggests, human service bureaucracies tend to become entrenched, because employees are likely to protect their own interests at the expense of those of their clients.

Total Institutions: An Extreme Form of Bureaucratic Organization

The total institution (Goffman, 1961) is an organizational form sometimes encountered in the field of human services. Like other forms of bureaucratic organization, it is based on differentiated statuses, arranged in a hierarchy, and on a strict system of rules. In addition to these characteristics, total institutions also have the following traits:

- Clients are "inmates"; that is, they reside at the institution that serves them.
- Inmates have restricted contact with the world outside the institution.
- "(T)here is a basic split between a large managed group (the inmates) . . . and a small supervisory staff. . . . Social mobility between the two strata is grossly restricted; social distance is typically great and often formally prescribed." (Goffman, 1961, p. 7)

Examples of total institutions in the human service field include mental hospitals, prisons, and nursing homes, among others.

Although the structure of specific institutions varies, in the mental hospital studied by Goffman, a ward system was used to organize the inmates. Clients were rewarded for what the professionals defined as appropriate behavior by being moved to more favorable wards, while noncompliant clients were relegated to the less desirable, back wards. As in the status inequality model described in Chapter

2, clients were expected to accept the professionals' definition of the situation, and lack of acceptance was labeled as denial.

Goffman was especially concerned with the effect of this organizational structure on clients' self-concepts. He concluded that, in the process of conforming to the views of the staff, clients lost whatever self-identity they may have had before entering the institution. Thus, like the hospital patient described earlier, a man who previously thought of himself as a carpenter, father, son, churchgoer, and golf enthusiast would come to see himself only as a resident of a particular ward. This merging of institutional and personal worldviews might actually hinder reintegration into society after the inmate leaves the institution. The role of the self-concept in professional–client interaction will be discussed further in Chapter 4.

Newer Organizational Forms

Because of the disadvantages of bureaucratic organization noted above, some human service agencies have been moving toward other organizational forms. In this endeavor, they have borrowed from the business world, where managers have learned that workers perform more productively when they are included in the decision-making process. Newer, "human relations" approaches (Lewis, Lewis, & Souflee, 1993) acknowledge the potential contributions of lower-level staff to organizational vitality.

In participatory management models, the "top-down" process of decision making is replaced by a more democratic version, in which all staff members have the opportunity to contribute to agency policy (see, for example, Toch & Grant, 1982). The client is likely to benefit from such a model, because the input of direct service staff is likely to be more relevant to the client experience than that of upper-level administrators. However, in the process, some efficiency may be sacrificed for effectiveness. Although participatory management is being used by increasingly more private, human service agencies today, the clients of public agencies tend to remain subject to the problems inherent in government bureaucracy.

In a review of the characteristics of successful human service programs, Schorr (1997) notes that such programs are "comprehensive, flexible, responsive, and persevering" (p. 5). She quotes a program representative who reports that "no one ever says, this may be what you need, but it's not part of my job to help you get it" (p. 5). In her travels around the country, Schorr encountered a number of programs that were successfully using this nonbureaucratic approach to serve clients.

Another recent trend in the organization of human service agencies has been the shift from nonprofit to for-profit management. In the past, human services were generally provided directly by the government or by private, nonprofit organizations that received both public and private funds. Those organizations typically provided services that were free, or they used sliding scales to charge clients according to their ability to pay. Because they were structured to break even, nonprofit agencies charged only enough to cover their operating costs.

However, analysts suggested that many nonprofit agencies operated inefficiently. In addition, representatives of for-profit corporations began to see the operation of human services as an opportunity to enter new markets. These representatives appealed to government officials with their proposals to manage services more efficiently and effectively and at lower cost. As a result, many prisons, rehabilitation facilities, schools, and other human service organizations today are operated as businesses. Even the welfare system has been experiencing a shift toward for-profit management as Temporary Aid to Needy Families (TANF) has replaced(Aid to Families with Dependent Children (AFDC). An article in *The New York Times* reported the following example:

> The newest and most formidable entrant in a field once left largely to local charities and several small companies is Lockheed Martin, the $30 billion giant of the weapons industry. A nonmilitary division, Lockheed Information Services, is bidding against Electronic Data Systems and Andersen Consulting to take over $563 million in welfare operations in Texas. (Bernstein, 1996, p. 1)

In addition to their profit-making orientation and their size, the newer managers include companies that are not necessarily based in the communities in which the services are provided.

What are the consequences of this shift for service users? Competition among service providers is not necessarily bad for clients. Just as businesses with superior products to sell are likely to attract more customers than those with shoddy merchandise, for-profit service agencies may be motivated to satisfy their clients in order to stay in business. However, the "clients" of service agencies are not necessarily the service users. Those who pay the bills may be third-party insurers or government agencies, whose interest is efficient operation rather than consumer satisfaction. In addition, the fate of service users who are poor but ineligible for government benefits may be grim in a for-profit system in which they are a liability for service providers.

Thus, the structure of human service agencies can affect the nature of the services that are provided. Client outcomes are likely to vary as a result. Consequently, professionals need to be aware of the impact of organizational variables on their clients during the intervention process.

Opportunity Structures: Preexisting Organizational Constraints Affecting Service Users

Just as the organizational characteristics of an agency may set the parameters of a service encounter, preexisting client characteristics may have a similar effect. As Fig. 3.1 indicates, one of those characteristics is the client's opportunity structure. Before they ever become clients of human service agencies, potential service users are subject to the opportunities and constraints of the societies in which they live. These opportunities include access to financial security, jobs, friendships, medical care, and other resources. Opportunities vary both between and within societies. Within society, access to opportunities may be determined by neighborhood of residence, family ties, race, religion, and other factors.

The term, "opportunity structure," was introduced by Cloward and Ohlin (1960) in their study of juvenile delinquents. Their work, in turn, was based on earlier work in the structural–functional school in sociological theory by Robert K. Merton and on the work of the "Chicago School" sociologist, Edwin Sutherland. They were interested in explaining why some youths in poor neighborhoods became delinquent while others did not. Their conclusion was that not all youths had access to the same opportunities.

They suggested that all youths occupy a place in two different opportunity structures: legitimate and illegitimate. The legitimate structure relates to opportunities to get a good education and establish a career. Some children in poor neighborhoods do in fact do well in school because of supportive teachers, family members, and other opportunities for success that are not available to all. Cloward and Ohlin suggest that access to illegitimate opportunities is differentially distributed as well. Some boys have the opportunity to become apprenticed to older professional criminals, who help them establish themselves in a career of crime; others live in more disorganized communities, where access to an established, criminal hierarchy is limited. The latter group may become "retreatists" and turn to drugs when legitimate opportunities are absent as well.

This theory of differential opportunity can be applied to other service users, in addition to juvenile delinquents. In my studies of parents of children with disabilities, for example, I learned that these parents have differential access to two different opportunity structures: "normal" society and a subculture of disability. Most parents have a goal of normalization, which includes appropriate child care and educational placements for their children, acceptance by their neighbors, and generally a lifestyle that is not significantly different from that of other families in the same social class who do not have children with disabilities. However, integration into normal society is often problematic for these parents for a variety of reasons, including social barriers such as stigma, physical barriers such as stairs and curbs, and economic barriers such as the high costs of treatment. On the other hand, normalization is fostered by opportunities such as supportive family members, understanding employers, and laws such as the Americans with Disabilities Act and the Individuals with Disabilities Education Act.

Some families who are not able to achieve normalization become integrated instead in a disability–advocacy subculture built around relationships with other families in similar situations. These families typically join national disability organizations, such as the ARC or the Spina Bifida Association of America, and local support and advocacy groups with names like Parent to Parent or Families Together. The subculture has its own literature, including *Exceptional Parent* magazine, various newsletters, and electronic mail lists and websites. However, not all parents have access to these opportunities, either. Some parents do not speak English; have disability-related limitations of their own; live in isolated, rural areas; are illiterate; or are simply poor and overwhelmed with the daily need to provide food, clothing, and shelter for their families. [For a further discussion of the opportunity structures of families of children with disabilities, see, Darling and Baxter (1996) and Seligman and Darling (1997).]

Different opportunity structures will be meaningful as well for other client populations. Human service professionals need to learn as much as possible about the clients they serve in order to understand the context within which they will be working. A sociological approach to human service practice requires that professionals help clients to change their opportunity structures. In the case of parents of children with disabilities just discussed, professionals in the past commonly used an approach based on status inequality and tried to change the parents, assuming that, without professional services, they would be unable to accept and cope with their situation. In the partnership model, which is becoming more common in this field, the focus of services is on expanding the parents' opportunities. Such opportunity expansion involves activities such as advocacy to promote the inclusion of a child with disabilities in a regular public school class (promoting opportunities for normalization), or the provision of information about Internet support groups to parents who were not previously aware of the existence of such groups (promoting opportunities for access to the alternative disability subculture).

How can professionals learn about the relevant opportunity structures for the clients they serve? The first step probably involves reading the literature about the population of interest, so that they will be familiar with the world of poverty, drug addiction, domestic violence, mental retardation, or whatever conditions characterize those who use their services. Literature written by clients, such as autobiographical accounts, is often the most enlightening. Such literature includes articles in newsletters published by consumer groups such as the Alliance for the Mentally Ill and the National Union of the Homeless, as well as magazines and books. The sociological methods of observation, interviewing, and questionnaire development are perhaps the best ways of learning about clients' opportunity structures. These methods will be discussed later in this volume.

Roles: The Expected Behaviors of Service Providers and Service Users

In addition to the concepts of social organization and opportunity structure, the concept of social role, which also derives from structural theory, can be used to better understand the client–professional encounter. Sociologists use the concept of role to describe the behaviors associated with a particular status, or place in society. Studies have shown, for example, that certain expectations have traditionally been associated with gender roles in American society, and knowledge of these expectations has been useful in understanding the behavior of men and women.

This section will be concerned with the cultural expectations associated with the roles of service provider and service user in American society. Much of the literature in this area comes from the field of medical sociology, in which the prototypical professional–client relationship is that between doctor and patient. This literature has relevance for other professional–client relationships in human services as well.

The Professional Role

The pattern variables discussed earlier in connection with bureaucracy also can be used to describe the ideal–typical professional role in American society. As Parsons (1951) has suggested, the professional role tends to be characterized by the traits of universalism, functional specificity, affective neutrality, achievement, and collectivity orientation. The first four were discussed in the section on bureaucracy above. Collectivity orientation (as opposed to self-orientation) suggests that professionals are expected to be altruistic, that is, they are expected to work toward their clients' well-being rather than toward their own self-interest.

Freidson (1970b) argues that Parsons's criteria could apply as well to nonprofessional service providers such as plumbers as to professional service providers such as physicians. He suggests that an additional criterion needs to be added: that of professional dominance. Physicians in particular are expected, because of their advanced training and presumed expertise, to exercise authority over their patients. This authority also contains elements of paternalism, so that when medical professionals make decisions on behalf of their patients, they are assumed to be acting in their patients' best interest. Typically, the patient shares this assumption. During my last visit to the dentist, for example, I overheard a discussion between a patient and a hygienist in the next room. The hygienist told the patient that it had been a year since her last X rays and asked her whether she wanted X rays to be taken again that day. The patient replied, "Whatever you say. You know what you're doing. As long as the insurance will pay . . ."

Freidson suggests that the basis for professional dominance is organized autonomy. He argues that the profession of medicine is self-governing, because its work tends to be too complex to be readily understood by others. Unlike bureaucrats, then, physicians operate somewhat independently from other structures. However, for the client, the consequences of professional dominance are very similar to those of bureaucracy, including depersonalization and compartmentalization.

One of the ways that physicians maintain their dominance over their clients is through information control. The literature in medical sociology contains many examples of how the medical profession maintains its dominance by keeping patients "in the dark" about their diagnoses and/or prognoses, especially in the case of chronic and terminal illness (Anspach, 1993; Clark & LaBeff, 1982; Glaser & Strauss, 1965; Quint, 1965) and permanent disability (Darling, 1979, 1994; Davis, 1960; Quine & Pahl, 1986; Svarstad & Lipton, 1977). In these cases, the physician's usual basis for authority—the ability to cure—is absent; the physician remains in control only as long as the patient (or patient's family) maintains hope (for a cure). As one physician remarked,

> I don't enjoy it. . . . I don't really enjoy a really handicapped child who comes in drooling, can't walk and so forth. . . . Medicine is geared to the perfect human body. Something you can't do anything about challenges the doctor and reminds him of his own inabilities. (Darling, 1979, p. 215)

Physicians use various techniques to control information, including denial of the truth, stalling, and "passing the buck" by making a referral to another physician. Sometimes, they do tell patients the truth but use technical jargon or euphemism, so that the patients do not understand what they have been told. For example, rather than using a commonly understood diagnosis like cerebral palsy or mental retardation, physicians have told parents that their children had "motor delays" or were "slow for their age" (Darling, 1994).

For patients, the primary consequence of information control is a feeling of *anomie*, which is characterized by both meaninglessness and powerlessness. Most studies indicate that patients suspect that something is amiss long before their physicians provide them with an accurate diagnosis and prognosis and experience considerable stress when their fears are not immediately confirmed. The result is often disillusionment with the medical profession. This account by the mother of a child with Down syndrome is illustrative:

> I asked what was wrong with her ears, and they said not to worry about it. . . . I always thought they told you the truth in the hospital and if you wanted to know anything you should ask. I really thought her ears looked funny and I had this funny feeling, so I asked the doctor, "Is there anything wrong?" and he looked right at me and said, "No." So I assumed she was O.K., and there was nothing wrong with her. . . . The next morning he told me she was retarded. . . . I was very bitter about it. . . . I had had the same pediatrician for six years, and he had always been truthful. I trusted him. . . . I guess he felt that I didn't need to know at that time. (Darling, 1979, pp. 131–132)

Although Freidson (1970b) suggests that medicine is the only profession characterized by professional dominance, elements of dominance, such as paternalism and information control, can be found in other helping professions as well. Such dominance is probably most pronounced when the difference in education between the client and the professional is great. Parents who did not graduate from high school themselves are likely to feel intimidated in conferences with their children's teachers and school officials, when those professionals use unfamiliar terms. And any parent is likely to be intimidated by the unfamiliar acronyms like IEP (Individualized Education Program) and MDT (multidisciplinary team) that are used so commonly in education and other human service fields today.

Wilensky and Lebeaux (1965) suggest that the field of social work is becoming more professionalized, as evidenced by its concern with maintaining authority. This concern is characterized by a movement toward credentialism. Social workers, psychologists, family therapists, and other helping professionals have been instituting processes for accreditation and licensing on both the national and state levels. These credentials are increasingly being recognized by various funding sources. In Pennsylvania, for example, Medical Assistance reimbursement is only available for services performed by licensed professionals. Thus, credentialed professionals become the gatekeepers of the human service system, and clients become dependent on their judgments.

The human service system today is characterized by conflicting tendencies. While professional dominance and the status inequality model from which it derives are being promoted through commonly used reimbursement systems such as Medical Assistance, they are at the same time being eliminated in many system sectors. As Chapter 2 suggested, newer approaches that promote partnerships between clients and professionals are becoming increasingly popular. Interestingly, some service models seem to be promoting both professional dominance and partnership at the same time (cf the example in Chapter 1 of the lay family service worker whose services were not billable in the state early intervention system). Changes in client and professional roles resulting from newer partnership approaches will be discussed later in this chapter.

When clients enter a new helping relationship, they are likely to have certain expectations about the professionals they will encounter, based on their past experience in society. They will probably expect these professionals to be universalistic, functionally specific, affectively neutral, and dominant and may be surprised (perhaps pleasantly surprised) by professionals whose behavior does not adhere to these traditional norms.

The Client Role

Just as certain expectations are associated with the roles of professionals in human services, clients are also expected to behave in prescribed ways. Again, the literature in medical sociology seems to say the most about these role prescriptions. Perhaps the best known client role in the literature is the "sick role," first described by Talcott Parsons.

Parsons (1951) viewed illness as a form of social deviance, because good health is generally regarded as normative. However, he suggested that illness is regarded as acceptable in society under certain conditions. According to Parsons, people who are ill are not blamed for their illnesses and are exempt from certain obligations, such as work, for a period of time. However, in return for this legitimization, they are expected to acknowledge that their illness is undesirable and must try to get well; further, they must seek competent help and cooperate in treatment.

Although the sick role seems to describe the norms associated with acute illness in American society, it may not explain other client roles. Freidson (1970b) suggests that the criterion of responsibility is important in distinguishing between medical and legal deviance (i.e., illness and crime). He argues that those who break the law are generally blamed for their actions and, as a result, may lose some privileges and acquire additional obligations, such as prison terms and fines. On the other hand, those who are ill tend to be excused from ordinary obligations such as work and may acquire additional privileges.

However, as noted in Chapter 2, the increasing medicalization of deviance has resulted in less blaming for some actions in society today, and both hereditary and environmental factors are held responsible for various forms of deviant behavior. In court, for example, defendants commonly argue that they are not responsible for their criminal acts because of extenuating circumstances in their backgrounds, such as having been abused as a child. In a recent case, lawyers for Jesse Timmendequas, who was found guilty of raping and murdering 7-year-old Megan Kanka in a well-publicized trial, argued that he should not be put to death because of "mitigating circumstances," including having been raised in an impoverished, dysfunctional family where abuse and neglect were rampant and having suffered from fetal alcohol effect and head injuries resulting from two car accidents. As Freidson suggested, being defined as "sick," rather than "bad," would, result in a lesser reduction of privileges or a lighter punishment.

On the other hand, today people are often blamed for conditions for which they were not held responsible in the past. Since the discovery of the link between smoking and lung cancer, for example, victims of that disease have sometimes been regarded with contempt rather than pity. Various diseases, including AIDS, venereal infections, drug addiction, and alcoholism, have long been associated with blaming and stigma for their victims. However, those with conditions such as heart disease and cancer, who used to be blame-free, are sometimes being stigmatized today when their diseases are preceded by sedentary lifestyles and high-fat diets. Similarly, drivers hurt in accidents while under the influence of alcohol may not receive much sympathy.

The legitimacy dimension of the sick role seems to apply best to acute illnesses, such as a cold or the flu, and to injuries, such as sprained ankles and broken arms, that result from accidents that could not have been readily prevented. The dimension is more problematic in the case of chronic illness and permanent disability. Human service clients often include individuals with "illegitimate" conditions, such as mental illness, mental retardation, and obvious physical disability. Legitimacy is determined by societal values. Because our society tends to value high achievement and physical attractiveness, these individuals are likely to have experienced stigma in the form of stares, taunts, jeers, physical avoidance, or job discrimination. Human service professionals may, as a result of their socialization in a stigmatizing society, tend to devalue these clients as well.

Client roles are also shaped by the human service system itself and by agency expectations for client behavior. Peter (1999) has shown how the lack of autonomy and responsibility sometimes exhibited by human service clients results more from agency socialization than from the clients' innate incompetence. She cites the example of a client with mental retardation who engages in various forms of "deviant" behavior, such as withdrawing from social involvement and engaging in self-abuse as a way of getting attention, and argues that these behaviors are adaptive in a context in which clients have little power to control their lives. She concludes that the service system encourages a client role that exaggerates incompetence. An understanding of the client role therefore requires an understanding of the power imbalance between service providers and service users that exists in service settings based on a status inequality model.

Conflict between Client and Professional Role Prescriptions

As noted earlier, the prescribed professional role in American society is characterized by the traits of universalism, affective neutrality, functional specificity, achievement, and dominance. On the other hand, the client role may be characterized by the opposite traits: particularism, affectivity, functional diffuseness, ascription, and submission to professional dominance. Whereas the professional is concerned with all clients equally, clients typically regard themselves and their needs as special. Although professionals try to maintain emotional distance between themselves and their clients, clients seem to appreciate professionals who "care." Whereas professionals focus on only some aspects of their clients' lives, clients regard themselves in a more holistic way. Professionals acquire their jobs through choice and achievement, whereas clients sometimes acquire their statuses involuntarily. Finally, while professionals expect, because of prescriptions inherent in their own role and in the sick role, to be dominant in their relationships with clients, clients expect to be submissive to professional authority. These differences can result in conflict between professionals and their clients.

The quotes from parents of children with disabilities presented earlier in this chapter suggest these parents' dissatisfaction with their physicians' failure to treat their children as diffuse individuals, rather than "things," animals, or "articles in a medical journal." Lack of emotional understanding also has been cited as a reason for dissatisfaction with medical professionals:

> Just going to ___ Children's Hospital was an emotional experience. I had never been exposed to the world of the handicapped. Seeing all those children in wheelchairs and braces made me think of Kathy. . . . I got the impression that (the doctor) didn't

> understand why I was so upset. He kept saying, "Why are you crying?" (Darling, 1979, p. 152)

On the other hand, the mother of a premature baby with serious medical problems told me that she had a much better relationship with the attending physician after an interchange in which he began to cry about the lack of improvement in the baby's condition.

Some parents in this situation blame professionals' lack of sensitivity on the fact that professionals view their work as a job, while families must live with their children's disabilities 24 hours a day. One mother who had four teenagers with the same cerebral-palsy-like syndrome attributed the victim blaming of the professionals she encountered to their achieved status:

> I told my doctor I was always tired, and he said, "It's your nerves." . . . It got to the point where I thought, "Nobody wants to help me." . . . I saw a psychologist on TV . . . and I called him. . . . He said, "Don't you think someone else could take care of your children as well as you can?" I said, "It's not a matter of someone else. It's a matter of being able to pay somebody." . . . He said, "Go to work." . . . I'm not qualified. I've been home for 20 years. . . . I'm seeing someone else now. He's kind of giving me the blame for the way I am: "It's your fault you feel the way you do about things." I don't want to feel this way. . . . He says, "you create your own problems." My problem is that I have four handicapped children, and that has nothing to do with the fact that I had an unhappy childhood. . . . I'm nervous because I have reason to be nervous. . . . That night we were supposed to go someplace, and the van at the CP [cerebral palsy] Center broke down, so suddenly we had four kids to worry about. . . . We had to change our plans. . . . That's the problem with these professionals. . . . They have a job. . . . They don't live with the parents 24 hours a day. What sounds nice at the office just doesn't work in real life. (Darling, 1979, pp. 179–180)

One of the most frequent complaints in this situation has related to professional dominance. Many parents come to resent professional control over their lives:

> The doctor said, "professionals, not parents, should decide on institutionalization." I didn't like that.
>
> [The obstetrician said,] "you cannot possibly take care of this child. I'll send the social worker up to you, and you can put him away." I was mad at the world and was determined I was going to get through it.
>
> At the beginning, I let (the doctors) rule me. . . . Now they do like I ask them to. . . . I used to be in awe of them. . . . Now I won't just sign anything. . . . I've complained to nurses. I've changed a lot. . . . We've had a lot of disputes. They would not give her a bottle in the hospital. They thought she was too old to have a bottle at two years. . . .
>
> We were always going back and forth to ___ Children's Hospital. . . . It was a constantly pulling away. We could never be a family. . . . It was always, "We have to go to the hospital." We had to go to doctors, doctors, doctors. . . . We never could get to know our child. . . . We got to the point where we hated doctors, we hated ___ Children's Hospital. (Darling, 1979, pp. 153–154)

Concern with professional dominance also has been present in other populations. For example, a man who spent a long time in a rehabilitation center and who applied for government benefits following a head injury experienced great difficulty in obtaining information from professionals. He writes:

> I've suffered years of the Do-gooders' afflictions. Their game is about wanting to be in control of other people's lives. You need some help, you had better be willing to give up your dignity and autonomy. And show some gratitude. (Golfus, 1994, p. 168)

Although professional dominance still exists, new roles have been emerging—for both clients and professionals—that are based more on mutual authority and respect. This change is discussed in the next section.

New Roles for Clients and Professionals

Ayer (1984) and others have suggested that the failure of professionals to meet family needs has resulted in self-help activities by families. Although most service users begin by acquiescing to professional authority, many come to play an entrepreneurial role (Darling, 1979, 1988) in order to secure appropriate services. This role includes: (1) seeking information, (2) seeking control, and (3) challenging authority.

When clients encounter difficulties in their interactions with professionals, they are likely to continue to search for appropriate services and helpful service providers. Negative experiences can be a catalyst for action. Pizzo (1983) argues that parent advocacy derives from "acute, painful experiences," and Haug and Lavin (1983) report that the most important variable in consumerist challenges to medical authority is the experience of medical error. Patients with chronic conditions that result in frequent contact with medical professionals are more likely than others to encounter errors or discrepancies in their treatment. The mother of a child with multiple medical problems explains her actions:

> There is so much confusion. Each doctor tells me something different. . . . I wish they would talk to each other. I have requested that all communication between doctors be carbon copied to me, in the hopes of deciphering what is being said. . . . I have purchased some medical dictionaries so I can better understand the terminology and discuss Michael's condition with my doctors on a more realistic level. I'm starting to wonder if perhaps Michael doesn't need to see some other specialists. . . . I keep asking my cardiologist, and he finally responds, "It's your dime. If you want to see one, go ahead." I want to trust him, but at the same time I don't feel that he is taking Michael's condition seriously enough. . . . I refuse to simply wait for him to die. (Spano, 1994, pp. 38–39)

Patients with chronic conditions and parents of children with chronic conditions are likely to encounter others in similar situations in the course of their treatment. Through interaction, they learn that their concerns are shared. They also learn about the possibilities for activism and advocacy from the experience of others; they learn about techniques that have worked and come to realize that authority can be successfully challenged. As an article about the Parents' Union of Philadelphia (Wice & Fernandez, 1984) noted, "Mrs. Thomas was powerful when she was linked to others through an alert advocacy group. . . . Alone, a parent may be tempted to give up. Together, parents have power" (p. 40).

Pizzo (1983) notes that many parents become involved in self-help groups after seeing something in the media. Beginning with the Civil Rights Movement of the 1950s and 1960s, modern advocacy movements have received considerable attention in the media, and groups ranging from gays and lesbians to persons with disabilities have become increasingly aware of the possibility of asserting their rights and challenging authority. As consumerism has grown, publications have appeared that have served as instruction manuals for empowerment in areas as diverse as women's health, educational advocacy, and automobile buying, among others. Many grassroots groups of human service consumers also have published newsletters that promote empowerment strategies.

As service users have become more outspoken, professional roles have changed in response. As noted in the two preceding chapters, many professionals have been moving toward a partnership model in human services. In this model, the professional is not dominant; rather, clients and professionals are viewed as equal partners. The professional's contribution to the relationship is specialized knowledge, based on training and experience, and the client contributes particularistic expertise, based on experience in his or her culture and daily routine. The professional acts as a facilitator or consultant to families, who then decide on a course of action. These descriptions by parents suggest professionals who subscribe to the partnership model:

> The important aspect of the doctor's presentation was that he involved us as equals in the decision-making process. . . . By involving us in the process and by giving us his professional opinion as an opinion, he returned to us our parental rights of making the important decision that would affect our child's life. *We were in control*, but we were no longer alone. (Stotland, 1984, p. 72, emphasis added)

> The staff at the early intervention center knew we wanted Aric to attend a regular kindergarten class. . . . They gave us ideas to get him into the setting. They never took control out of our hands, and we always did the steps ourselves. They were there as a resource and support. The staff at the early intervention center helped me to gel the vision. But it didn't take the Family and Child Learning Center to show me promise [in Aric]; I could see that when he was born. (Leifeld & Murray, 1995, pp. 246–247)

The Institute for Family-Centered Care published a checklist ("Families As Advisors," 1992) for professionals to help them determine whether or not they subscribed to the partnership model. Some of the items included:

- Do I believe that families bring unique expertise to our relationship?
- Do I believe in the importance of family participation in decision making at the program and policy level?
- Do I believe that families' perspectives and opinions are as important as professionals'?

- Do I work to create an environment in which families feel supported and comfortable enough to speak freely?
- Do I listen respectfully to the opinions of family members?

As noted in Chapter 2, newer training programs for physicians and other professionals are encouraging aspiring professionals to practice partnership skills prior to entering practice.

On the other hand, some professionals have argued that empowerment has gone too far and that professional dominance is still appropriate in human services. In a critique of client-driven services, Goodman (1994) argues that client direction disguises the essential inequality in the client–professional relationship: (1) The client is distressed; the professional is in control; (2) the client has a problem; the professional does not share the client's problem; and (3) the client needs help; the professional has resources and expertise to provide help. She argues further that the client has a choice and does not necessarily have to follow the professional's advice. Finally, she reaffirms the principle of affective neutrality with the suggestion that intimacy compromises objectivity.

In the same vein, a physician made the following comments on an e-mail discussion list:

> With all due respect to family centered care, there are parents who certainly know their children, but may not know what they need. In my practice, I see a significant number of families dealing with poverty, illiteracy, mental health disorders, substance abuse, incarceration of one or both parents, and more. They want the best for their kids, but may not have any idea what the options are or how to attain them. (Children with Special Health Care Needs List, November 2, 1996)

This critique seems to address a situation in which the client makes all treatment decisions without input from the professional. This situation does not occur when the model is truly one of partnership. In a partnership between client and professional, each contributes expertise. Professionals are important in such a relationship precisely because they have knowledge and resources that previously have not been available to the client. Once the client is informed, he or she can make any necessary decisions about treatment. Goodman, too, seems to suggest that the client–professional relationship is one-sided, rather than a balance between two complementary kinds of expertise. As Chapter 5 will explain, clients have expertise based on their life experiences. Professionals do not share this kind of expertise, which is essential to the application of the sociological perspective in human services.

Another critique of the client empowerment approach suggests that this approach may actually be dangerous. Gelles (1996) argues that, in the case of child welfare services, goals of family preservation and empowerment and of child protection can come into conflict with each other. He suggests that attempts at partnership with abusive parents have not prevented child maltreatment and death.

Certainly some of the causes of child abuse are often rooted in societal conditions that are beyond the ability of families and human service professionals to control (see Chapters 9 and 10 for a further discussion of the limits of human service work). Some cases of imminent risk may indeed require child protection efforts that deny empowerment rights to families. On the other hand, the overzealous removal of children from abusive situations that was practiced in the past did not prevent families from continuing the same practices with other children born into the family, and some situations defined by professionals as dangerous were merely culturally different. Some potentially dangerous situations can be changed through the introduction of different opportunity structures. Professionals need to exercise caution in making judgments about the appropriateness of their interventions, whether those interventions are based on a status inequality or a partnership model.

Chapter Summary

This chapter, the first of two providing a theoretical foundation for a partnership model in human services, has presented several concepts derived from structural–functional theory in sociology. Structural theories suggest that human behavior can be explained in terms of the organization of society. As the chapter has shown, clients may be affected by whether an agency is structured bureaucratically or uses a participatory management model of organization. Similarly, client outcomes will depend to some extent on their location within various opportunity structures.

Furthermore, social structures are associated with cultural expectations regarding appropriate behavior. People who occupy different positions in society are expected to play different roles. In our society, professionals are expected to achieve their positions through their own efforts and to be universalistic, functionally specific, affectively neutral, and collectivity oriented. Until fairly recently, they also were expected to be dominant in their relationships with clients. With the advent of newer partnership approaches in the human services, these role expectations have been changing.

Role-Play Exercise

The following exercise may be helpful in exploring the differences in interaction style that might accompany an approach involving professional dominance as opposed to one involving an egalitarian relationship between professional and client. This activity is appropriate for use with groups in a classroom situation, and students may enjoy acting out the scripts after they have written them. The purpose of the exercise is to reinforce understanding of the status inequality and partnership models in human services and to encourage students to think about the connections between role prescriptions and interactional outcomes. After completing the exercise, the actors may want to discuss how they felt during the different scenarios.

Write two scripts (2–3 minutes each) for each of the following human service situations. The first script should be based on a model of professional dominance and the second on a partnership model:

1. **Physician–patient.** The patient is at the doctor's office with the complaint of recurring headaches.
2. **Drug counselor–drug addict.** The addict has just entered a treatment program and is being interviewed for the first time.
3. **Marriage counselor–husband and wife.** The couple is at the counselor's office for the first time. They are seeking counseling because of frequent arguing.
4. **Professor–college student.** The student has come to see the professor during office hours because he is failing the course.
5. **Caseworker–parent accused of child abuse.** The caseworker has made a home visit to investigate a neighbor's complaint of child abuse.

Suggestions for Further Reading

Cloward, R.A., & Ohlin, L.E. (1960). *Delinquency and opportunity: A theory of delinquent gangs*. New York: Free Press.

Freidson, E. (1970). *Professional dominance*. Chicago: Aldine.

Garson, B. (1988). The automated social worker. In *The electronic sweatshop: How computers are transforming the office of the future into the factory of the past* (pp. 73–114). New York: Penguin.

Goffman, E. (1961). Asylums: Essays on the social situation of mental patients and other inmates. Garden City, NY: Doubleday Anchor.

4

Theoretical Foundations II

Social Process

In the previous chapter, the structural characteristics of both service users and service providers were described. Knowledge of these characteristics is important for understanding the context of human service work. Within this contextual framework, however, every interaction that occurs between any particular service provider and any given client is unique. An understanding of these interactional outcomes depends on knowledge of social process. As Fig. 2.1 suggested, social process is what occurs *between* interacting individuals, in this case, professionals and clients. The sociological perspective I will use to explore social process is symbolic interactionism. This chapter will provide an overview of the process of symbolic interaction using the client–professional encounter as the prime example. The concept of definition of the situation, which derives from symbolic interaction theory, will be highlighted, because of its central role in the partnership model that underlies this volume.

Symbolic interactionism owes its greatest debt to the early work of the American sociologists, George Herbert Mead, Charles Horton Cooley, and others. These theorists conceptualized society as a network of interacting individuals. Because interaction occurs continuously, society is constantly undergoing change. As a result, individuals must continually adjust their thinking and behavior to take the actions of others into account. The structural perspective employed in the last chapter provided insight into the relatively static aspects of client–professional interaction. Symbolic interactionism provides a framework for understanding the dynamic aspects of that interaction and helps us analyze what occurs in any particular human service situation. Figure 4.1 illustrates the relationship among the interactionist concepts that will be discussed in this chapter.

Definition of the Situation

Prior to their coming together, both client and professional have expectations about the human service situation. The professional has been socialized, both in school and on the job, to expect the client to act in certain ways. For example, he or she may expect the client to play the classic "sick role" described in the last chapter and to defer to the expertise of the professional. The client, on the other hand, will have some preconceived notions about the professional, based on his or her previous experience in the human service system or on what he or she has read or heard from others. In addition to these preconceived notions, both professional and client have preexisting worldviews, including norms, values, and beliefs derived from their previous interactions within their own cultural group. Diverse worldviews will be discussed further in Chapter 5.

Any human service situation has two components at the outset: (1) the preexisting ideas brought by both client and professional and (2) the setting. In the status inequality model, the setting for most human service interactions was the professional office or clinic. With the growth of partnership models in recent years, more interactions have been taking place in settings such as clients' homes, schools, community centers, child care centers, and other locations that are more "natural" to the client. The nature of the setting is likely to affect the client's perception of the situation. Generally, clients will feel less unsure about what is occurring in naturalistic settings than in less familiar professional environments.

When clients enter a new human service setting, they engage in a thinking process labeled by the sociologist W.I. Thomas as the definition of the situation. Thomas's (1928) well-known quote, "If men define situations as real, they are real in their consequences," suggests that human action is based more on what people think about a situation than on any objective conditions.

The process of defining the situation involves asking oneself the question, "What is going on here?" Typically, this process occurs at a subconscious level. In familiar situations, people do not spend much time thinking about what is happening. The process becomes more conscious, however, when events do not pro-

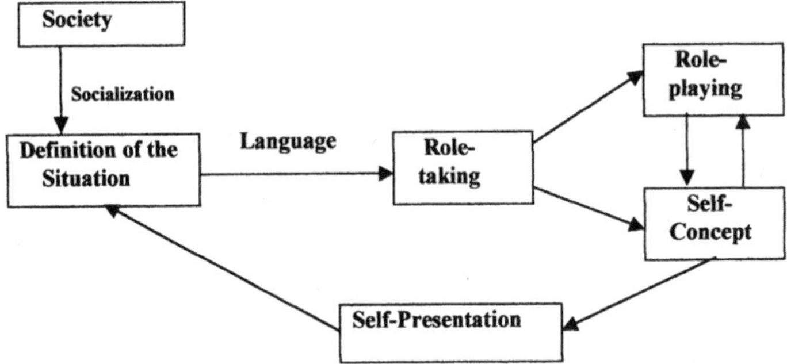

Figure 4.1. The process of symbolic interaction.

ceed as expected or when a similar situation has not been encountered in the past. Actors also are more likely to be conscious of the definitional process in situations that they perceive to be highly consequential, such as job interviews or meeting the parents of one's boyfriend or girlfriend for the first time.

In human services, the most important elements of a client's definition of the situation when he or she begins to interact with a professional for the first time are: (1) his or her definition of the agency and the professional and (2) his or her definition of the problem, or the reason for seeking help. Each will be discussed in turn.

Definition of the Agency

The client's definition of the human service agency is likely to be based primarily on previous experiences with human services and on information obtained through the media and through interaction with others who may have been clients of the agency in the past. Some clients will have had a considerable amount of human service experience, whereas others will have had very little or none. Commonly, clients of lower socioeconomic status tend to have more experience than those of higher status.

The agency that I directed for 15 years served families with young children through supportive home visiting, and, except for some court-ordered cases, all services were voluntary. Some families were referred by the local child protective service agency, and often these families were reluctant to participate in the services offered by our agency. When we were successful in enrolling these families, they eventually became more receptive to our home visits, which they came to define as helpful. Apparently, their initial hesitancy resulted from their fear that our staff, like the child protection caseworkers at the referring agency, had the power to remove their children and place them in foster care. Thus, their definition of the situation, which was based on experience rather than fact, made it difficult for us to establish a working relationship with them.

Thus, if professionals want to be truly helpful to their clients, they need to develop methods to gain insight into how their clients define them and the agencies for which they work. The methods of observation, interviewing, and questionnaire administration that will be discussed in later chapters are very useful in this regard. Professionals also need to learn as much as possible about the kinds of worldviews and definitions of the situation that are typically encountered in the client groups they serve.

From where do our definitions of the situation come? As suggested, they are the products of our past interactions in society. Client and professional definitions are most likely to be incongruent when their backgrounds differ significantly. In the example above, the professionals were (as most professionals are) from middle-class backgrounds, whereas the clients were of lower socioeconomic status. Misunderstandings are also common when clients and professionals are ethnically different. These differences and potential misunderstandings will be discussed further in Chapter 5, and techniques will be suggested for learning about the kinds of definitions that tend to prevail in various cultural groups.

Definition of the Problem

Professionals and their clients also may have different definitions of the reasons why clients are seeking help. An example from the agency cited above involved some self-referred families of lower socioeconomic status. These families wanted their children enrolled in our early intervention program for children with developmental delays. However, testing indicated that their children were functioning at or above their chronological age levels, making them ineligible for services. Our staff assumed that parents would not want their children to have a negative label and so questioned these parents about why they wanted so much to have their children labeled as developmentally delayed. In response, the families revealed to us that they knew (usually from interacting with other families) that developmental delays qualified as disabilities that would entitle them to receive Supplemental Security Income (SSI) payments from the government. These poor families realized that their neighbors who received SSI payments seemed much better off financially than they were. Their definition of the situation was that having their child labeled as disabled was a necessary condition for being able to adequately feed, house, and clothe their families. After this revelation, our staff was better able to understand behavior that had previously seemed inexplicable.

A similar case of definitional incongruity between client and professional was related to me by a colleague. She told me about a Head Start teacher she knew who had been having difficulty with a particular family. This family never seemed to follow through with any of the activities the teacher had left at their home, and the children seemed to be regressing developmentally. After several months of home visits with this "noncompliant" family, the teacher finally said in frustration, "I've been coming here for months leaving activities for you to do with your children and I can see that you never do them. Obviously, what I'm doing isn't meeting your needs. Tell me what you want from me." The mother then surprised her with this response: "You can get me a refrigerator." Apparently, the family's refrigerator had not been working for some time, and the mother was spending much of her day walking back and forth to a distant store (the family lived in a rural area) to buy milk and other perishable items. Her priority was feeding her children, and that took precedence over "playing games" with them. A similar case is described by another Head Start teacher and reported by Chafel (1993, p. 1):

> They lived in a trailer that had no screens. The first home visit was in August . . . I estimated 500 to 600 flies in the trailer. The mother . . . had a gallon of milk sitting on the counter. When I asked if she wasn't afraid it would sour, she said, "Yes, but it's just too hard to get it in the refrigerator." So, I said, "Why?" The refrigerator in the trailer did not work . . . the refrigerator that was working was outside, down an embankment with the

> door tied shut and a heavy box pushed against it. I took the milk to the refrigerator and it took me 12 minutes from the time I left the trailer with the milk 'til I got back.

In the first example above, the teacher called some used appliance stores and managed to get a working refrigerator donated to the family. The grateful family then came to define the teacher as someone who cared about them and began listening more closely to what she was saying about their children's development. Thus, their definition of the situation became more congruent with that of the teacher and they became more involved in the teaching activities that were suggested to them.

A somewhat different example involves a homeless woman at a shelter who was meeting with a social worker in an attempt to find a job and a permanent place to live. The social worker, who apparently had been trained in a status inequality perspective, seemed more interested in talking with the woman about her past:

> To Winnie, the questions were so distant from what she understood as her needs that she suspected they served only the prurient interests of the questioner. She voiced a common complain about social workers and others who presented themselves as helping professionals. Winnie said she needed help in reapplying for SSI (she had been injured in an auto accident), help in getting to and from job interviews, and help in finding a place to live. But the social worker just wanted to talk, again, about her personal (sex and drug) life before she came to the shelter. (Liebow, 1993, p. 137)

As in the previous examples, the professional's priorities were different from the client's, and this definitional incongruity resulted in services that were ineffective. Almost never have professionals been able to impose their definitions on their clients. As voluntary actors, clients usually reject courses of action that do not fit their own definitions of the situation. The result, in the status inequality perspective, is labeled as "noncompliance." A partnership perspective is often more productive, because the professional works alongside the client until they share a common definition of the situation. When a shared definition is not possible, services may be a waste of time.

Sometimes, the problem is not an incongruent definition but rather the lack of any definition at all. The sociological concept that describes this situation is anomie, or normlessness. Anomie occurs when individuals have difficulty making sense out of events, because they do not fit into any known pattern. For example, if a student were to come to class at what he believed to be the usual class meeting day and time but found the classroom empty with no explanatory note on the blackboard, he would not be able to readily define the situation. Anomie occurs most often in new situations that have not been experienced in the past. When individuals encounter a problem in their lives that is different from other problems they have known, they often look to human service agencies for help.

Anomie has two components: meaninglessness and powerlessness (McHugh, 1968). Meaninglessness relates to the inability to make sense of a situation; powerlessness suggests the feeling that accompanies this inability when no immediate course of action is apparent. Sometimes individuals look to human service providers to help them regain control over their lives. However, providers sometimes make the situation worse with professional dominance (see Chapter 3).

In fact, professionals sometimes *create* anomie by withholding information from their clients. For example, in the case of the parents of young children with disabilities cited in the last chapter, the quest for a diagnosis is a search for meaning. The effects of prolonged anomie in this situation are evident in the following description:

> The mother was a nurse and had a considerable amount of experience caring for normal infants. When her second child, a girl, was born, she became concerned because the baby would not nurse. She also noticed that the baby's eyes were always crossing "and she always seemed to be looking at her right side." The mother also wondered whether her daughter could see or hear, and she related her concerns to her pediatrician. The pediatrician assured her that nothing was wrong.
>
> The mother became further alarmed when, at 3 months, the baby seemed to be constantly falling asleep. Once again, her pediatrician assured her that nothing was wrong.
>
> At 5 months, the baby began to have seizure-like periods, but the pediatrician continued to deny any problem. Her husband also refused to agree that a problem might be present. He said, "I thought she was a little paranoid about it. . . . When you're not home all day you don't see the [baby's] lack of activity or anything like that." Because she received no support, the mother tried to rationalize her feeling that something was wrong by blaming herself for not spending enough time with the baby.
>
> Finally, when the baby was 6 months old, the mother "broke down and started crying" in the pediatrician's office. She insisted that something was wrong with the baby, and the physician reluctantly agreed to initiate diagnostic tests. When the child was eventually diagnosed as mentally retarded, the mother was more relieved than upset by the diagnosis. (Darling & Darling, 1982, p. 121)

When such families finally do receive a diagnosis, they still may feel powerless because they do not know what to do next. Typically, when a baby is born, parents receive even more advice than they may want from grandparents, neighbors, parenting magazines, and Dr. Spock. When a baby is born with disabilities, however, friends and relatives may stay away, and ordinary parenting guides say little about caring for children with special needs. In the past, physicians did not provide much guidance in this area either, resulting in extended periods of powerlessness. Today, referrals to early intervention programs are being made more promptly, allowing families to regain control over their lives while their children are still infants.

A concept related to the definition of the situation is awareness context. Glaser and Strauss (1965) introduced this concept to describe the situation in which physicians withheld information about prognosis from dying patients. They found that sometimes patients did not guess their true prognosis ("closed" awareness), but commonly patients became suspicious as a result of clues issued by family members and medical personnel. Interestingly, these patients, who knew they were dying, would not admit their suspicions and would continue to act as though they would get well ("pretense" awareness) to make interactions with doctors and relatives easier.

Pretense can create a barrier for professionals who wish to learn their clients' true definition of the situation. Pretense is perhaps most likely to occur in human services when clients believe they have "something to hide" from the professional. For example, clients are unlikely to admit child abuse, drug abuse, or probation violation when such acts are likely to result in punishment or other negative consequences. In some cases, cultural norms relating to "losing face" may preclude the admission of potentially stigmatizing behaviors or conditions (see Chapter 5 for a further discussion of such norms). In other cases, pretense may result from misunderstanding a professional's expectations: clients tend to tell professionals what they think the professionals want to hear. Pretense is a form of self-presentation, which will be considered more fully later in this chapter.

Eliciting the Client's Definition of the Situation

The first step, then, in using a partnership approach to providing human services should be to try to elicit the client's definition of the situation, including both the definition of the agency–professional and the definition of the presenting problem. The following are some examples of questions to elicit the client's definition of the agency:

- How did you first hear about this agency?
- Have you been here before?
- Have any of your friends or family been here?
- Have you seen our brochure?
- Have you been involved with any other agencies? Which ones?
- What did [referral source] tell you about our services?
- What have you heard about the services we provide?
- What made you choose this agency?

Developing questions to elicit the client's definition of the problem will be discussed in depth in Chapters 7 and 8.

As the client and professional continue to interact, their definitions of the situation will change. The process through which these changes occur will be the subject of the following sections.

Language: The Basis for Understanding

Language refers here to the symbolic exchange between the professional and the client and includes gestures and "body language," tone of voice, and interactional style, along with spoken language. The purpose of language is communication, and people generally assume when they speak that others can understand what they say. However, this assumption can be problematic. A language, or a system of symbols, is arbitrary: nothing about the letters, d-o-g, suggests a furry animal with four legs and a tail; in fact, speakers of other languages might call the same animal a *chien* or a *pero*. However, meanings are consensual, that is, they are generally accepted and shared by the members of a cultural group.

Intergroup interaction poses the most difficulties for symbolic understanding. The greatest difficulty usually involves interactants from completely different cultures. Obviously, if an English speaker does not understand any German, he or she would not be able to communicate very well with a person who spoke only German. Gestures sometimes have very different meanings as well, as the following example illustrates:

> On my first trip to the Middle East, my Arab business contact and I toured the city, walking along the street visiting customers. He wore his long robe, the air was hot and dusty, a priest chanted the call to prayers from a nearby minaret, and I felt as far away from my American home as one could possibly be. At that moment, my business friend reached over, took my hand in his, and we continued walking along, his hand holding mine.
>
> It didn't take me long to realize that something untoward was happening here, that some form of communication was being issued . . . but I didn't have the faintest idea what that message was. Also, I suddenly felt even farther from home.
>
> Probably because I was so stunned, the one thing I didn't do was pull my hand away. I later learned that if I had jerked my hand out of his, I could have committed a Sahara-sized *faux pas*. In his country, this act of taking my hand in his was a sign of great friendship and respect. (Axtell, 1991, pp. 42–43)

Even within the same culture, subcultural diversity affects the language that people use. Some of the common bases for language differences within American culture are suggested below:

1. *Gender*. As Deborah Tannen (see for example, Tannen, 1994) has suggested in several recent bestsellers, men and women use English differently, both at work and at home. For example, women's vocabularies tend to be richer in words relating to color: What my husband calls "blue" I may call "aqua," "chartreuse," or "navy." These differences tend to reflect different worlds of experience.
2. *Race*. As recent debates over "Ebonics" have suggested, African Americans and European Americans sometimes use grammar differently. Some scholars (see, for example, Dillard, 1972) have shown how "black English" has its own linguistic structure and is not simply a corruption of "white English." As in other cases of language variation, black–white differences are a product of social learning in communities that are separated to some extent.
3. *Ethnicity*. As Chapter 5 will suggest, people from different cultural backgrounds tend to have different communication styles. For example, some maintain eye contact with those to whom they are speaking; others tend to avert their gaze. Some groups, such as Asian Americans, tend to be re-

served in conversation; others, like Italian Americans, are more likely to be highly verbal. Again, these characteristics are learned through intragroup interaction.

4. *Education*. College graduates tend to have larger vocabularies than those with an eighth-grade education. Grammar also tends to be more "correct" among those with more education. The educational experience exposes us to reading material and interpersonal interactions that broaden and refine our use of language.
5. *Age*. Many words and phrases, especially slang expressions, tend to be generational. For example, what my peers might have called "groovy" or "sharp," my children call "cool." Teens today use a variety of expressions that may not be understood by older adults, for example, "chill" (calm down); "clueless" (out of touch); "bogus" (really great or terrible). Tomorrow's teens in turn will have their own vocabulary. These terms are learned through interaction within peer groups.
6. *Region*. People from different parts of the country might use different words or expressions for the same item or concept. The item I called a "pocketbook" while growing up in New York is known elsewhere as a "purse." The sandwich my neighbors in Pennsylvania call a "hoagie" or "sub" is known as a "grinder," a "hero sandwich," or an "Italian sandwich" in other states. Accents also differ from one region of the country to another, and New Englanders and Southerners sometimes seem to have particular difficulty being understood in other places. Once again, language socialization occurs within groups of people who interact frequently with one another.

Thus, when professionals and their clients differ in gender, age, social class, or other characteristics, they may have communication difficulties. The result may be a poor understanding of the client's definition of the situation by the professional and misunderstandings about the professional's point of view by the client. In addition, professional jargon and acronyms can be confusing to clients. Recently, the Secretary of the Department of Education in Pennsylvania initiated a "jargon jar," into which staff were required to deposit a dollar any time they used an acronym such as MAWA (mutually acceptable written agreement) or MOU (memorandum of understanding) that was not understandable by the general public. A common language is necessary for role-taking to occur.

Taking the Role of the Other

While the client is talking, the professional is taking the role of the client; while the professional is talking, the client is taking the role of the professional. Role-taking is a term used by symbolic interactionists to explain the thinking process that occurs during interaction. In order to communicate, we need to understand the discourse of the other person in the same way that he or she understands it. Thus, role-taking depends on a common language. Role-taking is sometimes described as "stepping into the other person's shoes"; it is the understanding that occurs on the part of the listener while another person is communicating.

Role-taking can be problematic in client–professional interaction, because the backgrounds of clients and professionals often differ. Typically, professionals are more highly educated than their clients and may come from different social class and ethnic backgrounds. The example of the homeless woman cited earlier suggested poor role-taking by the social worker: The woman wanted help with transportation and housing, but the social worker persisted in talking about sex and drugs. Role taking is usually most effective when the client and professional come from the same background.

How can role taking between professionals and clients be improved? One approach that has been successful in many programs is the use of indigenous professionals or paraprofessionals. In programs that serve Latino communities, for example, staff may be Latino as well, and programs that serve drug addicts or victims of domestic violence may use staff who are ex-addicts or abuse survivors. Sometimes, though, professionals cannot be easily recruited from the client community, or the population served by an agency is more diverse than the pool of available professionals, especially when an agency is small. Thus, all professionals need to work toward becoming better role-takers.

Role-taking ability can be learned, and practice in listening is valuable. Professionals also can try to learn as much as possible about their clients' cultures and lifestyles by spending time in the community and reading autobiographical literature by clients. Prepractice internships also are valuable. The observation techniques described in Chapter 6 may be especially useful in learning about the contexts of clients' lives.

Role-Playing

In the last chapter, role was used to describe the expected behaviors that accompany the statuses of client and professional in American society. Although clients and professionals are expected to act in certain ways, no two individuals play their roles in exactly the same manner, and the same individual will play his or her role differently, depending on the situation. In this section, I will consider the variability that occurs within the professional and client role from an interactionist perspective.

Whereas role-taking is a thinking process, role-playing involves action: It is what professionals and clients do when they interact with one another. Role-playing consists of actions such as speaking, gesturing, or maintaining a certain posture, which serve to communicate an actor's meanings to other people. These actions derive from an actor's definition of the situation and involve the use of language. In a human service interaction, while the client is playing the role of client, the professional is taking the role of client, and vice versa. When one person acts, the other person tries to make sense of that action. Thus, role-playing and role-taking occur simultaneously. Role-playing is based on role-taking: Each actor continually adjusts his or her behavior according to his or her perception of the response of the other. For example, a professional may realize that a client is becoming upset by a particular line of questioning and, so, may change the subject. Some of the elements of professional and client roles that are subject to situational change will be described below.

Playing the Professional Role

The professional role involves a number of actions, including introductory activities, asking questions, and giving advice. Each of these will be discussed in turn.

Introductory Activities

Professionals begin playing their roles even before they begin talking with their clients about the reasons they are seeking help. When interaction takes place in client homes especially, professionals need to be sensitive to family norms. For example, several years ago, I made home visits to a family living in a housing project and noticed a mat outside the door with shoes on it. I assumed that family members and guests were expected to take off their shoes before entering and did so. I was glad I had because on my next visit I saw a sign on the door that said, "Don't bother coming in if you don't take your shoes off first!"

Once, at a professional meeting, a teacher who had just begun making home visits after working in a classroom setting for many years asked me a question. She wanted to know what I did about family members who smoked. She said, "I tell them they can't smoke while I'm there. When I'm in their house, their home is my classroom, and I don't allow smoking in my classroom." I do not like working around people who smoke either but told her that I thought it was important to respect the family's right to establish the rules in their own environment (even if that meant a few minutes of inhaling second-hand smoke). Partnership-based practice suggests that the professional abide by the norms that generally apply in the service environment.

Other issues that often arise during home visits include the propriety of accepting food and drink that is offered and of asking family members to turn down the volume of the television. Most of the time, the professional would probably be wise to accept any food that is offered. Families seem to appreciate the opportunity to reciprocate in small measure for the services they are receiving and might be insulted if their offer were refused. (I have refused food in some especially dirty homes but have always felt guilty as a result!) The situation of a loud television is a little different from that of the smoker described above. Sometimes a television can be disruptive, especially when the client's attention is totally on the program being broadcast and not at all on what the professional is saying. In such situations, the professional may want to ask the family whether a different appointment time that did not conflict with a favorite program might be preferable.

Asking Questions

Before a professional can be helpful to a client, he or she needs to understand why the client is seeking services, which, as noted earlier, is part of the client's definition of the situation. Human services typically begin with an intake interview designed to elicit this information. Chapter 7 will provide guidelines for this and other types of interviews. Here, I will simply list some basic principles of interviewing using a partnership model:

- Because the interview is intended to elicit the client's definition of the situation and not to diagnose some predefined pathology, most questions should be open-ended and nondirective.
- The purpose of the interview is to help the client focus attention on his or her presenting problem, so that he or she may "fine tune" his or her definition of the situation and communicate it to the professional in a way that will maximize the professional's ability to help.
- The professional does not have a right or a need to know anything that the client does not wish to share.
- The interview should help the professional achieve a better understanding of the client's social situation and opportunity structure.
- The interview should be designed to maximize the client's ability to recall relevant information.

Although a general format may be used, no two interviews will proceed in exactly the same way. The nature of social interaction suggests that questions and responses will be shaped by the ongoing process of role-taking and that each question will be determined to some extent by the response preceding it.

Giving Advice

From a sociological perspective, the professional's role needs to include suggestions for expanding the client's opportunity structure. This aspect of the role is totally dependent on the preceding one: asking questions. Because advice must be based on the client's definition of the situation, the professional needs to completely understand that definition before providing suggestions. The type of help that is provided will be determined by the needs and concerns expressed by the client, as follows:

When the client is concerned about:	*The professional will provide (or refer to a provider of):*
Material needs (food, clothing, shelter, etc.)	Things
Service (action) needs	Services
Emotional needs	Support
Needs that cannot be met	Advocacy

Some examples of the types of help typically offered by human services in these situations are illustrative. "Things" may include food from food banks or information about applying for food stamps, accessing public transportation or housing. "Services" include child care, medical care, respite care, personal assistant services, job training, and numerous other types of activities that people need. "Support" can be provided either informally by family and friends or formally by agencies and professionals and may range from simple listening to professional counseling. "Advocacy" involves the use of techniques such as legal suits, lobbying, and other activities that create new services. These examples are provided only to illustrate aspects of professional role-playing; these forms of professional action will be considered in much greater depth in Chapter 9.

Playing the Client Role

Some of the variables affecting client roles include: (1) duration (Some people play the client role only sporadically during their lives, whereas others become committed to long-term client "careers"), and (2) setting (In individual settings, the client role only involves the professional, but in group settings, clients play different roles in relation to other clients as well as to professionals). These variables will be discussed in the following sections.

Duration

Role-playing by the client is likely to change over time. Commitment to a role depends on feedback from other people and is related to the concept of self, which will be discussed later in this chapter. Career is a symbolic interactionist concept that refers to a pattern of increasing role commitment. The concept is usually attributed to Becker (1963), who looked at careers of marijuana users, among others. Usually, a career involves a series of stages that last for varying periods of time. To understand a client's situation, a professional may need to know at which point on a career trajectory the client is located.

In a study of homeless men, for example, Snow and Anderson (1993) found that their subjects typically passed through the following stages: Job loss → marital strain → divorce or separation → recently dislocated → straddlers → outsiders. At each stage, some men left the career path, that is, they found jobs and/or returned to conventional lifestyles. However, as men moved along the path, they found that leaving the street became increasingly difficult. The recently dislocated still harbored hopes of returning to their former lives and did not think of themselves as homeless. These men were likely to use whatever services, such as soup kitchens and shelters, were available. After a period of time, those who were not able to resume their conventional lives became more adapted to living on the street and less dependent on human services. Eventually, those termed "outsiders" no longer had any illusions about finding a job and a permanent place to live.

Using a similar model, Aneshensel et al. (1995) looked at the careers of people caring for chronically ill relatives. They suggest that the caregiving career includes three sequential stages—role acquisition, role enactment, and role disengagement—and involves "a recurrent redirection and reorganization of one's life" (p. 349). Movement through the stages is associated with a series of decisions designed to cope with increasing stress, with nursing home placement serving as a turning point for many.

The concept of turning point (Strauss, 1962) is valuable in understanding movement from one career stage to another. For example, a turning point in the lives of late-marrying bachelors (Darling, 1977) was the death of a parent or a job change resulting in relocation; these events provided the impetus for marriage in some cases. Charmaz (1991) notes the case of a chronically ill woman who blamed herself for her pain until she took a class in existentialism and realized she could have a life beyond pain. In my studies of parents of children with disabilities (Darling, 1979), the receipt of a diagnosis was the turning point that enabled families to move from anomie to "seekership," a stage in which they searched for treatment programs for their children. In human services, encountering a helpful professional can be a turning point that enables a client to move from seekership to the solution of a problem.

Sometimes, though, unhelpful professionals can prolong problem careers. Scheff (1966), Goffman (1961), and others have explored this phenomenon in the case of mental patients. Both have noted a career path that begins with a person who does not define him- or herself as "crazy." With time, the responses of others—both family and professionals—cause this self-definition to change. After the person is admitted to a mental hospital, he or she realizes the necessity of either playing the role of a crazy person or being defined by the staff as "in denial."

Scheff (1966) suggests that the role is not difficult to play, because each society socializes its members in the cultural norms associated with craziness. He suggests that this socialization occurs through the media, with its stereotypic depictions of crazy people, as well as through other means. Even at early ages, children play-act the crazy role. Further evidence that the role is learned comes from observations of other cultures, as the behaviors associated with craziness vary considerably from one culture to another.

Goffman (1961) describes the "moral career of the mental patient." After being admitted to a mental hospital, the patient is socialized into the norms of the institution and learns to act as the staff expects. Patients learn that they must appear to accept their "illness" and cooperate with treatment in order to progress through the ward system. After they are released, however, they may have difficulty returning to the role of a "normal" person, because ex-mental patients are still expected to act crazy in our society. Compliance with these expectations is likely to result in a cyclical career path, with readmission following release from the institution.

Setting

While the mental patients studied by Goffman were learning to play the role that professionals expected, they also were being socialized by the other inmates. Goffman (1961) differentiates between primary and secondary adjustments. Primary adjustments relate to the "official" roles that patients play. Secondary adjustments, on the other hand, are part of the "underlife" of the institution: the interactions managed by the inmates themselves. Goffman found, in the institution he studied, that the inmates had organized an intricate system of social relationships and norms governing those relationships. Secondary adjustments included "working the system" to obtain forbidden goods; "make-dos," such as using a radiator to dry clothing; "stashes," or secret hiding places; and "free places," where inmates could escape from the ever-present surveillance of the staff. He argues that these adjustments made life in a total institution (see Chapter 2) bearable for the inmates. Similar adjustment systems have been found as well in other total institutions in the human service system, such as prisons and youth detention centers.

In any human service setting where clients closely interact with other clients, role-playing is likely to vary depending on who is present. Professionals who work in group homes, residential treatment centers, and institutions of various kinds need to understand this variability in their clients' behavior. In a school for delinquent girls where I once worked, the girls had created a "make-believe family," with some girls playing parent roles and grandparent roles and other girls playing the role of children. Those in grandparent and parent roles had higher status than the others, and the "children" would typically defer to them in group interaction, even when staff members were present. On the other hand, when their "elders" were not present, the "children" often acted in more dominant ways. Knowledge of the underlife of this institution was helpful in understanding such behavior.

The Client's Self-Concept

Components of the Self-Concept

One component of a client's definition of the situation is his or her definition of him- or herself. The concept of self is central in symbolic interactionist theory, because it represents the primary individual component in the society–individual relationship. The client's self-concept is important in human services, because role-playing and self-concept are closely related. A person who defines herself as crazy, for example, is likely to play the role of a crazy person. The converse is also true: If a person plays a role long enough, he or she is likely to incorporate that role into his or her self-concept. The self-concept, then, is the basis for action. Professionals who want to broaden the role repertory available to their clients need to be sure that their clients' self-concepts will accommodate the new roles. For example, a client who continues to define himself as a drug addict, even after completing a treatment program, may not be able to take advantage of new role opportunities that do not involve drugs.

As Cooley (1964) classically stated, the self-concept is a reflected appraisal of the definitions received from others, or a "looking-glass self." In other words, through the process of role-taking, we come to see ourselves as others see us, and the self-concept is a product of symbolic interaction. A child who is constantly told that he is bad will come to think of himself as a bad boy. A student who consistently receives A's is likely to think of himself as a good student. However, not all definitions are weighted equally; variations in definitional impact will be discussed shortly.

Knowledge about a person's self-concept is not always immediately apparent. Some people are self-effacing even though they think highly of themselves, whereas others may play roles competently even though they feel insecure. Because the self-concept is not visible, sociologists have developed a number of techniques to gain insight into what people think about themselves. One such technique is the "Twenty Statements Test" (Kuhn & McPartland, 1954), or TST. This simple test uses a form with the question, "Who am I?" at the top and numbers from 1 to 20 down the left side. Respondents are asked to answer the question in 20 statements beginning with, "I am."

Administrations of the TST and other measures with large samples suggest that the self-concept has two components: consensual and subconsensual. Consensual statements, which are usually listed first on the TST (and are therefore believed to be most salient or important), include factual or cognitive information about which no disagreement would be likely, for example, "I am a woman"; "I am a student"; "I am a father." Subconsensual statements are evaluative and involve judgments about the self that could be open to question, for example, "I am beautiful"; "I am a good student"; "I am a terrible athlete." The evaluative component is commonly known as self-esteem. Numerous studies have suggested that high self-esteem (favorable self-definition) is associated with behaviors such as good school performance, career success, satisfaction in interpersonal relationships, and disease recovery (see, for example, Coopersmith, 1967; Rosenberg, 1965). On the other hand, low self-esteem seems to be correlated with behaviors such as juvenile delinquency, school failure, and poor health. Of course, these correlations do not indicate the direction of effect. In fact, success may lead to high self-esteem, rather than high self-esteem's leading to success. Most likely, self-esteem can be both cause and effect in these cases.

High self-esteem commonly has been viewed as a desirable outcome in human service work. Recently, some have criticized esteem-promoting approaches for being based on an overindividualized view of problem causation. In a sense, the promotion of esteem enhancement is related to victim-blaming, discussed earlier in this volume. In this view, individual traits are seen as the cause of problems; thus, low self-esteem is viewed as an etiologic factor. When problems are in fact socially caused, esteem enhancement is not a productive solution because the source of the problem does not reside in the individual. Hewitt (1998) argues that the current emphasis on self-esteem in the helping professions and other areas derives from the value that Americans place on individualism and "the pursuit of happiness." He suggests that such an emphasis can be counterproductive to promoting social responsibility and the betterment of society as a whole.

As noted earlier, not all definitions of the self are weighted equally. In the process of role-taking, some definitions may be heard but discounted, and others may not be heard at all. Some of the factors that seem important in determining attention to and acceptance of the definitions of others include source, frequency, intensity, duration, and recency/primacy.

Source

People tend to pay more attention to definitions from others who are important to them, that is, their significant others (Sullivan, 1947). Typically, significant others include family members and close friends, as well as "experts" of various kinds, including physicians and members of the clergy. Numerous studies have indicated strong correlations between the opinions of children and those of their parents. Adolescents are likely to go to their parents for advice on some matters, such as career choice, but to use their peers as significant others in other areas (e.g., what to wear to a dance).

A concept that is closely related to that of significant others is reference group (Shibutani, 1961). Reference groups are those from which we derive our perspectives. High school students, for example, are likely to evaluate their grades in terms of the grades their friends receive. Thus, a student with a C average might not be upset if most of her friends had similar averages. However, a student with a C average whose friends all received A's might feel a need to improve her performance.

As Chapter 5 will show, significant others vary among social groups. For example, African Americans are more likely than European Americans to include members of the clergy among their significant others. Similarly, helping professionals are likely to vary in degree of significance. Freidson (1970a) suggests, for example, that some patients are more likely to listen to members of their "lay referral structure" than to their physicians, resulting in lack of compliance with "doctors' orders." Obviously, human service professionals cannot be very helpful if they are not perceived as significant others by their clients.

Various instruments have been designed to determine the members of an individual's "reference set," or network of significant others. One simple method would have the individual list "those persons who are important to you and whose opinion you value." Presumably, those persons who are listed first would be most salient to the individual.

Frequency, Intensity, Duration, and Recency/Primacy

As Kinch (1968) and others have suggested, other factors, in addition to the significance of the other, are important in determining which definitions will be incorporated into the self-concept. Definitions heard more frequently and over a longer period of time are more likely to have an impact than those heard only occasionally and during a brief period in a person's life. Similarly, those that are issued more forcefully are more likely to be heard than those issued weakly or in jest. Thus, brief contact with a professional may sometimes be less effective than a relationship of longer term.

Some psychoanalytic theorists have suggested the importance of primacy and argued that the definitions received earliest in life are weighted more heavily than those received later. On the other hand, symbolic interaction theory suggests that people continually redefine the situation and that the past is constantly being redefined in terms of the present. The discussion of turning points presented earlier would support this suggestion. Thus, recency also seems to play a role in self-definition.

Labeling and Stigma

Clients of the human services are perhaps more likely than others in society to have low self-esteem. They have been defined as "people with problems," a kind of negative label. Labeling is the process of applying negative definitions (Becker, 1963), and the labeling concept is closely tied to the concept of self in symbolic interaction theory. Gans (1995) suggests that labeling in human services can lead to an assumption that all clients are alike, resulting in an inappropriate application of punitive actions. Numerous studies in the sociology of deviance (see, for example, Becker, 1963; Lemert, 1967) have suggested that deviant careers are likely to result from labeling. The mental patient discussed earlier might have a career path that looked like this: Acts of norm violation → labeling as "crazy" by friends and family (significant others) → self-definition as crazy → continued acts of norm violation (role-playing). Thus, deviant careers involve commitment to a (negative) self-concept, along with commitment to a role. The deviant accepts the label that has been applied by others, incorporates it into his or her self-concept and plays the expected role.

A related concept is stigma, which describes a condition that results from labeling. Goffman (1963) suggests that stigma is a discrepancy between "virtual and actual social identity." Individuals who are labeled are generally regarded as morally inferior to others and are treated accordingly. Stigmatization occurs in everyday social interactions, through mechanisms such as ostracism, avoidance, or "fictional acceptance" (Davis, 1961), and in more formal interactions, such as the refusal to hire an otherwise qualified person for a job. Stigmatization characterizes many groups of clients in the human services, including criminals, drug and alcohol abusers, and people with mental illness and mental retardation, among others. Members of all of these groups occupy devalued statuses in American society and are likely to have experienced stigma in one form or another.

In fact, receiving treatment in the human service system may be more stigmatizing than the condition that led to the treatment-seeking. In American society, for example, "mental patients" and even "ex-mental patients" are sometimes stigmatized more than people who simply act in unusual ways. A clinical diagnosis can serve as the basis for stigmatization. The process leading to the application of such clinical labels can be conceptualized as "status degradation ceremonies" (Garfinkel, 1956), in which the individual and his or her actions are made to seem "out of the ordinary." The denouncer, on the other hand, is vested with the authority to represent the values by which the degraded person is being judged. Stigma often lingers after treatment is completed. In a recent study, for example, Link, Struening, Rahav, Phelan, and Nuttbrock (1997) found that men who had had dual diagnoses of mental illness and substance abuse but who were now symptom-, drug-, and alcohol-free continued to experience relatively strong effects from stigma a year after their treatment had been completed.

A series of studies of persons diagnosed with mild mental retardation, who had been released from a large institution (Edgerton, 1993), indicated that the effects of stigma were greatest shortly after release. The ex-residents used various techniques to try to hide their institutional past in order to form social relationships or to be hired for jobs. Eventually, as they approached retirement age, their past became less relevant and some were able to achieve some degree of normalization.

Professionals also can play a role in reducing labeling and stigma. Because deviant careers result from societal reactions, they can be changed. Professionals can affect reactions in a number of ways. They can (1) create opportunities for different reactions to occur by helping the client move to a new situation; (2) try to change the current situation by changing the frequency, intensity, and duration of negative definitions that are occurring; or (3) become a significant other for the client and provide new, positive definitions. Each of these methods will be briefly discussed.

Facilitating a Move to a New Situation

The following letter appeared in "Dear Abby":

> My heart goes out to "Mike," the son of "Worried Mom in Virginia." I have walked in his shoes. Starting in the fourth grade at a private school in Atlanta, I was taunted and teased by many of my peers for reasons I was unable to understand. I was neither ugly nor pretty, fat nor thin, rich nor poor, but nonetheless, I was called names too mean-spirited to repeat.
>
> I transferred to a "better" private school, but since some of the same kids were there who knew me from my former school, the ostracism followed me. These kids were so vicious, they even picked on a very nice, soft-spoken Italian boy in my class because his English was poor. They singled us out because we were "different."
>
> Then a miracle happened. Because my grades were poor, my mother no longer wanted to spend all that money for a private school where I was miserable, so she sent me to a public school where I knew no one, and no one knew me.
>
> My grades went up; I had boyfriends and girlfriends. I had not changed, my environment had. . . . ("Past harassments," 1995, p. B2)

The "miracle" was of course a turning point that allowed this individual to receive new definitions of herself and to develop in turn a more positive self-concept (through role-taking).

The situational nature of behavior already has been suggested. As the letter above clearly shows, entering a new situation is likely to result in the acquisition of new significant others, who in turn will offer new definitions of self. Situational change is already a commonly used intervention in human services. When clients move from their home environment to a residential treatment setting, they are likely to encounter new definitions. This approach is commonly used for juvenile and adult offenders, substance abusers, and people with mental health diagnoses. Such programs tend to have high short-term success rates. However, when clients return to their home environments, they commonly resume their former behaviors.

Ray (1961) looked at this phenomenon in the case of heroin addicts. He found that when they left a treatment program and returned home, addicts were likely to experience rejection from nonaddicts and acceptance from friends who were still addicted. This account is illustrative:

> When I got home I stayed off for two months but my mother was hollering at me all the time and there was this one family in the neighborhood that was always "chopping me up." I wanted to tell this woman off because she talked all right to my face but behind

> my back she said things like she was afraid I would turn her son on because I was hanging around with him. . . . Finally I just got disgusted because nobody wanted to believe me and I went back on. (Ray, 1961, p. 137)

Thus, in the home community, the ex-addict is likely to encounter interaction situations in which a nonaddict identity is difficult to maintain. Ray suggests that these experiences create a sense of social isolation and lead to a "recaptured sense of the meaningfulness of experience in the social world of addiction" (p. 139).

Thus, simply removing a client from his or her environment for a short period of time is not likely to prevent recidivism or relapse upon return to that environment. Professionals need instead to assist clients in moving to new situations. For children, options may include school transfer or foster care. For adults, turning points may include finding a new job, joining a new church or social group, or even separation or divorce. Professionals may be able to support clients who are contemplating such changes.

Changing the Current Situation

Often, moving the client to a new situation is not feasible. Opportunities for moving to a new house or a new job may simply be unavailable, or the client may not choose to take advantage of opportunities that do exist. In such cases, the professional may want to explore the possibility of changing the nature of the definitions the client receives in the current situation.

One option may be to change the client's daily routine. For example, the frequency of exposure to negative definitions may be reduced if a client spends less time with the friends who issue those definitions. Work schedules sometimes can be changed, as can meal times, sleep schedules, and the timing of leisure activities.

Sometimes introducing new interactional possibilities into a situation is also helpful. "Big Brother" and "Big Sister" programs are built on this principle, as are other mentoring programs. These interventions add new significant others who provide positive definitions to balance other negative definitions that the client may be receiving.

Becoming a Significant Other

As noted earlier, the professional must become a significant other for the client, or the client will not take his or her advice seriously. When professionals are significant others, their definitions can have an impact on their clients' self-concepts. Professionals who provide positive definitions can empower their clients and encourage them to take advantage of existing opportunities or to create new opportunities for themselves.

This intervention is not a permanent solution, however. Clients' involvement with human service agencies is usually time-limited. When that involvement ends, the client needs other, supportive significant others to provide positive definitions. Otherwise, the pattern of recidivism or relapse noted earlier is likely to occur. Some of the newer, community-based interventions (see Chapter 2) seem promising in this regard. Rather than working with a single client or family, the professional works with an entire community, helping to create support networks within existing relationships. Then, when the professional intervention ends, a client can continue to find support from friends and neighbors, the church, or the local family center.

Self-Presentation by Clients and Professionals

As noted above, the self-concept is invisible. In an interaction situation, people cannot see each other's self-concepts; each sees only how the other person chooses to play his or her role. Part of role-playing involves self-presentation or impression management. Self-presentation is the deliberate act of trying to influence another actor's role-taking through one's actions. Goffman (1958), using a dramaturgic analogy, suggests that people are like stage actors who try to create certain impressions on their audiences.

In the human service situation, clients may present themselves in one of two ways:

1. They may present their "true" selves, that is, they will not try to impress the professional and will act in much the same way they would if they were with friends or family. Such a presentation is sometimes related to a definition of the situation in which the service is not regarded as being potentially helpful. This definition may occur in situations in which the service is involuntary, such as imprisonment or court-ordered counseling, or among clients whose prior experience with human services has been negative. In these cases, the client may not care what the professional thinks and may feel that nothing will be lost if he or she presents a sullen or indifferent demeanor.
2. They may engage in "impression management" and try to create an image of pleasant compliance. The following example suggests that some clients may be very aware of the impressions they are trying to create:

   > I was conscious of the need to make these doctors identify with us as strongly and as quickly as possible. . . . I made sure that Julian and I dressed in a way that we imagined the doctor's family might dress. We were meticulous about showing up for appointments, at least 15 minutes early, to prove that we were concerned, responsible parents. We paid our bills promptly at the end of each visit. I tried to elicit personal comments from the doctor by referring to topics that might interest him. . . . Finally, I worked with David to make sure he was a cooperative and likable patient. (Stotland, 1984, p. 72)

In general, self-presentation is likely to be most conscious when people feel that much is at stake. Court appearances and first dates are situations that are likely to give rise to deliberate impression management, as are intake interviews at human service agencies that provide goods or services that clients really want.

Impression management also is likely to vary by sociocultural background. Middle-class people are sometimes more concerned than members of the lower class with making a good impression on others, professional or otherwise. People of higher socioeconomic status also are more able to dress "in a way that we imagined the doctor's family might dress" and to use a more "professional-sounding" vocabulary. In addition, people of different cultural backgrounds might be more or less cautious about revealing their "true selves" to others. These differences will be discussed further in Chapter 5.

Professionals also engage in self-presentation. They may try to appear "professional" to convince clients of their expertise, or they may deliberately create an impression of informality and camaraderie to put their clients at ease. Some agencies have dress codes that require professional staff to dress in business suits. On the other hand, one antipoverty agency I know requires their staff to dress in jeans in order to make their clients feel comfortable. Lower-socioeconomic status clients have told me that they felt intimidated by well-dressed professionals; however, middle- and upper-class clients might define casually dressed agency staff as unprofessional. In general, professionals should probably be guided by what they believe will best foster a partnership relationship with their clients.

Impression management by the client, then, is an attempt to influence the professional's definition of the situation, and the professional's impression management is designed to affect the client's definition of the situation. Thus, the process of symbolic interaction is circular. Definitions of the situation change constantly throughout the course of interaction, based on the behavior and appearance of the interactants.

Chapter Summary

Figure 4.1, which was presented at the beginning of this chapter, breaks down what occurs during the course of human interaction into component parts. The outcome of professional–client interactions will be determined to some extent by what each person knows from past experience in society, but will be shaped as well by what takes place during the current encounter. To review:

The process of symbolic interaction consists of an alternation between external and internal elements. The external elements—society (people interacting with one another), language, role-playing, and self-presentation—are visible and audible and consist of what people do when they interact. The internal elements—definition of the situation, role-taking, and self-concept—cannot be seen or heard because they occur in people's minds; they make up what people think when they interact.

People's initial definitions of the situation, then, are based on their prior interactions in society. These definitions are subject to change through subsequent social encounters. Human interaction occurs through the medium of language. People can understand what is said to them because of their role-taking ability. Based on that understanding, they will come to see themselves as others see them and to play the roles that they have learned. During their role-playing they will present themselves in a way they believe will create the desired impression on the other person. Society is made up of people playing roles and presenting selves. Thus, the process is circular, and each interaction that takes place changes society to some extent. Each person's experience of society is the sum total of all the interactions that person has had. This chapter has shown how the process of symbolic interaction can explain the client–professional encounter and has suggested some ways in which professionals can act to influence their clients' definitions of the situation. The next chapter will look at how each person's experience, or "social world," varies according to structural and cultural characteristics.

Suggested Exercises

These exercises may help students better understand the concepts of symbolic interactionism through the process of applying them to actual human service situations.

In each of the following situations, use an interactionist perspective to suggest some actions that the professional might take to assist the client:

1. You work for a family preservation program. A new client has come to your office. During the intake interview, he seems very uncomfortable. He does not say much in response to your questions and keeps looking at the floor. He is shabbily dressed, and his language suggests that he is not highly educated. He was required by the court to come to your agency following an incidence of child abuse. You need to develop a working relationship with him. Suggest some strategies you might use, incorporating your understanding of the following concepts: definition of the situation, role-taking, and role-playing.
2. You are employed at a shelter for abused women. Your client is a woman who has been at the shelter several times. Each time, she has returned to the same violent home situation. She says she does not want to return this time but she is afraid of living on her own. She is concerned because she has no job skills. When you suggest returning to school, she says that she was not a good student and never finished high school for that reason. She

has never worked and is afraid that she would not be capable of holding a job. She says, "I am a failure. I've never been very good at anything." How might you go about changing her self-concept?

3. You work at a health center that serves a lower-socioeconomic status Latino community. Your client has just been diagnosed with AIDS. You have the responsibility of discussing this diagnosis with him and providing information about treatment options. However, when you try to talk with him about the seriousness of his situation, your client insists that he does not need treatment; his cousin "had the same thing, and he got better without any medicine." You do not know whether he does not understand what you are saying or simply refuses to believe the diagnosis. How might you learn more about his definition of the situation?

Suggestions for Further Reading

Becker, H. (1963). *Outsiders: Studies in the sociology of deviance*. New York: Free Press.

Goffman, E. (1958). *The presentation of self in everyday life*. Edinburgh: University of Edinburgh Social Sciences Research Centre.

Liebow, E. (1993). The servers and the served. In *Tell them who I am: The lives of homeless women* (pp. 115–147). New York: Penguin.

Ray, M. (1961). The cycle of abstinence and relapse among heroin addicts. *Social Problems, 9*, 132–140.

Scheff, T. (1966). *Being mentally ill: A sociological theory.* Chicago: Aldine.

II

The Client's Social World and Methods for Discovering It

5

The Social World of the Service User

As the last two chapters suggested, professionals in human services need to learn as much as possible about the opportunity structures and definitions of the situation of their clients. Although no two individuals or families will have exactly the same opportunities or definitions, the situations of people in similar circumstances are likely to create shared conditions of life and common ways of thinking. Because professionals typically interact in social worlds that are different from those of their clients, they may not understand "where their clients are coming from."

Because a partnership approach to human services requires that the client's definition of the situation be the operative one, this chapter will assist professionals in understanding service users from diverse backgrounds. The first part of the chapter will suggest the elements of the client's social world that are important for the professional to understand. The second part of the chapter will then illustrate the variations in service-related definitions and opportunities commonly found in different socioeconomic and ethnic groups.

Clients' Resources, Concerns, and Priorities: Areas for Professional Focus

In the terminology of human services, opportunity structures provide the framework for the strengths or resources that clients possess. Typically, clients from higher socioeconomic groups have greater access to material resources, such as money and comfortable housing, than clients of lower status. However, all clients have some resources. Those who are poor may have access to good support from family or church or to government benefits that provide for education or child care. Using the client's existing resources is an important part of providing services from a partnership perspective. Sometimes, family or neighborhood groups can be mobilized to provide what clients need in a natural way that does not then require the further intervention of professionals. Thus, identifying available resources is usually an early step in service provision.

As noted in the last chapter, an important part of the client's definition of the situation is the definition of the "problem," or reason for seeking help. In human services today, "problem," a term from the status inequality literature, is being replaced by "concern." The term, "concern," suggests that clients' reasons for seeking help are legitimate and also shifts the focus from the professional's definition to the client's. As Chapter 9 will suggest, some client concerns can be alleviated by human service agencies through the provision of goods or services; however, other concerns may require advocacy by professionals to create opportunities that do not currently exist.

In the client's mind, some concerns are likely to be more pressing than others. For example, not having any food in the house may take precedence over wanting to learn parenting skills. Generally, concerns can be ranked in order of their importance or temporal priority for the client. If the client's definition is to prevail, the professional will want to work on the clients' concerns in priority order.

Resources and concerns can be categorized into a number of areas that may be relevant for human service intervention. These include information, material support, informal support, and formal support. Each will be discussed in turn. Throughout the discussion, the voices will be those of service users rather than those of service providers, in keeping with the partnership perspective being applied here.

Information

Information or knowledge can be both a resource and a concern. Some clients with prior experience in the human service system already know a considerable amount about help-seeking procedures before they encounter a new professional. Others may know very little about where to turn for the kinds of help they need.

The kinds of information that clients want vary. Most clients want to know as much as possible about the issues that concern them, especially if they are in a state of anomie (cf Chapter 4). Sometimes, because of previously encountered professional dominance or a concern that is new, a service user's priority may be to better define what is troubling him or her. In the medical and mental health realms especially, clients usually are looking for an accurate diagnosis and prognosis in order to know how to proceed with treatment. As one parent of a child with mental retardation said,

> When the doctor told us, he couldn't believe how well we accepted the diagnosis. All I can say is that it was such a relief to have someone finally just come out and say what we had feared for so long! We felt that now we could move ahead and do the best we could for Timmy. (Dickman & Gordon, 1985, p. 31)

A number of studies (see, for example, Darling & Baxter, 1996) have indicated that the desire for information is the most salient concern among parents of children with disabilities, and the concern is clearly a priority among other client groups as well.

Some service users have good research skills, a resource in the information area. These individuals may have access to good libraries or may be skilled at using the Internet to secure information. Typically, research skills are commensurate with education, and clients who are college graduates may be better at finding information on their own than those who did not graduate from high school. On the other hand, individuals with considerable experience in using human services, regardless of education level or social class, may be quite adept at using the telephone and locating knowledgeable experts in their area of concern.

Once a concern has been defined, clients typically seek information about available services. The role of the professional in providing this kind of information will vary according to the agency of employment. Sometimes, the agency with which the client is already involved may provide the kinds of services the client wants. Often, though, the professional will need to make a referral to a different agency. For this reason, human service professionals need to be knowledgeable about all the services located in the community. Many communities maintain directories of human services, and networking through councils and consortia of agencies is also helpful.

Material Support

Like information, material support can be both a resource and a concern. Material support refers to goods or things (as opposed to services) that a client might have or want. Some common examples of material support include money, government benefits, food, clothing, shelter, furnishings, medical equipment, a means of transportation, and toys and leisure items. Clearly, material support is a more common resource among the rich than among the poor and, conversely, a more common concern among the poor. For the poorest families, material support is likely to be the concern of highest priority. Material support may be provided informally, through friends or relatives, or formally, through human service agencies, such as food banks and homeless shelters, or government programs such as subsidized housing or Medical Assistance. The effect of material resources on priorities is clear in the following statement:

> You're always thinking about your expenses. There's no cream on top. Actually, now that I'm getting child support, there is some cream. . . . Ice cream used to be a real luxury. Soda was a luxury. Cable TV. I used to not go out. To go out to a movie? Well, [try] to justify spending $7 for a movie, when you can just go down to the store and rent one. But the car insurance, the rent, the utilities, and the food were number one. I always kept those up. And then everything else came after that. (Berrick, 1995, p. 62)

At the time of this writing, a major concern related to material support is the change in people's opportunity structures that may result from recent welfare reform legislation. New federal legislation requires that welfare recipients find work and leave the welfare rolls within 5 years. In areas of the country with few employment opportunities, many individuals are concerned about the availability of jobs paying a living wage. Other concerns relate to lack of transportation and affordable or safe child care that would enable parents of young children to work.

Education is often touted as the key to ending welfare dependency. However, at least some individuals without advanced job skills seem to have limitations in their ability to succeed academically:

> "How much longer will you be in school?" I ask.
> After I pass that test. I never pass the test. The only problem I have is I don't know my time tables that well. . . . I have to get out the times board or count and she'll be tellin' me that I've run out of time if I'm takin' a test. . . . I don't know what it is, I'll cry 'cause I can't do certain things. . . . [My teacher] tellin' me, "You could do it, Cora." I just got to get those time tables. But when I come home and then the babysitter will leave, so then the house is a mess, and I got to get my kids something to eat and I can't study with them in the house, you know. I tell my teacher, I say, by the time they go to bed and sleep, I start studying and next thing I know I'm asleep too. . . . If I don't pass the test, I don't know what's going to happen. (Berrick, 1995, p. 137–138)

Mothers such as this one have significant concerns relating to their ability to provide for their children after their benefits expire.

Because of the priority of material support, human service professionals will usually want to identify the nature of their clients' resources in this area, regardless of the reason why the clients were referred to them. For example, a family may have been referred to an agency because of a child's poor performance in school. If the parents are struggling to make ends meet, however, they may not be as concerned about their child's school performance as they are about their financial situation. On the other hand, asking questions about finances may be regarded as intrusive by a family for whom material support is not a major concern. In fact, in my experience in human services, some middle- and upper-class families refused services rather than disclose information about their financial status. Appropriate methods for obtaining information about material support and other sensitive areas will be addressed in Chapters 6, 7, and 8.

Informal Support

Informal support refers to the assistance people receive as a result of their relationships with their primary groups—family, friends, neighbors, fellow churchgoers or clergy, and co-workers. This support may take the form of assistance with material needs as discussed in the last section, with service needs such as the need for child care or with emotional needs through simply listening or otherwise acknowledging the validity of an individual's concerns.

Some individuals have extensive support networks, whereas others have few people they can rely on for assistance when needed. In a study of one group of single, African-American mothers in a poor neighborhood (Cook & Fine, 1995), for example, the women "felt bereft of positive social networks. . . . They reported being 'the sickly sister who stayed in the neighborhood,' 'The kid they thought was slow' " (p. 126). These women provided considerable support for children, parents, and neighbors but could not identify anyone who regularly supported them.

Variations in informal support are reported by Antonucci and Depner (1982). Men report being more satisfied with their networks than women. However, women rely on their networks for more kinds of support than men: "Whereas men's social networks tend to be large and diffuse, the networks of women are smaller and more intense" (p. 244). They report that some research indicates that men tend to rely on one key relationship, usually their spouse. With respect to age, "older people tend to provide less support to their network members and receive more support than they provide" (p. 245).

Perhaps the people with the least informal support in society are those who are homeless. Numerous studies of homeless individuals (see, for example, Kozol, 1988; Liebow, 1993) have suggested that many people become homeless when they are rejected by their families. A typical career path of homeless families includes varying periods of time during which the families live with relatives after losing their own homes. Homelessness commonly occurs when these relatives are no longer able or willing to house these families.

Usually, the main source of support is an individual's immediate family. Consequently, professionals need to look most closely at the relationships among these individuals. The literature in the field of family systems theory and methods (see chapter 2) can be valuable here. In addition, the concerns of family members other than the client are important. For example, a woman who is caring for her chronically ill mother may not have the time or emotional energy to help her child with the school difficulties that brought the family to the attention of an agency. Concerns involving other members of the family can compete with the concerns for which clients are referred for help. Also, when other family members have concerns of their own, they are not likely to be able to provide support to the client.

Barrera (reported in Pecora, Fraser, Nelson, McCroskey, & Meezan, 1995) describes three different forms of social support:

- Social embeddedness: connections people have with significant others in their immediate environment.
- Perceived social support: levels of confidence of individuals about the amount of support that would be available if needed.
- Enacted social support: actual support provided through actions such as listening, expressing concern, lending money, helping with a task, offering suggestions, giving advice, or showing affection.

Some researchers have looked closely at the characteristics of social support networks. Kazak and Marvin (1984) and Kazak and Wilcox (1984), for example, have suggested the importance of concepts such as network size, network density, boundary density, network reciprocity, and network dimensionality. These concepts describe the structure and function of networks for their members. These researchers applied the concepts to families of children with disabilities. In relation to reciprocity, for example, they write, "Asking a friend to watch a child requiring specialized care may contribute to network drain and may not be matched by requests of a similar magnitude from the network" (Kazak & Wilcox, 1984, p. 649). Many studies suggest that large and active support networks can be extremely important in helping individuals cope with stressful situations (see, for example, Cameron & Vanderwoerd, 1997).

Cameron and Vanderwoerd (1997, pp. 21–23) suggest the following structural dimensions of support networks:

- Range of supports available (the types of available support, such as material, emotional, or service).
- Levels of support available (the adequacy of supports in buffering the effects of stressors).
- Length of commitment.
- Reciprocity.
- Technical expertise.
- Openness to all in need (availability to stigmatized and other "undesirable" cases).
- Availability in a crisis.
- Motivation and skill requirements (willingness and ability to help).

Even people with few material resources may have resources in this area. Thus, informal support can be a resource as well as a concern. Kozol (1995), for example, shows the role played by a church in supporting residents of a poor community in the South Bronx. St. Ann's provided food and after school activities in addition to religious functions, and its minister, Reverend Overall, was clearly a significant other for families in the community. In another example, the women in a homeless shelter, who generally had truncated networks of support, were still able to find friendship and solidarity in the other residents of the shelter:

> The most powerful force for group cohesion and solidarity grew out of the realization that "we're all in this together," that for better or worse, we share our lives, and for the present at least, we share a common fate. (Liebow, 1993, p. 210)

Such solidarity may be enhanced by a group's stigmatized status (Goffman, 1963).

In the case of deinstitutionalized individuals with mild mental retardation, Edgerton (1993) found that informal support was essential for successful adaptation to life in the community. "Benefactors"—usually employers, spouses or lovers, neighbors, or landlords—helped the ex-patients cope with the demands of everyday life by filling out forms, answering the door, and helping with tasks involving reading and writing. The assistance of these benefactors enabled the ex-patients to pass as "normal."

Human service professionals can assist their clients by helping to mobilize existing networks of support. In one case (Capossela & Warnock, 1997), a woman dying of cancer was encouraged by a professional to organize her friends into a helping network. These friends then agreed to take turns providing services such as child care and transportation to medical appointments. Professionals also can assist with community organization to expand informal helping networks. Activities of this kind will be discussed further in Chapter 9.

Formal Support

Formal support becomes important when opportunities for informal support are limited. In a study of parents of children with intellectual disabilities, Baxter (1987) found that those parents experiencing the highest levels of stress expressed the greatest need for professional help. In these cases, human service professionals may be able to provide the assistance that is needed. In addition, professionals, because of their training and experience, may be better equipped than laypersons to provide some technical services, such as medical care. Formal support refers to services provided by agencies and professionals and includes emotional, technical, and service support.

Emotional support involves the provision of empathy and assurance to individuals who do not have sufficient support within their primary groups. A common mechanism for the provision of such support is support groups. These are usually professionally organized groups of individuals with similar concerns that meet on a regular basis. Through these groups, individuals come to realize that their concerns are shared. The groups also serve as forums for the exchange of information as well as sources of role models for the members. As reference groups (see Chapter 4), these groups also provide bases for comparison, as these comments by the mother of a child with a disability suggest:

> I was in a once-a-week mothers' group, and it was very helpful. You find out you're not the only person with this problem. You don't feel sorry for yourself when you see some children that are just vegetables. (Darling, 1979, p. 161)

The counseling literature contains much information on organizing and conducting support groups. Many professionals prefer to gradually turn the control of the group over to the members, and many successful groups have been organized by clients themselves, without any professional intervention at all.

Technical support refers to services such as medical and dental care, education, legal services, therapy, and other specialized forms of treatment for conditions such as lack of job skills, illiteracy, disability, addiction, or acute illness. These services are designed to improve the functioning of the individuals they serve and generally require specialized training on the part of service providers. Because of the specialized skills required, these services typically cannot be provided through informal support alone. Technical support is often provided within a status inequality framework; however, it also can be provided within a partnership perspective when a concern in this area is client defined and not merely professionally diagnosed.

Finally, service support includes the provision of services such as child care, adult day care, sheltered employment, organized recreational programs, foster care, assisted living, and other services to meet client-defined needs when appropriate informal supports are not available. As noted in the Information section above, professionals may be able to provide needed services directly or they may have to refer clients to other agencies. When needed services are not available or are available only on a limited basis in a community, professionals may need to become advocates for their clients in an attempt to secure additional funding or to otherwise lobby those in positions of power to expand service offerings. Such activities will be discussed further in Chapter 9.

As in the other areas that have been discussed, formal support can be both a resource and a concern for clients. Some clients are satisfied with the services they are receiving; others may be dissatisfied or even disillusioned with what they have received (or not received) from agencies and professionals. The following is a description of the successful provision of formal support:

> Kathy Young stayed a shut-in for almost one year after separating from her husband. . . . She had no means of supporting herself and had no high school diploma to fall back on. . . . At 35, she felt she was at a dead end. . . .
>
> But in January 1994, she found . . . , a family support program. . . . Within one year, Young said, she began to turn her life around with the help of programs, staff, and therapists. . . .
>
> Young took the GED exam in November 1994, and the next month learned she had gotten a score "five points away from the highest score on the national." She enrolled in community college to study business. Her long-term goal is to become a paralegal. . . .
>
> "My self-esteem has boosted immensely," she said. ("Family Support Center," 1995, pp. 6–7)

Sometimes an agency can be both a resource and a concern for a client. Schools are valuable resources for students and their families because of the educational services they provide. In addition, as discussed in Chapter 2, schools are increasingly providing services such as meals, child care, and adult education that are welcomed by the families they serve. However, as Kozol (1991) and others have shown, many schools are failing in their efforts to educate children. Kozol cites many examples of school buildings in poor communities with old, poor quality or no equipment or books, unmotivated teachers, and locations next to toxic waste sites. The safety of school buildings is also questionable, as the number of violent incidents on school grounds seems to be increasing. Families whose children attend these facilities are likely to have concerns about this form of formal support.

Similarly, homeless shelters can be resources for their clients, yet the poor quality of some shelters has been a concern for many. For example, Kozol (1988) describes a converted hotel serving as a shelter with no running water, rats, filth, and other safety concerns. Some homeless people choose to live on the streets rather than resort to such facilities.

In identifying their clients' resources and concerns in this area, agency staff will need to determine which services clients are already using and whether they are satisfied with those services. After this determination has been made, the staff can assist clients in exploring concerns that are not currently being met. Finally, they can try to match these concerns with existing services. Techniques for performing these activities will be discussed further in Chapter 9. Chapters 6, 7, and 8 will suggest techniques for helping clients identify their resources, concerns, and priorities in the areas of information and material, informal, and formal support.

Socioeconomic and Subcultural Diversity

Resources, concerns, and priorities will vary from one client to the next, even among clients from similar social backgrounds. However, a better understanding of those backgrounds can be helpful to professionals in focusing on some common characteristics they are likely to encounter. The life experiences of people from the same social class or ethnic background often result in similar resources and shared concerns. In addition, racism and sexism can be important in limiting resources and increasing concerns. The following sections will explore some of the service-related characteristics often found in members of some of the more common socioeconomic and ethnic groups in American society. These characteristics include attitudes toward problems and toward receiving help from agencies and professionals, as well as differential opportunities and lifestyle differences that need to be taken into account in the development of service plans.

A Note on Gender

Regardless of social class, race, or ethnicity, the experiences of women typically differ from those of men, and consequently their definitions and attitudes are likely to differ as well. In particular, sexism is likely to play a role in limiting the opportunities available to women in education, employment, and other areas of life (see, for example, Reskin, 1993; Sadker & Sadker, 1994). Thus, human service professionals need to keep gender in mind when working with women of any socioeconomic or ethnic background.

The Influence of Social Class

Although human service professionals tend to come from middle-class backgrounds, their clients are often of lower socioeconomic status. Economic changes resulting in a decreased need for semiskilled labor and low wages for unskilled jobs during the past few decades have led to an increase in young families living in poverty. Poverty rates are highest in single-parent families, and approximately one in three children in mother-only families lives in poverty (Zinn & Eitzen, 1993). Poverty severely limits the lifestyle choices available to families, and most of the attitudes and behaviors attributed to lower-class families in the literature are best explained by limited opportunities. Earlier theories suggesting a distinct "culture of poverty" (see, for example, Lewis, 1959) are being questioned today, as many researchers agree that lower-class lifestyles result more from different resources than from different values. Thus, the source of socioeconomic diversity is unlike that of the ethnic diversity that will be discussed in the next section.

Lower-class families seem to have a higher tolerance for "deviance" than middle-class families. The lower-class parents of children with mild mental retardation discussed in Chapter 2 did not define their children as pathological. Similarly, Guttmacher and Elinson (1971) found that upper-class respondents were more likely than lower-class respondents to define a series of behaviors that deviated from the norm as illness. Various "social problems," such as teen pregnancy, drug abuse, domestic violence, and juvenile delinquency, tend to be viewed as more devastating when they occur in middle-class families than in lower-class ones. Although poor people definitely would define such occurrences as problems, the magnitude of their concern may be lessened by the survival mentality necessitated by their life situation.

The nature of family interaction, especially interaction between parents and children, also seems to vary by social class. Laosa (1978) found, for example, that in a group of Chicano families, mothers with more formal education tended to use inquiry and praise in teaching their children, whereas mothers with less education were more likely to use modeling as a teaching technique. Sometimes middle-class professionals tend to assume that middle-class techniques and interaction styles are better and therefore intervene to teach these techniques and styles to their lower-class clients. Such professionals need to be careful about imposing their definition on a situation in which it might not be appropriate.

Lower-class families also may have less informal support than others. Dunst, Trivette, and Cross (1988) found that low-socioeconomic status (SES) families of children with disabilities had less family support than a higher-SES group. Similarly, Colon (1980) has suggested that the multiproblem poor family has a truncated life cycle, with a greater loss of family members and greater shortening of life stages than the middle-class family. Even when poor people have family members who want to help them, those family members are likely to be poor themselves and to have few resources to share.

On the other hand, a strength of many poor families is their ability to survive through mutual support networks. In a study of poor African-American families, Stack (1974) found networks spread over several kin-based households. Friends included in these networks were sometimes defined as kin. Networks provided a means of survival through the exchange of goods, such as food, clothing, and furniture, and services, such as child care and housing. One common service was "child keeping," an informal system of foster care in which children moved from one household to another as family situations changed. These families resented the interference of human service agencies in such child-keeping arrangements.

Roschelle (1997) suggests that such support networks may not be as strong in lower-class minority communities today as they were in the past. Similarly, George and Dickerson (1995) found that the high rates of poverty that currently prevail among some African-American single mothers may be depleting the resources that grandmothers traditionally provided, resulting in a weakening of the extended family in some communities. Roschelle (1997) notes that immigrants tend to be less involved in support networks than native-born individuals.

A lifestyle characteristic that tends to vary by social class is the organization of time. People who work every day have daily routines that are structured by their work schedules. People who are unemployed, on the other hand, do not necessarily rise early in the morning or eat three meals a day. Consequently, early morning appointments are sometimes missed. Professionals need to take their clients' routines into account when scheduling services.

A different kind of scheduling issue may also arise. The clients with whom I worked were commonly sent to a hospital in the nearest large city for consultations. Buses, the only available form of public transportation, ran between our city and the hospital city twice a day, with the earliest bus of the day arriving at noon. This hospital routinely scheduled appointments for these clients at 8:00 AM. Clients who could afford private transportation generally kept these appointments, either by leaving early in the morning or by staying at a hotel in the city the night before. Poor clients, on the other hand, sometimes skipped their appointments entirely. At least one poor family I knew (a mother with two young children) took the bus and then spent the night at the bus station in order to arrive at their appointment on time.

In general, the characteristic of lower-SES clients that is most relevant for human service providers is a chronic shortage of cash. Such a shortage is likely to restructure the priorities of these individuals and to shift their focus from the professional's definition of the problem to issues of survival. Thus, before addressing other concerns, professionals need to help such clients with issues of material support.

Ethnic Variation

An ethnic group has been defined as "those who conceive of themselves as alike by virtue of their common ancestry, real or fictitious, and who are so regarded by others" (Shibutani & Kwan, reported in McGoldrick, 1982, p. 3). Ethnic identification may be based on race, culture, or national origin. Census data from 1989 indicated that the population of the United States consisted of ethnic groups in the following proportions (Harry, 1992a):

Group	*Percentage of population*
Black	12.0
Hispanic (of any race)	8.3
Asian, Pacific	2.8
Native American	0.7
White	84.1

These data represent a decrease in the white population in proportion to the other groups, compared with data from the previous census. Chan (1990) notes that shortly after the year 2000, one third of the projected US population will consist of people of color, and the white population of the state of California will be in the minority. Among whites are people with various ethnic identifications, including Irish, Italian, Jewish, and German. Members of some ethnic groups identify very strongly with the group, whereas others think of themselves more as Americans than as ethnics.

Because attitudes toward problems and toward professionals vary by ethnicity, professionals should be aware of their clients' ethnic identifications. The following discussion is not intended to be an exhaustive or definitive review of the literature on ethnic groups, but rather to suggest the kinds of ethnic differences that may be relevant to the provision of human services.

African-American Subculture

Much of the literature on African Americans has focused on social class rather than ethnicity. Consequently, many of the patterns that have been suggested have been socioeconomic, based on the overrepresentation of blacks in the lower social classes. However, Tolson and Wilson (1990) and others have shown that black families are not homogeneous and that considerable diversity exists among two- and three-generational families of varying socioeconomic levels. Many studies suggest that an African-American subculture exists apart from socioeconomic status; professionals need to be careful to distinguish these ethnic patterns from characteristics associated with poverty. In addition, the effects of racism, although not subcultural, are relevant for the provision of services to African Americans of all social classes.

Because African Americans are disproportionately poor, they tend to be overrepresented in the human service client population. Infant mortality and low birth weight, both consequences of poverty, are twice as high for blacks as whites (Edelman, 1985). Teen pregnancy, another consequence of poverty, is also more common among African Americans (Franklin & Boyd-Franklin, 1985). However, informal support is often high in such families. Dodson (1981), Franklin and Boyd-Franklin (1985), Harrison, Serafica, and McAdoo (1984), and others have suggested that childrearing in African-American families has historically been a communal process, with a high level of involvement by the extended family. Staples (1976) suggests that the "attenuated extended family," consisting of a single adult and her children as well as additional relatives in the home, is a common family form. This family is likely to be surrounded by a large kin network, including fictive kin as well as blood relations. A system of informal adoption also exists (Hines & Boyd-Franklin, 1982). On the other hand, material support from family members is more likely to be lacking among blacks than among whites because of higher levels of poverty (Edin & Harris, 1997).

Racism is at least partially responsible for the large proportion of African Americans found among students labeled as "educable mentally retarded" (EMR) in the public schools and among the inmates of correctional institutions. Moore (1981) found that black children constituted 45% of EMR enrollment nationally. Poor school performance seems to result in a much greater likelihood of labeling among these students than among comparable white students. Similarly, 32.2% of young black men in comparison with 6.7% of young white men are either in prison, in jail, or on probation or parole (Davis, 1997). Further, Kilty and Joseph (1997) have noted that 55% of those convicted and 74% of those imprisoned for illegal drug use are black males, even though this segment of the population makes up only 13% of all users.

Although racism and high levels of poverty are important intervening variables in defining the role of African Americans in the human service system, some writers have suggested that cultural factors also need to be taken into account in service provision. Although many African Americans probably have more cultural characteristics in common with European Americans than with other African Americans, some differences have been noted. Boykin (1988) suggests, for example, that African Americans of all social classes share a distinctive subculture consisting of characteristics such as communalism, expressive individualism, and orality. Such a subculture may give rise to distinctive communication patterns. One report (University of Pittsburgh Office of Child Development, 1991) suggests, for example, that, compared to whites, blacks may use more hand and body gestures, avoid eye contact, and wait short times before speaking, resulting in overlapping speech patterns. European American professionals unfamiliar with these patterns might have difficulty taking the role of their African-American clients and incorrectly assume that they are rude or uninterested.

Other researchers have noted distinctive social patterns. Manns (1981) found that African Americans of all social classes have more significant others than European Americans. When asked to name a significant other, blacks are more likely than whites to name a relative. Sudarkasa (1981) suggests that the roots of the black family system lie in the African principle of consanguinity, which emphasized the extended family over the conjugal relationship.

In naming a nonrelative significant other, half the black respondents in Manns's (1981) study mentioned a minister. Other studies (Franklin & Boyd-Franklin, 1985; Hines & Boyd-Franklin, 1982) also have mentioned the relative importance of religion in African-American family life at all social levels. Hines and Boyd-Franklin (1982) have written:

> In the Baptist church, a Black family finds a complete support system including the minister, deacons, deaconesses, and other church members. Numerous activities . . . provide a social life for the entire family, which extends far beyond the Sunday services and provides a network of people who are available to the family in times of trouble or loss. (p. 96)

Some writers have suggested that African Americans also have characteristic nuclear family patterns. Several researchers (Bartz & Levine, 1978; McAdoo, 1981) have noted that black parents tend to be more authoritative with their children than white parents. Studies (Bartz & Levine, 1978; Polk, 1994) also suggest that African-American parents encourage earlier independence training in their children than other parents. Professionals from other ethnic groups may need to recognize these as cultural differences rather than pathological variants.

Latino Subculture

Latinos constitute the second-largest ethnic minority in the United States. Harry (1992a) suggests that although intragroup diversity exists, Latinos share a common language (Spanish) and worldview based on Catholic ideology, familism, and values of personalism, respect, and status. Although similarities exist among various groups of Hispanic origin, Mexican Americans, Puerto Rican Americans, Cuban Americans, and other Latinos do have separate identities and subcultures. Socioeconomic status also varies, with recent immigrants having the highest poverty rates (Beinart, 1997). Ortiz (1995) reports that Puerto Ricans have been more affected than other Latino groups by the changing economy and showed a decline in socioeconomic status during the 1980s. She notes that Puerto Ricans also have more female-headed households than other Latinos. Because of the great variability among Latino families, Massey, Zambrana, and Alonzo Bell (1995) suggest that programs for this group need to be community based.

As in the case of African Americans, socioeconomically based lifestyle characteristics among Latinos are sometimes incorrectly attributed to cultural difference. Like other groups with high levels of poverty, Latinos may not have a regular source of health care and may experience barriers to service use such as lack of child care, lack of transportation, lack of knowledge, lack of insurance, or inability to pay. Zambrana, Dorrington, and Hayes-Bautista (1995) note that Latinos are even more likely to be uninsured than other groups in poverty. They cite evidence, however, to suggest that the problem is structural, not cultural.

Most of the human service-related literature on Latinos has focused on Mexican Americans and Puerto Ricans, who together have had the highest levels of poverty in the Latino community and have constituted the largest Latino groups in some areas of the country.

Mexican Americans tend to be geographically concentrated, with most living in the Southwest. Wendeborn (1982) has written of this population:

> Unlike the early European immigrants who were cut off from their prior homelands by the vast Atlantic Ocean, the Hispanic patient of Mexican heritage still has access to Mexico. Many still have immediate families and other relatives in Mexico. This proximity to Mexico lends itself to retention of the Mexican culture—thus the Hispanic of Mexican heritage is in many ways a bicultural person. (p. 6)

Because of their cultural differences and the effects of racism, Mexican Americans and other Latinos, like African Americans, tend to be overrepresented among labeled populations in the public schools and the criminal justice system.

Mexican culture is marked by language and lifestyle differences from the mainstream. As a result, Mexican-American families who do not speak English or are not familiar with the larger American culture may find interactions with professionals difficult and may be uncomfortable in institutional settings. Stein (1983) reports that Latino parents do not participate as actively in the development of their children's educational plans as do Anglo parents or parents in general. Both schools and medical settings tend to be intimidating. Azziz (1981) notes that, to Latinos, hospitals are places where the sick go to die. Hospital visiting rules, which exclude some family members, also are foreign to them. In addition, the Spanish-speaking person may have difficulty distinguishing among various hospital personnel and may pay more attention to a technician who speaks Spanish than to a physician who speaks only English. Romaine (1982) notes, too, that time has a different meaning in Mexican culture, and Mexican Americans may not keep appointments, creating scheduling problems for professionals. Quesada (1976) mentions the concept of *dignidad*, a kind of reticence, which may result in a paternalistic dependence that is misunderstood by professionals.

Value differences can also pose difficulties for professionals. Latinos with disabilities, for example, may be reluctant to use personal assistance services because they view the body as private ("Adapting Research to Cultures and Countries," 1995/96). For these individuals, the use of family providers might be preferable to the employer–employee model usually espoused by the Independent Living Movement.

Latinos who are undocumented are especially unlikely to turn to human services for help because of fear of deportation. In a study of battered women who were incarcerated, Bonilla-Santiago (1996) found that, in comparison with European-American women, Latinas were less likely to have received assistance or protection from police, legal aid, welfare, family counseling agencies, or community mental health centers. The women in her sample cited threats from their partners to call the US Immigration and Naturalization Service. They also feared leaving their partners more than the European-American women did, because language and legal barriers made them less employable.

The traditional Mexican family has been characterized as having values of familism, male dominance, subordination of young to old, and person orientation rather than goal orientation (Alvirez & Bean, 1976). Guinn (reported in Williams & Williams, 1979) notes a number of additional differences between Mexican-American and Anglo values: Mexicans stress being, and Anglos stress doing; Anglos value material well-being more than Mexicans; Mexicans have a present time orientation, and Anglos have a future orientation; Anglos value individual action, and Mexicans value group cooperation; Mexicans are fatalistic, whereas Anglos value mastery of the universe.

The implications of such value differences for human services are suggested by different definitions of domestic violence by Latina and Anglo-American women. Bonilla-Santiago (1996) found that the Latina women in her sample were more tolerant of wife abuse than their Anglo counterparts because of their acceptance of differences in power between men and women. Acts such as verbal abuse and failure to provide food and shelter were considered abusive by the Anglos but not by the Latinas, and acts such as hitting had to occur more frequently before the Latinas considered them abusive.

On the other hand, traditional gender role expectations have been changing among Latinos as more women have been working outside the home (Vega, 1995). Coltrane (1998) reports shared decision making and participation in housework in a sample of dual-earner Chicano couples, and Powell (1995) reports that Latino fathers willingly participated along with their wives in a parent education and support program. Thus, professionals need to be careful about making assumptions about cultural differences as more groups become acculturated to mainstream norms and values.

The importance of the extended family in Mexican culture has been noted by many writers. Heller (reported in Williams & Williams, 1979) states that the web of kinship ties imposes obligations of mutual aid, respect, and affection. Falicov (1982) notes that the family protects the individual and that extended family members may perform many parental functions. Cousins may be as close as siblings. In addition, *compadres*, or godparents, play an important role. Lieberman (1990) also mentions the *madrina*, who is selected by the parents to share the responsibility for the child. In a study of the extended family as an emotional support system, Keefe, Padilla, and Carlos (1979) found that Mexican Americans consistently rely on relatives more than friends, regardless of geographic proximity. Both Falicov and Karrer (1980) and Keefe and colleagues (1979) note that Mexican women have a strong tendency to confide in female relatives. At the same time, the closeness of family members can be perceived as a problem, and Keefe and colleagues note that their respondents sometimes resented their relatives' intrusion into their personal affairs.

In a study of independent living services for individuals with disabilities ("Adapting Research to Cultures and Countries," 1995/96), the usual model of providing support only for the individual was found to be inappropriate for Latinos. Because decisions in this population are typically made by the family as a group, independence is defined differently, and support services need to be provided to the entire family.

Mexican-American attitudes toward child rearing sometimes differ from those of the cultural mainstream. Falicov (1982) and Falicov and Karrer (1980) note a relaxed attitude toward the achievement of developmental milestones and self-reliance, along with a basic acceptance of the child's individuality. Such attitudes could result in differences between parents and professionals in definitions of child pathology.

Although folk beliefs diminish as succeeding generations become increasingly acculturated in the mainstream, some Mexican Americans and other Latinos may continue to hold traditional beliefs about the nature of disease and disability and may continue to rely on *curanderos*, or folk healers. Some common Mexican folk beliefs include *mal ojo* (the evil eye) as a cause of illness and a susceptibility to *susto*, a severe fright (Prattes, 1973). Folk healers are sometimes preferred over professionals because of their warmth and personal relationship with the family. Recommendations made by professionals are usually also discussed by the entire family and second opinions are commonly sought (Schreiber & Homiak, 1981; Wendeborn, 1982). Professionals may need to acknowledge their clients' needs in this regard and not attempt to impose their views.

Puerto Ricans also have been shown to rely heavily on the family as a source of strength and support. Garcia-Preto (1982) has written:

> In times of stress Puerto Ricans turn to their families for help. Their cultural expectation is that when a family member is experiencing a crisis or has a problem, others in the family are obligated to help, especially those who are in stable positions. Because Puerto Ricans rely on the family and their extended network of personal relationships, they will make use of social services only as a last resort. (p.164)

Differences in meaning in Latino groups can produce role-taking difficulties for professionals. Harry (1992b) has noted that the low-income Puerto Rican families in her study did not accept professional definitions of their children's disabilities because of different meanings they attached to terms such as handicapped or retarded. One parent said, "They say the word 'handicap' means a lot of things. . . . But for us, Puerto Ricans, we still understand this word as 'crazy'" (p. 31). These parents "felt that the school's labeling process did not recognize the child's individuality and family identity"(p. 32).

On the other hand, professionals should not assume that culturally different clients have different definitions of the situation. One study of poor Mexican mothers (Shapiro & Tittle, 1986) found, for example, that like their Anglo counterparts these respondents perceived their children's disabilities as causing stress and the disruption of family functioning. Similarly, a study of amniocentesis decisions by Mexican-origin women (Browner, Preloran, & Cox, 1999) found that health-care providers incorrectly assumed that decisions would be governed by "deep-rooted, cultural givens," such as opposition to abortion. In fact, these womens' decisions were related more to such variables as their understanding of risks and their faith in their doctors.

Asian-American Subculture

Just as one should not necessarily generalize from one Latino group to another, one must be careful not to assume that all Asian subcultures are alike. In addition, immigrant family concerns differ from those of American-born Asian families (Bromley, 1989; Timberlake & Cook, 1984). Most of the literature focuses on Japanese and Chinese Americans, and some similarities exist between these groups that may be generalizable to other Asian Americans.

Like other ethnic groups, Asian Americans value the family very highly. In traditional Asian families, family problems are regarded as private, and bringing them to the attention of outsiders is considered shameful (Shon & Ja, 1982). However, reticence in revealing coping difficulties does not necessarily mean that a family will not accept technical support in the form of medical, educational, or therapeutic services. Harry (1992a) has written that the essence of Eastern cultures is collectivism and harmony, and that modesty is important. She notes that Asians sometimes regard disabilities as bringing shame to the family and may not seek professional help for that reason. Yee (1988) has noted that denial of a child's disability is common in Asian families.

In Chinese, Japanese, and other Asian families, obligation to the family is important and may supercede individual needs. Japanese children are expected to be respectful and considerate toward their parents and to have a high degree of self-control (Harrison, Serafica, & McAdoo, 1984). Huang (1976) notes that Chinese children usually grow up in the midst of adults and are not left with babysitters.

Lee (1982) writes that the mother–son relationship is particularly close in Chinese families, even after a son marries. The oldest son usually has more responsibilities than other children in the family.

Kitano and Kikumura (1976) note that the Japanese are taught to defer to those of higher status, and open confrontation is avoided. As a result, members of this group are unlikely to challenge a professional, even when they do not agree with a recommended course of treatment. Similarly, Chan (reported in Harry & Kalyanpur, 1994) suggests that the mandate that parents participate in their child's educational planning may be "both alien and threatening" to those with a traditional Asian background. Thus, the client empowerment movement in human services (cf. Chapter 2) may be culturally inappropriate in some cases. Fong (1994) suggests that the partnership model in general may be inappropriate for some Asian families. As in the case of other ethnic groups, however, considerable intragroup variability is likely to be present among Asian-American families, especially those with long exposure to mainstream American culture and its emphasis on consumerism.

Native American Subculture

Because of intertribal variation, Native Americans cannot be regarded as constituting a single subculture. In some ways, however, various tribes seem to be more like each other than like the cultural mainstream. Attneave (1982), Harrison and colleagues (1984), and others have listed the following differences in values between Native Americans and the American middle class:

Native American	*American middle class*
Cooperation	Competition
Harmony with nature	Control over nature
Adult centered	Child centered
Present time orientation	Future time orientation
Expression through action	Verbal expression
Short childhood	Extended childhood
Education for knowledge	Education for grades

Because they are more accepting of fate and less achievement oriented than most middle-class, European Americans, Native Americans tend to be more tolerant of deviance and disability. Locust (1988) has noted that among the Hopi some of the gods are in fact disabled and that the Native American belief system stresses the strengths of individuals rather than their disabilities. Harry (1992a) has observed that most Native American languages do not have words for disability.

Native American families also are likely to have good informal support when coping with family problems. Traditionally the extended family shares in child rearing, and Native American children tend to be treated permissively and loved by everyone in the family (Williams & Williams, 1979). Anderson (1988) has suggested that grandparents may be even more important in child rearing than parents.

Professionals involved with Native Americans should be aware of a tendency toward reticence. Interactions may be marked by long silences and little self-disclosure (Attneave, 1982). In addition, professionals need to accept the fact that some Native Americans still use traditional healers, such as medicine men and shamans. Spector (1979) also has noted that Native Americans may be offended by direct questions or note taking by professionals.

Because of past experiences of discrimination or inappropriate labeling by European American professionals (White, 1995), Native American clients may be reluctant to seek help from human service agencies or may be suspicious of practices they encounter there. Several years ago, I field tested a questionnaire in various locations. The questionnaire contained codes (e.g., *IS* for informal support; *I* for information) beside each item to assist professionals in categorizing client responses. The only respondents to question these codes were a group of Native Americans in Wisconsin who were suspicious about their meaning. (As a result, the codes were removed from the questionnaire.)

A recent report ("Developing Systems of Support," 1998) describes a culturally appropriate service delivery model being used with Native American families in Wisconsin. This model reverses the Western system of "one serving many" (e.g., one physician seeing many patients) by using a principle of "many serving one" (e.g., many women baby-showering one pregnant woman). In this model, the entire community is mobilized to provide the services needed by an individual or family.

Other Ethnic Subcultures

African Americans, Latinos, Asian Americans, and Native Americans are all generally regarded as minority groups in American society. Because of past experience with racism and powerlessness, members of these groups are more likely to be passive in their interactions with European American professionals than members of the majority. Harry (1992a) notes that, in comparison with majority group parents, parents from these groups have exhibited the following characteristics when interacting with professional educators:

- Lower level of involvement.
- Less awareness of procedures, rights, and services.
- Expressed sense of isolation and helplessness.
- Low self-confidence.
- Stressful life circumstances that are overwhelming.
- Greater need for logistical supports such as transportation, respite, and child care.

- Culturally based assumptions of deference to authority and noninterference in educational matters.
- Professionals' implicit or explicit discouragement of parents' participation in the educational process.

Similarly, Sontag and Schacht (1994) found that minority (Latino and Native-American) parents reported less participation than European American parents in their children's early intervention programs.

Although ethnic variation is also present among the European-American majority, value differences from the cultural mainstream may not be as pronounced, especially among the third, fourth, and fifth generations. One exception may be more insulated groups such as the Amish. With regard to expectations about health care, McNeal and Leach (1997a) note that the Amish believe that illnesses such as measles and chicken pox and dental cavities are normal and that immunizations are unnecessary. Preventive care is generally regarded as unimportant, and medical insurance is nonexistent. Homeopathic remedies are commonly used. The following are some suggested strategies for health care professionals who provide services in the Amish community (McNeal & Leach, 1997b):

- Don't be afraid to give them literature, but ask whether anatomically explicit literature would be offensive.
- Seek out trusted "English" people, such as a community friend, a driver with whom they contract for transportation, or a shopkeeper. These people can introduce you to community leaders, such as bishops and schoolteachers.
- Dress conservatively. Women should not wear jeans or slacks.

Among more mainstream ethnic groups, some differences in values and beliefs are sometimes still present. For example, both Jewish Americans and Italian Americans may value the family more than their Anglo-Saxon counterparts (see, for example, Herz & Rosen, 1982; Rotunno & McGoldrick, 1982). Because of strong family support, Italian families may make less use of professional support services than other groups. On the other hand, Jewish Americans may tend to be more favorably inclined than other ethnic groups toward reliance on professional "experts." Although third- or fourth-generation Italian or Jewish clients may not have these characteristics, they may experience conflict with parents and grandparents who do not approve of their help-seeking behavior.

Implications for Professionals

Human service professionals should be aware of subcultural differences. However, the professional must be careful not to stereotype service users on the basis of social class or ethnic identity. Within most subcultures, a considerable amount of intragroup variation exists. Professionals should not assume that individual members of a group will share all the values and beliefs commonly held by the group as a whole. In a study of lower-class black mothers' aspirations for their children, for example, Bell (1965) found aspirations varied within a group, which was homogeneous in both social class and race. The value of subcultural studies, then, is in making professionals more aware of possible characteristics their clients may exhibit and in helping to explain some of the characteristics they may encounter.

The need for a better understanding of subcultural differences is demonstrated by a number of studies that reveal misunderstandings between professionals and clients of a different cultural background. One study of mental health therapists and their Spanish-speaking patients (Kline, Acosta, Austin, & Johnson, 1980) found that the therapists did not accurately perceive the patients' wants and feelings and instead projected their own wishes onto the patients. Such misperceptions may persist even when interpreters are used. Marcos (1979) found, for example, that clinicians evaluating non-English-speaking patients through an interpreter made "consistent, clinically relevant, interpreter-related distortions, which may give rise to important misconceptions about the patient's mental status" (p.173). Fein (1997) reports that because the number of languages spoken in large cities like New York is increasing, volunteer interpreters are being used by health care facilities, resulting in instances of serious communication difficulties.

Studies with Mexican-American groups (Ada, reported in Harry, 1992a; Delgado-Gaitan, reported in Harry, 1992a) have shown that passivity can be overcome by professional techniques that are inclusive rather than exclusive. The individuals in these studies were empowered by the realization that their nonacademic skills were valuable. Thus, the process of encouraging minority service users to share their concerns and priorities may require special techniques. A number of recommendations emerge to guide professionals who work with culturally and socioeconomically different clients:

- *Do not overlook resources or overemphasize concerns.* Particularly in the case of clients of lower socioeconomic status, professionals may tend to focus on their clients' deficits rather than their strengths. All clients have strengths, but professionals may have to work harder to discover them when clients feel as though they have no power. VanDenBerg and Grealish (1997, p. 2) suggest some questions that are useful in strengths discovery:
    - If you could say one good thing about yourself, what would it be?
    - I like your (hair, makeup, clothes, etc.). Did you come up with that yourself?
    - What do you do for fun?
    - Who has been the biggest influence on your life?
    - What are the best things about your family? Your community?

- *If at all possible, the professional should speak the family's native language.* As Laosa (1974) and others have suggested, abandonment of one's native language may imply abandonment of one's entire culture. Hanson (1981) and others have noted the importance of providing written materials in the client's native language. Fracasso (1994) has suggested the technique of "back translation," whereby materials that have been translated be translated back to English by an independent translator, to assure that meanings have not been changed. As Harry (1992a) has noted, interpreters should be bicultural as well as bilingual to avoid misunderstandings caused by nuances of meaning.
- *Indigenous professionals, paraprofessionals, and consultants should be used as much as possible.* Although professionals can learn about the cultural backgrounds of the people they serve, they can never acquire the cultural worldview to the same extent as one raised in the culture. Service users also are likely to feel more comfortable interacting with their peers. Quesada (1976) thus recommends that community members be hired by provider agencies, either as professionals, paraprofessionals, or consultants. Harry (1992a) suggests that information be disseminated through traditional community supports such as churches or through community leaders.
- *Scheduling should be flexible.* As noted earlier, transportation and child care barriers may prevent some service users from keeping appointments. Quesada (1976) notes, too, that people working on an hourly basis may not be able to spend long periods of time at an agency. In some cases, home visits may be preferable to office appointments.
- *Attempts should be made to elicit the family's definition of the situation.* Although important for all professional–client interactions, this guideline is especially important in the case of the culturally different service user. Professionals can take certain steps to better educate themselves about the subcultures of the people they serve. Harry, Torguson, Katkavich, and Guerrero (1993) describe, for example, a teacher training program that requires students to spend time with a culturally different family, including interviewing the parents and participating in a community-based activity.

Wayman et al. (1991) suggest a series of questions for home visitors in early intervention to ask themselves as an aid to understanding a family's values and lifestyle. Among others, these include:

- Who are the members of the family system?
- Who are the key decision makers?
- Do family members all live in the same household?
- Who is the primary caregiver?
- Is there an established bedtime?
- What are the parameters of acceptable child behavior?

- From whom does the family seek help?
- Is the family proficient in English?

Methods for acquiring such information will be discussed in Chapters 6, 7, and 8.

- *Survival issues should take precedence over other intervention issues.* As noted earlier, individuals or families with major concerns about food, clothing, shelter, or health care may not be interested in addressing other concerns. Assistance with clients' material concerns is important for all professionals, even those with specialties in other areas.
- *When possible, professionals should adapt their communication style to the expectations of the family.* Kavanagh and Kennedy (1992) suggest numerous strategies for communicating with culturally different families. Some examples follow:
  - Do not discredit folk theories or remedies unless you know they are harmful.
  - Establish a personalized relationship by means of disclosing selected, culturally appropriate personal information.
  - If appropriate, acknowledge unfamiliarity with the family's culture.
  - Ask direct questions only if appropriate to the family's cultural and linguistic expectations. (Direct questioning should be avoided with some Asian, Latino, or Native American families.)
  - While showing respect for the family's views, openly acknowledge differences between your views and theirs.
  - Adjust the tone of your voice and your body position to synchronize with those of family members.
  - Include extended family members or others in an interview if they are normally part of the family's support system.
  - Apologize when you make an error.
  - Temporarily reverse roles, that is, allow the family to teach you about their culture.
  - Be able and willing to tolerate periods of silence.

The authors recommend role-playing and other exercises to practice these techniques before they are needed in an interaction situation.

Chapter Summary

This chapter has explored the social worlds of service users in terms of their differing social class and cultural backgrounds. The chapter introduced the concepts of resources, concerns, and priorities as components of clients' opportunity structures and the definitions of the situation that result from them. In a *Verstehen* approach, service providers must work to understand the context of their clients' lives, which includes both what they already have and what they think is lacking. The chapter showed how resources, concerns, and priorities may differ among various groups in American society and suggested some ways that human service professionals could work more effectively with members of these groups.

Suggested Exercises

The following exercises may be helpful to students or professionals who wish to develop a better understanding of the social worlds of service users and to enhance their role-taking ability prior to interacting with actual clients:

1. *Write a sociological autobiography.* Think about your own background and the experiences that have shaped your attitudes. Have you had any experiences with members of the socioeconomic or cultural group from which your clients are likely to come? What did your parents, friends, and other significant others tell you about members of this group? Think about strangers you have seen in public places or on television who might have been members of this group. What did you think about them? Have you ever deliberately avoided interacting with a member of this group? Why do you think you acted in this way? Make a list of all of your group affiliations and experiences with members of other groups and examine how each has affected your attitudes. Use your list to write an autobiography that traces your experiences and shows how they shaped your present attitudes.
2. *Get to know some members of different groups.* If you are a student, you may want to volunteer or to do an internship that involves helping a community group with some local project. Grassroots and self-help organizations provide better opportunities to get to know people than professionally run agencies. In a professionally run agency, you may learn more about the values and behavior of professionals than those of the people they serve. Spending time at a local community center where people "drop in" for social activities rather than keeping appointments for specific services also can be valuable. Another beneficial activity would be interviewing members of other groups or participating in their gatherings. Most college campuses have organizations for members of various racial, ethnic, and religious groups. If you are European American, attend a service at an African-American church or go to a NAACP meeting. If you plan to work with people with disabilities, spend some time at a group home for people with mental retardation or mental illness, or

attend meetings of groups such as the local chapter of the United Cerebral Palsy or Spina Bifida Association.

3. *Read some personal accounts by members of the groups that interest you.* Many service users and former service users have written books and articles about their experiences. You will find autobiographies written by mental patients, drug abusers, homeless individuals, and many other people who have had the kinds of concerns you are likely to encounter in human service work. Some examples from the disability field include Susana Kaysen's (Kaysen, 1993) *Girl Interrupted* (by an ex-mental patient) and Nancy Mairs's *Waist-High in the World* (Mairs, 1996), and John Hockenberry's *Moving Violations* (Hockenberry, 1995) (by individuals with physical disabilities).
4. *Read consumer-oriented literature.* Two types of literature are available. First, many organizations publish newsletters for their clients. Articles written by professionals may not be very valuable for this purpose, but most newsletters also include articles and letters written directly by service users. These often contain "tips" for other service users derived from personal experiences and sometimes involve complaints about difficulties in obtaining services. The second type of literature consists of newsletters published directly by consumer groups. These are even more likely to include articles about bad experiences in the human service system and to suggest advocacy techniques.

In actual professional practice in the human services, general knowledge about the characteristics of diverse groups is useful as background information. However, the professional cannot make any assumptions about a particular client based on his or her group memberships. Each new client must identify a unique set of resources, concerns, and priorities. The most important professional function in sociological practice is assisting clients with this identification process. The next three chapters will discuss techniques for carrying out this function.

Suggestions for Further Reading

Cook, D.A., & Fine, M. (1995). "Motherwit": Child rearing lessons from African American mothers of low income. In B.B. Swadener & S. Lubeck (Eds.), *Children and families "at promise": Deconstructing the discourse of risk* (pp. 118–142). Albany: State University of New York Press.

Harry, B. (1992). *Cultural diversity, families, and the special education system: Communication and empowerment.* New York: Teacher's College Press.

Lynch, E.W., & Hanson, M.J. (Eds.). (1992). *Developing cross-cultural competence: A guide for working with young children and their families.* Baltimore: Paul Brookes.

6

Identification Techniques I

Observation

The preceding chapters have created a background for practitioners interested in using a sociological approach to provide human services from a partnership perspective. As noted throughout, the emphasis has been on a *Verstehen* approach, in which the definition of the situation of the service user guides any professional intervention that occurs. Thus, the practitioner must come to understand this definition as thoroughly as possible. The traditional sociological research methods of observation, interviewing, and questionnaire administration can be adapted for use by human service professionals to increase their understanding. This chapter will present the method of observation and will show how practitioners acting as partner observers can learn more about their clients' opportunity structures and definitions of the situation.

Prior to any intervention in the client's social system, the professional must understand the client's concerns and priorities, as well as the resources that already exist to address those concerns. Thus, the first step in providing services from a partnership perspective is to identify the client's resources, concerns, and priorities. In status inequality approaches, this step is usually called assessment. During assessment, the professional "diagnoses" the client's problem. In the partnership approach being advocated here, professional activities focus on assisting the client in a process of identification. This process is similar to traditional assessment processes; the change in terminology is used to suggest that the client and the professional are working together to clarify the definition of the situation in preparation for a plan of action to address identified concerns.

Various methods are available to assist professionals and their clients in identifying clients' resources, concerns, and priorities. Some of these methods were originally developed for research purposes. Sociological researchers who have taken a *Verstehen* approach have been interested in understanding the meanings of participants in various social situations (see, for example, Taylor & Bogdan, 1984). Methods for learning about participants' meanings are relevant for practitioners concerned with their clients' definitions of the situation. Monette, Sullivan, and DeJong (1994) have noted further that parallels exist between stages in social research and steps in human service practice, in that both involve a problem-solving process. Thus, the next few chapters will borrow heavily from the research literature in sociology. Although the goal here is service provision rather than research, the techniques that will be discussed are equally appropriate for both endeavors.

Lofland and Lofland (1995) suggest that sociological researchers obtain data through a combination of looking, listening, and asking. The research methods that are most applicable to human service work—observation, interviewing, and questionnaire development—are based on these activities. Each will be discussed in a separate chapter. Chapters 6, 7, and 8 will explore these methods as tools for assisting with the process of identifying client resources, concerns, and priorities. Chapter 11 will explore the same methods as tools for assisting agencies in the evaluation of existing services and the initiation of new services.

Ethical Issues

The process of identifying concerns, priorities, and resources involves obtaining information that may not have been disclosed previously. Professionals involved in this process therefore must balance their need to know with their clients' rights to privacy and autonomy. Thus, while engaging in observation, interviewing, or questionnaire administration, professionals need to be sensitive to their clients' wishes and concerns. A number of principles that commonly guide practice in the human services are relevant here.

The Principle of Confidentiality

Most human service agencies require that all personally identifiable information about clients be kept within the agency. Restrictions are typically placed on which staff members are allowed access to client files, and those who do have access are expected to refrain from discussing such information with others. Any release of information to individuals outside of the agency generally requires written consent from the client.

The reasons for such confidentiality policies are clear. First, the ethical principle of personal autonomy suggests that, unless others have a compelling need to know, individuals retain ownership of all information about themselves. Beyond this ethical imperative, the sharing of confidential information can be harmful. In some cases, the harm results from the embarrassment or ostracism that may follow the revelation of characteristics associated with stigma in our society, such as a criminal record or a history of mental illness. In even more serious cases, the unwarranted release of information, such as the whereabouts of a woman seeking refuge from domestic violence, could be dangerous or life threatening.

Some human service situations create ethical dilemmas for professionals. In many areas of human service work, professionals are regularly subpoenaed to provide testimony in custody hearings, criminal trials, and other court proceedings. Although legally bound to comply, practitioners commonly recognize that, by releasing confidential information in court, they are likely to lose their clients' trust. Often that trust has not been easily acquired.

Another situation requiring the breaking of confidentiality is child abuse reporting. Although professionals recognize the need to report abusive behavior by their clients, they are often reluctant to do so, because they fear losing the positive client–professional relationship they have managed to develop. Most situations of child abuse or neglect are not clear-cut. Most human service professionals only rarely see obvious cases of physical or sexual abuse or serious neglect. More typically, they see parents who love their children but who discipline them a little more severely than they should or whose housekeeping standards are below their own. In these cases, they must make difficult decisions about balancing the client's right to self-determination against the welfare of the child.

An example of the difficulty involved in such decisions is illustrative. When I was a human service administrator, one of my staff members came to see me after completing a home visit with a young family. She reported that when she arrived at the home she was greeted by the family's 4-year-old daughter. The child's 6-month-old brother was asleep in a crib. The staff member asked the girl whether her parents were at home, and the child replied that her father had gone to the store. The children were alone in the house. The staff member entered the home and waited for the father to return. He arrived about 15 minutes later. The staff member recognized the danger involved in leaving such young children unsupervised, even for a relatively short time, but was reluctant to report the family to the local child protection agency. She said that she had worked very hard over a period of a year to develop a relationship of trust with this family and believed that the parents truly cared about their children. She preferred to simply discuss the problem directly with the family and to try to help them understand the danger involved in leaving their children alone. The staff member and I discussed the fact that, under the law, she had no choice but to report the family, and she did so. First, though, she called the father and explained to him what she needed to do and why. Fortunately, in this case, the professional was able to reestablish a positive relationship with the family, but in other cases, the violation of confidentiality does negatively affect future client–professional interactions.

The principle of confidentiality is compatible with a partnership approach in human services, because this approach is based on respect for the service user and his or her way of life. The practitioner would want to be especially careful about assuring the client that the process of information gathering is intended to assist the client in identifying resources and concerns and not to provide information to outsiders. However, clients also should be informed, at the outset, that in some situations professionals are required by law to report certain information to authorities.

Client Autonomy in Special Situations

In general, service users have the right to self-determination and professionals do not have the right to make decisions for them, no matter how paternalistic their intentions. In some cases, though, the ability of clients to make appropriate choices on their own behalf is questionable. These cases typically involve children, people with mental retardation or some mental health diagnoses, or older people with dementia. Some recent examples of cases that have come before the courts include parents who, because of their religious beliefs, have denied medical treatment to their children and parents who have had their adult children with mental retardation sterilized. Human service professionals need to be careful in obtaining informed consent from individuals with limited cognitive abilities. Certainly, many individuals with mental retardation are capable of making choices (cf Perske, 1972) about the receipt of services, and professionals can establish partnership relationships with them. In some cases, though, caregivers or specially appointed advocates may need to be consulted on behalf of certain clients.

The Right of Refusal

A partnership approach assumes that services are voluntary. Of course, in actual human service practice, services are sometimes court-ordered, as a result of legal action stemming from child abuse or other crimes or offenses. However, even in such cases, the professional can consult with the client in determining which methods to use and in the application of chosen methods. All clients should have the right to refuse to answer some questions, to object to being observed in some situations, and to terminate a session. Clients also should have the right to question the relevance of any particular question or method. Observations and questions not directly relevant to a client's stated concerns are intrusive and an invasion of privacy.

Choosing a Method

Qualitative versus Quantitative

Generally sociologists classify methods using a qualitative–quantitative dichotomy. Qualitative methods include observation and depth interviewing, and sociologists who prefer *Verstehen* approaches commonly use these methods, which contribute to a deeper understanding of people's lives. Quantitative methods include some surveys and questionnaires from which data can be scaled for comparative purposes.

Qualitative approaches are usually regarded as more subjective. Because the observer or interviewer may act differently in different observation or interview situations, to some extent the outcome is dependent on the identity of the observer or interviewer and on the situation. In contrast to the questions on a standard survey form, for example, the questions in a depth interview will vary somewhat from one respondent to another, because questions are derived from previous answers. Thus, the nature of qualitative methods is determined to some extent by the people being observed or interviewed and allows for some flexibility. Such methods have both advantages and disadvantages.

The advantages of qualitative methods in human services relate to the need to obtain in-depth information about service users. Surveys and other quantitative methods typically capture only one point in time without providing any context for a respondent's answers. If a client responds, "Yes," to a question that asks about a need for child care services, for example, the professional does not have any way of knowing whether the client already has approached family members or contacted child care providers in search of these services. In an in-depth interview, on the other hand, the professional could ask additional questions to provide clarification. In addition to clarifying context, depth interviewing and observation also can reveal a sequence of events that could help to explain a client's behavior. Qualitative methods thus are valuable for making sense of client responses. For this reason, they are sometimes used in combination with more quantitative strategies.

Another potential advantage of qualitative methods relates to their appropriateness for particular clients. Written questionnaires require certain levels of literacy that some clients may not possess. Further, for clients who do not speak English, observation is sometimes the only method that can be used. Also, as indicated in Chapter 5, cultural preferences for various methods will differ from one group to another. Members of some groups may be uncomfortable with written forms and may prefer more informal methods such as observation.

The disadvantages of qualitative methods relate to time, intrusiveness, and observer or interviewer bias. Generally, observation and depth interviewing take longer than questionnaire administration. Human services today are often subject to timelines issued by funding agencies. Government regulations may require, for example, that a service plan be in place 30 days after a client is enrolled in an agency. Thus, even when qualitative approaches may be "best practice" in a given case, more quantitative methods may have to be used to meet administrative deadlines. The rapid initiation of services also may be in the client's best interest in some cases. A family that has no food in the house, for example, cannot wait for a lengthy identification process to be completed before being referred to a food bank.

Another disadvantage of qualitative methods involves their intrusiveness. Clients may feel uncomfortable with an observer watching their activities of daily life or with an interviewer who asks what are perceived to be personal questions. Written instruments, by contrast, seem more anonymous, and refusal to answer a particular question is not met with a disappointed look on the face of an interviewer. Further, as noted in Chapter 5, cultures differ in their attitudes toward privacy.

Finally, subjective methods like observation and depth interviewing are especially subject to questions about validity and reliability. Because information is filtered through an observer or interviewer, it is subject to his or her interpretation and may not reflect the "true" meaning or intention of the client. In contrast, written instruments do not change from one client to the next and can be more readily tested for accuracy and response consistency.

As suggested above, the advantages of quantitative methods are related to the disadvantages of more qualitative approaches. Written surveys generally require little time to complete and they are (when constructed well) usually simple to administer. Whereas qualitative methods require long training periods for those who use them, almost anyone can administer a questionnaire. Questionnaires also can be checked for validity and reliability through comparisons using large numbers of clients or the same clients over time. Finally, as already suggested, written instruments are usually regarded as less intrusive than observation or depth interviewing.

On the other hand, the disadvantages of quantitative methods relate to the advantages of qualitative approaches. Information obtained through questionnaires and similar techniques is often devoid of context, which may be essential in human services for a complete understanding of a client's situation. Questionnaire responses are subject to misinterpretation. Sometimes, a client simply misunderstands a question. For example, the Parent Needs Survey, which will be discussed in Chapter 8, contains the item, "More friends with a child like mine," as part of a checklist of needs for parent support. The social worker at the agency I directed reported that, when questioned, some parents who checked this need said they thought it meant, "More friends for my child." Clearly, the difference in interpretation would be important in intervention. Thus, when possible, quantitative methods should be supplemented with qualitative ones to help assure validity. Questionnaires can assist professionals in focusing on areas of concern and provide the basis for interview questions.

Which Method Should be Used?

Ideally, because they produce different kinds of information, both quantitative and qualitative methods should be used. However, in actual practice the use of a combination of methods can be time consuming, and, as noted earlier, funding, policy, and ethical constraints may require an abbreviated identification process. Whenever possible, best practice would dictate flexibility in choice of methods based on three factors: client preference, cultural considerations, and relevance and appropriateness.

Client Preference

In partnership-based practice methods should not be selected by the professional alone. Rather, practitioners should explain the various methods to their clients and then ask them which method(s) they would prefer. Some clients may be uncomfortable with observation or may perceive a depth interview as overly intrusive. Others, especially those who do not read well, may not be comfortable with a written questionnaire. Usually, with careful explanation and assurances about confidentiality, most clients will be receptive to most methods. However, they always should be aware of any method being used (including observation) and they should always have a choice.

Cultural Considerations

As Chapter 5 indicated, members of some ethnic groups are comfortable with verbal communication with professionals, whereas members of other groups feel uneasy about revealing personal information in this way. Some Native Americans, for example, might prefer observation to direct communication. Group differences in literacy levels or in ability to speak English also would be important to consider. When practitioners are unsure about cultural or social preferences, they should ask their clients prior to initiating the identification process.

Relevance and Appropriateness

Any method that is chosen should yield information that is relevant to addressing the client's concerns. Methods chosen for any other reason are likely to unnecessarily invade the client's privacy. Before asking personal questions or observing situations of family intimacy, the professional should carefully evaluate the necessity of obtaining information of this kind. Although practitioners who use a status inequality approach routinely obtain personal information from clients, partnership-focused professionals generally should consult with their clients about the relevance and appropriateness of such information for addressing client-defined concerns.

The ethical basis for the use of any method, then, is the desire to help the client. Information that is gathered is to be used only for the purpose of expanding

Activities of Daily Living

Select codes representing what client does with reasonable safety.

CODES for level of ADL functioning

1. Independent. Performs safely without assistance.
2. Uses assistive device, takes long time, or does with great difficulty
3. Does with some help
   - 3A. Does with supervision, set-up cueing or coaxing only
   - 3B. Does with hands-on help
4. Does with maximum help or does not do at all. Helper does more than half of all of the activity

CODES for bowel & bladder management

1. Independent. No accidents
2. Self care devices or ostomy/no accidents
3. Does with some help
   - 3A. Does with supervision, setup, cueing or coaxing/assist with equipment/infrequent accidents
   - 3B. Does with hands-on help and/or accidents less than daily
4. Does with maximum help and/or daily accidents

Questions 1–8: Describe the client's ability to perform the following activities.

ACTIVITIES OF DAILY LIVING	Code for level of functioning	If coded 2–4, describe how client currently manages	Describe additional help needed
1. Bathing			
2. Dressing/Undressing			
3. Grooming			
4. Eating			
5. Transferring in & Out of Bed or Chair			
6. Toileting			
7. Bladder Management			
8. Bowel Management			

Figure 6.1. Part of a client assessment instrument from an aging services agency.

the client's opportunity structure by building on the client's existing resources. In order to build, the practitioner must understand the foundation. The construction of new opportunities is most likely to occur when professionals and their clients work as partners and collaborators.

Suggested Exercise

Figure 6.1 is used by an agency that serves older clients. In order to determine the kinds of assistance that clients may need, caseworkers determine their clients' ability to perform various activities of daily living (ADLs). This information is then used to determine whether the clients are eligible for the various services that the agency provides. Possible methods for obtaining needed information include observation, interviewing (verbal questioning) of the client or family members, and asking clients or family members to complete a written questionnaire. Think about the best ways for obtaining the information necessary to complete the form. Why do you think that these methods are better than the others in this situation?

Observation in Practice

Observation can be the least intrusive and most unobtrusive of all the methods being described here. In addition, some have suggested that observation is the most complete method for understanding human behavior. Becker and Geer (1967) have written,

> The most complete form of the sociological datum, after all, is the form in which the participant observer gathers it: an observation of some social event, the events which precede and follow it, and explanations of its meaning by participants and spectators, before, during, and after its occurrence. Such a datum gives us more information about the event under study than data gathered by any other sociological method. Participant observation can thus provide us with a yardstick against which to measure the completeness of data gathered in other ways, a model which can serve to let us know what orders of information escape us when we use other methods. (p. 109)

As a sociological research method, observation commonly has taken the form of participant observation, which Becker and Geer (1967) describe as follows:

> By participant observation we mean that method in which the observer participates in the daily life of the people under study, either openly in the role of researcher or covertly in some disguised role, observing things that happen, listening to what is said, and questioning people, over some length of time. (p. 109)

Participant observation is a naturalistic method that occurs in the ordinary settings in which people live and work. As the name suggests, the observer actually takes part in the activities being observed, becoming, at least for awhile, a member of the group under study. This method has been favored by qualitatively oriented sociologists, as well as by anthropologists who have studied primitive societies.

In human services, community-based practitioners may not have the opportunity for long-term participant observation in their clients' natural settings. However, this method can be valuably approximated during the course of professional–client interaction in the form of *partner observation*. As a partner–observer, the professional spends as much time as possible in the client's natural environment and tries to blend into that environment without actually living in it. Observation can be used throughout the identification process, but is perhaps most useful at the beginning, when the professional has little knowledge about the service user. The following sections will suggest techniques for implementing this method.

Entering the Setting

Observation occurs naturally and automatically whenever professionals and clients interact. Observant professionals will notice their clients' dress, posture, and interactions with others who are present in the situation. However, when such observation occurs in professional settings such as offices and clinics, the amount of information the professional gains will be limited. In general, practitioners can learn considerably more about their clients by visiting the clients' homes, workplaces, and other settings that are normally part of their clients' life activities. In fact, home visiting has become the method of choice in many human service organizations today (see Chapter 2).

Initially, the goal of the professional should be to help the client feel comfortable with his or her presence. The practitioner might say, "It would be helpful to me to learn more about the ordinary things you do every day, to see what a typical day is like for your family." As Taylor and Bogdan (1984) note, all the participants in a setting should receive an explanation of your presence to avoid any misunderstandings. In the collaborative model being advocated here, each participant also should consent to the observation before it begins.

The observer's role also should be negotiated with participants. As Gold (reported in Monette et al., 1994) notes, in a research context the researcher primarily is either an observer or a participant. Gold suggests three variants:

1. The complete participant role. In this variant, the observer simply participates in ongoing social interaction without revealing to participants that he or she is also observing (and using information obtained from the observation). This role is never appropriate in collaborative practice.
2. The participant-as-observer role. Here, the observer's intentions are known to the other participants. The observer participates in their routines but is never mistaken for a member of the group being observed. This role

variant usually takes place over an extended period of time and may not be feasible in most human service situations.

3. The observer-as-participant role. This case is similar to the one above, except that the observer spends less time with the group being observed, sometimes as little as a few hours or a day. An example of this role in a prepractice situation is the assignment of first-year medical students to a family for a semester. Lewis and Greenstein (1994, p. 79) have described this assignment as part of a goal of having the students "learn the patient's perspective in health and illness before they even put on their white coats to become immersed in the technical skills of clinical medicine." Students are matched with families that include a member with a chronic health condition and are required to make six to eight home visits to this family. They are encouraged to attend their "patient's" medical appointments and to observe children at school when appropriate. Many become involved in helping the families they observe with babysitting and other activities. This variant of the participant observer role is probably the most used and most useful in human service practice in general. While spending time in clients' homes, practitioners can participate in activities such as watching television, eating meals or snacks, playing with children, or helping with the dishes. The extent of participation will vary, because clients' comfort with including a stranger in their activities will differ from one family to another.

Observation without participation also is possible and may be most appropriate with families who are uncomfortable with direct participation in their activities. Simple observation also may be the most appropriate method in settings such as school classrooms or work situations, where participation by the observer might be regarded as intrusive. In both participant and nonparticipant observation, however, the observer tries not to guide or interfere with the behavior of participants in any way, allowing them to act as normally as possible. On the other hand, the observer should act naturally and may respond to questions or enter into ongoing conversations when appropriate.

In observation, as well as in other methods, the professional will learn more (and ultimately be more helpful to clients) if he or she is able to establish rapport early in the process. Taylor and Bogdan (1984) describe rapport as follows:

- Communicating a feeling of empathy for [clients] and having them accept it as sincere.
- Penetrating people's "defenses against the outsider." . . .
- Being seen as an "OK" person. . . .
- Sharing in [clients'] symbolic world, their language, and perspectives. . . . (p. 36)

Taylor and Bogdan (1984) suggest that rapport can only be established if observers accommodate themselves to the routines of the people they are observing. If clients normally watch a particular television show at the time of a scheduled observation session, the professional should watch it with them. If the professional wishes to observe other activities, he or she should schedule a visit at another time.

Other methods for establishing rapport include casual conversation and helping out. When clients mention concerns regarding their children, professionals can certainly say they have had similar concerns with regard to their own children (if such a statement is true). Sharing selected bits of personal information can put clients at ease by helping them to define the professional as "someone like them." Getting involved in activities also can help to "humanize" the professional. For example, if nursing home residents are engaging in a craft activity, the observer can help the residents with that activity. On a home visit, an opportunity to help may be provided by a situation in which a mother is attempting to fix dinner and to respond to a fussy toddler at the same time. (One of my staff members once found herself following a family to the barn to assist in the delivery of a calf!)

Taylor and Bogdan (1984) suggest, however, that participation should be limited in some circumstances. They suggest, for example, that observers should not place themselves in a competitive situation with those they are observing. In addition, observers should not engage in activities that make them feel uncomfortable. Several years ago, one of my students, who was observing in a group home for adults with mental retardation, was asked by a resident to help her take a bath and complied with this request even though she "felt funny" about doing so. This student probably should have told the resident that she could not help with this activity and would wait outside until the woman was finished bathing (she also could have alerted a member of the staff to the resident's need for assistance, if necessary). Young female observers also have sometimes reported being harassed by males in a setting where they were observing. Certainly, an observer should leave any situation that seems threatening.

Although formal interviews should not be conducted during an observation session, observers acquire information both by watching and by listening. Information can be obtained through listening either by *eavesdropping* or *situational conversation* (Schatzman & Strauss, 1973). Eavesdropping occurs naturally when the observer is in a setting. In a family home or work situation, one is likely to overhear direct conversation and telephone conversation. In eavesdropping, the observer does not participate verbally. In situational conversation, or "incidental" questioning, on the other hand, the observer may ask some questions that seem appropriate in the context of what is being observed. For example, if a neighbor stops by during a home observation and offers to pick up some items at the store for your client, you could ask the client whether the neighbor often offers to help in this way. A child drawing a picture might be asked, "What are you drawing?" In general, the observer should keep such questioning to a minimum to avoid unduly interfering in the natural flow of events.

What to Observe

Observation in human services can be either *casual* or *focused* (Darling & Baxter, 1996). Casual observation occurs naturally while a professional is engaged in other activities with clients as well as during sessions specifically scheduled for that purpose. During casual observation, the professional generally does not have a specific agenda but merely wishes to learn as much as possible about the client's way of life. Casual observation may be scheduled early in the professional–client relationship. Focused observation, on the other hand, is usually scheduled after a client has expressed some concern. For example, an adolescent client may indicate that he or she is having difficulty during a particular activity at school. The professional would then arrange to observe that activity in order to better understand the client's concern. Both casual and focused observation can be used to provide information about a client's resources and concerns.

Observing Resources

Earlier chapters have noted the importance of identifying both concerns and resources. In relation to involvement in educational programs, Stoneham (1985, p. 462) has written, "Every family has strengths and, if the emphasis is on supporting strengths rather than rectifying weaknesses, chances for making a difference in the lives of children and families are vastly increased."

Resources in the areas of informal support and material support are typically the most readily observable during home visits. In addition, an observer is likely to see evidence of a client's knowledge and skills when observing the client's interactions with others. Specifically, the observer may wish to pay attention to the following:

- *Informal support.* Household composition; relatives, friends, and/or neighbors who visit; telephone conversations; family photographs that are displayed; religious pictures and symbols; supportive interactions among family members.
- *Material support.* Quantity and quality of furniture, cars, clothing, toys, food, and other items; type of housing; type of neighborhood.
- *Knowledge and skills.* Parenting skills; housekeeping skills; skill in managing difficulties as they arise; communication skills; occupational skills;

knowledge revealed in conversations; demonstrations of technical knowledge, such as the performance of physical therapy exercises; literacy skills; skills in using special equipment, such as computers.

Observing Concerns

Needs or concerns in the same areas also become apparent during the course of observation. The observer may notice:

- *Informal support.* Arguments among family members or others; lack of help in the performance of activities such as child care or household chores; absence of visitors or callers over a long period of time.
- *Material support.* Absence or poor quality of needed household items; lack of food, clothing, shelter, or a means of transportation.
- *Knowledge and skills.* Inability to handle family conflicts; apparent inability to perform ordinary activities such as grooming, cooking, or moving about the house; expressed concerns about lack of knowledge in any area.

Observing Routines and Norms

As indicated in Chapter 5, individuals and families differ considerably in values, beliefs, and lifestyles. In order to appropriately address a client's concerns, the practitioner needs to understand their context. Observation in a client's home provides an opportunity to get to know a way of life that may not be familiar. Wayman et al. (1991, pp. 62–63) suggest some questions that home visitors might ask themselves during their observations:

- Who are the key decision makers?
- Who is the primary caregiver [of children]?
- What are the mealtime rules?
- What types of foods are eaten?
- Does the infant sleep in the same room/bed as the parents?
- Is there an established bedtime?
- What are the parameters of acceptable child behavior?
- What form does the discipline take?
- Do they rely solely on Western medical services?
- What are the general feelings of the family when seeking assistance—ashamed, angry, demand as a right, view as unnecessary?
- To what degree is the family proficient in English?
- Does the family tend to interact in a quiet manner or a loud manner?
- Do family members share feelings when discussing emotional issues?

In general, observation is the best method for learning about interaction styles and daily routines. Extended observations can reveal how people structure their lives and can answer questions about behavioral norms and favored activities. Such information can be invaluable in planning interventions when the observer remains nonjudgmental and respectful toward the client's beliefs, values, and lifestyle choices (see, for example, Dilsworth-Anderson, Burton, & Turner, 1993).

Recording Observations

In general, note taking while observing in a partnership context is inappropriate. Clients are likely to feel uncomfortable and may not act naturally if they see their words and actions being recorded, either in writing or by audio- or videotaping. In addition, an observer who is busy writing may miss some of the action or may not be able to participate fully in an ongoing activity. On the other hand, videotaped information is accurate and complete and is available for later review. Videotaping is sometimes the best method for sharing an observation experience with other members of a human service team who were not present in the setting. When the advantages of sharing the observation in this way outweigh the disadvantages that recording usually entails, the observer should discuss the value of videotaping with the people being observed and secure their consent before proceeding. Taylor and Bogdan (1984) suggest, with regard to research, that "researchers should refrain from taping and taking notes in the field at least until they have developed a feel for the setting and can understand the effects of recording on the informants" (p. 57).

Although recording during the observation is usually not wise, writing *field notes* immediately after the observation, when memory is fresh, is important. Monette et al. (1994, p. 233) state that all field notes should include five elements:

1. A *running description*, which is simply the record of everything that occurred.
2. *Accounts of previous episodes that were forgotten or went unnoticed* but were remembered while the observer was still in the field.
3. *Analytical ideas and inferences* based on what was observed.
4. *Personal impressions and feelings*, in order to suggest any biases that may be involved.
5. *Notes for further information*, including plans for future action.

The description component should be as factual as possible and should include descriptions of both the setting and the people who were present. Sometimes, a diagram or picture is helpful. Following this physical description, the observer should record, in chronological sequence, the events and interactions that occurred.

Quotation marks should only be used when exact quotes are remembered. In general, most conversations will be paraphrased rather than recorded exactly. Evaluations and judgments should be avoided. For example, a person might be described as "quiet" but probably should not be described as "shy."

The following is an example of a descriptive note based on a home visit with a client, Beth Johnson, age 12, and her family. Beth has been referred to a home visiting program by her school guidance counselor because she is frequently absent and has been falling behind in her schoolwork.

> I arrived for my initial visit with the Johnson family on October 21, 1997 at 3:00 PM. The home is located in a rural area, at least 5 miles from any stores and commercial development. A few other homes are located nearby, and all appear to be small and shabby. The Johnson home is an older trailer. A car with a missing tire is parked in front.
>
> I was greeted at the door by Mrs. Johnson, who said that the children had not yet arrived home from school. We sat at the kitchen table and talked about my difficulty in finding the home from the directions I had been given. The home appeared to be clean and furnished with inexpensive furniture, some of which was broken. I did not see a telephone in either the kitchen or the living room. Mrs. Johnson appeared to be very thin and pale, and she had a bruise on her cheek. She was dressed in jeans and a T-shirt that appeared old but clean.
>
> The children—Beth and a younger brother—arrived shortly. Both were wearing jeans and sweatshirts that appeared clean and relatively new. They dropped their school bags on the floor and turned on the television. I joined them in the living room and asked what they were watching. They replied briefly but did not seem interested in having a conversation.
>
> Mrs. Johnson went outside to take some wash off the line, and I went with her. She said her husband should be home soon and explained that he had gone out with a friend to try to find a tire for the car. We went back inside, and Mrs. Johnson folded the laundry, while the children continued to watch television. The children did not speak to each other or to their mother. Mrs. Johnson asked me some questions about the family's referral to my program. She said she was concerned about Beth's failing grades. She said that in prior years Beth had always gotten B's and C's.
>
> Mrs. Johnson began to prepare spaghetti for dinner and repeated that her husband should be home soon. She seemed quiet, but not unfriendly. I noticed when she opened the refrigerator that it only contained a few items. The cupboard seemed to contain only a few cans and boxes.
>
> When I left at 4:30, the children were still watching television, Mrs. Johnson was cooking, and Mr. Johnson had not yet returned home.

In addition to this descriptive summary, the observer would include a section of analysis and impressions, such as the following:

> Observer's Comments:
>
> *Information–knowledge:* Mrs. Johnson appears to have some housekeeping skills. I could not tell much about concerns relating to information during this visit.
>
> *Material support:* This family appeared to be of low socioeconomic status. They did not have a reliable means of transportation and may not have had a telephone. Their food, clothing, and furniture, and the condition and location of their home suggested that they might have some material needs.

Informal support: I could not tell much about the relationship between Mrs. Johnson and her children. She seemed to care about them, but they seemed rather distant. There are some nearby neighbors, but I do not know about their relationship with the Johnsons. Mr. Johnson's father probably lives nearby and may be a source of transportation.

Formal support: I did not learn anything about the family's involvement with other agencies or services during this visit.

Other family members: I was concerned about Mrs. Johnson's health and well-being. I wondered about the possibility of domestic violence. I need to learn more about Mr. Johnson.

Possible misinterpretations: My presence in the home may have changed this family's behavior. Perhaps both the children and Mrs. Johnson are more talkative when they are alone. My suspicions about domestic violence may be totally unfounded. Beth's problems at school may be the result of something in the school situation and have nothing to do with events at home.

Based on these interpretations, the observer would also make some notes about areas to be covered in a subsequent interview with family members:

Areas for Further Exploration:

1. Employment or other source of income. (Does either parent work?)
2. Transportation. (Does the family rely on relatives or others? Can they get the car fixed?)
3. Family roles. (What role does Mr. Johnson play?)
4. Family interaction. (How do the children normally interact with each other? With their parents? How do Mr. and Mrs. Johnson interact with each other?)
5. Relationships with neighbors, relatives, and friends. (What kinds of help does the family usually receive?)
6. Parents' knowledge about the school situation and about available services. (Has Beth talked about problems at school? Is the family aware of tutoring services? Have the parents met with Beth's teacher?)
7. Advocacy skills. (Do the Johnsons feel comfortable about talking with school personnel about their concerns?)
8. Beth's definition of the situation. (What is Beth's explanation for her difficulties at school?)

Advantages and Limitations of Observation

Observation is helpful in establishing the parameters of a situation and in providing a context for further work. Specifically, observation is valuable in human services because it:

- Occurs naturally.
- Is unobtrusive and nonintrusive.

- Requires no special materials.
- Is not dependent on a client's literacy or ability to speak English.
- May be more acceptable to the client, especially in some subcultures.
- May foster acceptance of the service provider.
- May disclose information that the client is not able or willing to share in other ways (Becker & Geer, 1967).
- May foster an appreciation of the client's situation.
- Provides a qualitative sense of a client's lifestyle and family interactions (when observations occur in a home setting).
- Avoids the distortions of meaning that may occur in direct questioning (Becker & Geer, 1967).
- Clarifies meanings, which can be learned more precisely when they occur in context (Becker & Geer, 1967).
- Permits the acquisition of some kinds of information that may not otherwise be available, such as information about family routines, material resources, and subcultural norms.

On the other hand, the usefulness of observation is limited by a number of factors:

- Observation is always subjective; that is, it is biased by the observer's own viewpoint. "Eyewitness" accounts of the same event by different observers typically vary. Monette et al. (1994) and others have suggested that people's perceptions are influenced by their expectations. Thus, the validity of observations as accurate accounts of events is questionable.
- People who are being observed are likely to engage in self-presentation (see Chapter 4). Although impression management is likely to decrease as the observer becomes more familiar, people who are being watched are likely to act differently from usual. Monette et al. (1994) refer to this phenomenon as *reactivity*. One of my students once reported that a family she was observing appeared to "stage" an argument for her benefit. A client who wishes to qualify for certain services may try to appear dysfunctional. On the other hand, I once made an unscheduled home visit to a family served by the human service program in which I worked. During all my previous, scheduled, appointments, the house had been immaculate. When I arrived unexpectedly, however, dishes filled the sink and toys were strewn about the floor. The mother was obviously embarrassed, and I realized that in the past she had always cleaned the house prior to my arrival. Once again, then, information learned through observation may not be a valid representation of what is ordinary for a client or family.
- A brief observation only reveals a small sample of a client's life. This sample may or may not be representative of a typical day. Thus, information obtained from observations may be unreliable.

- Misunderstandings can occur, especially in observation with culturally different clients. An observer who is unfamiliar with the culture may not understand the true meaning of observed objects or activities. Differences in interaction styles also may be misinterpreted. Some families communicate loudly with much shouting and arguing, whereas others are quiet. Members of loud families do not necessarily dislike or disrespect one another but could be perceived in that way by some observers.
- Some people are not comfortable with being observed. Although observation is generally less intrusive than direct questioning, under some circumstances it can be more intrusive. When being interviewed or completing questionnaires, people can control the nature and amount of information that they disclose. They may have less control over the natural course of events in a home or work setting. They also may be embarrassed, as the mother in the last example, by the condition of their home or workplace and prefer to meet with the professional elsewhere.

In research, the validity and reliability of observed data are important (see, for example, Kirk & Miller, 1986). In human service practice, validity and reliability are probably more important in a status inequality than in a partnership approach. In the former, the professional would want an accurate and consistent way of assessing a client. In the latter, however, as noted throughout this volume, the perspective of the service user is more important than that of the professional. Validity in this context means understanding the service user's perspective as clearly as possible. Observation thus becomes a valuable tool for increasing this understanding.

However, because of the limitations of observation, this method almost always should be supplemented by other methods. Observers will need to become interviewers to clarify the impressions they have gained through observation. Because observation is time limited, observers will need to ask questions to "fill in the gaps" and understand whether observed behaviors and routines are typical. Answers to direct questions can also provide a history and a context for what was observed. More quantitative measures can be used to counteract any observer bias that may have occurred. The next two chapters will explore the most valuable methods for supplementing observation: depth interviewing and questionnaires.

Chapter Summary

This chapter introduced the methods that can be used by human service practitioners to help their clients identify their resources, concerns, and priorities. The chapter then discussed some of the ethical issues involved in the identification process, including the principles of confidentiality, client autonomy, and the right of refusal. The advantages and disadvantages of both qualitative and quantitative methods were then considered. The remainder of the chapter presented the method of partner observation, a variant on the traditional sociological research method of participant observation. The discussion focused on observer behavior, the kinds of information that observation provides, and the process of recording and using observational data. An example of an observation report was provided.

Suggested Exercise

Students may wish to practice observing a family referred by a local human service agency. This observation should occur in the family's home (and with their permission) and should last for approximately 1 to 3 hours. Upon completion of this observation, the student should write a report based on the following guidelines:

1. *Description of setting*
   a. Background: Who/what is being observed and why? How did you make contact with the people being observed?
   b. Physical description: Date, time, and length of observation; location; location of observer in relation to people being observed; description of physical setting (furniture, number of people present, etc.)
2. *Description of events*. What happened? (Direct quotes are not necessary, but you may want to paraphrase what the people in the setting said.) This section should be written according to the chronological sequence of events and should provide the reader with the "story" of what transpired on this occasion.
3. *Analysis*. Based on the observation described above, describe your impression of this individual's or family's resources and concerns in all the following areas:
   - Information
   - Material support
   - Informal support
   - Formal support

   All these areas should be addressed. If you do not think you learned anything about a particular area during your observation, you should say so.
4. *Discussion and summary*. State whether or not you think this observation was an "accurate" reflection of this individual's or family's situation. Why or why not? What additional methods would you recommend to more completely identify their resources, concerns, and priorities? Summarize what you have learned from this observation and how this learning might be helpful in assisting this individual/family in addressing their concerns.

Additional guidelines:

1. The report should be three to ten double-spaced, typewritten pages in length.
2. The people observed should be identified by pseudonyms only.

Suggestions for Further Reading

Becker, H.S., & Geer, B. (1967). Participant observation and interviewing: A comparison. In J.G. Manis & B.N. Meltzer (Eds.), *Symbolic interaction: A reader in social psychology* (pp. 109–119). Boston: Allyn & Bacon.

Schatzman, L., & Strauss, A.L. (1973). *Field research: Strategies for a natural sociology*. Englewood Cliffs, NJ: Prentice-Hall.

Taylor, S.J., & Bogdan, R. (1984). *Introduction to qualitative research methods: The search for meanings.* New York: John Wiley & Sons.

7

Identification Techniques II
Interviewing

Interviewing is a commonly used method in all human service fields, including social work, nursing, and counseling. In status inequality approaches, interviewing is used as part of the process of client assessment. In this process, the professional asks the client questions in order to evaluate the client's situation and to determine an appropriate course of treatment. Interviewing also is a useful technique in the partnership approach being advocated here. When used in a partnership context, interviewing is a way of learning more about a client's definition of the situation and a means of clarifying the client's definition of concerns, resources, and priorities.

This chapter will discuss the use of interviewing in the identification process. The construction of an interview schedule will be considered, along with the development of questions that provide useful information. The interview process will then be explored in depth, with attention to issues such as establishing rapport and encouraging responsiveness. Some special interviewing situations also will be considered. Finally, the advantages and disadvantages of interviewing in relation to other methods will be discussed.

The type of interview best suited for a partnership approach is the *depth* or *in-depth interview*. Like observation, depth interviewing is a qualitative technique, designed to establish a contextual basis for understanding. As in the case of observation, much of the relevant literature on depth interviewing comes from qualitative research in sociology and anthropology. The *Verstehen* approach taken by qualitative researchers has produced techniques that are valuable in encouraging respondents to discuss their views and concerns—a major focus of the sociologically oriented practitioner in human services.

With respect to research, Rubin and Rubin (1995) have written:

> . . . qualitative interviewing is more than a set of skills, it is also a philosophy, an approach to learning. One element of this philosophy is that understanding is achieved by encouraging people to describe their worlds in their own terms. . . . In qualitative interviews you listen so as to *hear the meaning* of what is being said. (pp. 2, 7)

They suggest that in qualitative research, the interviewee is not just the object of research; rather, the interviewer and the interviewee are "conversational partners."

This description also applies to interviewing in partnership-based human service work.

As the last chapter suggested, some informal "interviewing" may take place during observation. Observers typically "eavesdrop" (Schatzman & Strauss, 1973), as well as engage in casual questioning with the people they are observing. Such activities are not planned; rather, they occur naturally during the course of participation in a setting. The techniques to be discussed in this chapter, on the other hand, are based on the advance construction of an *interview schedule*, which lists questions or topics that will guide the discussion. Thus, formal interviewing is a way of focusing a conversation in order to elicit relevant information.

Unlike observation, which is controlled by the people being observed, interviewing is controlled by the person asking the questions. Observation usually leaves many questions unanswered. A postobservation interview can clarify observed events as well as introduce subjects that were not directly observed. Whereas observation is time-limited, interviewing can address a long period of time and provide a historical context for observed events. Interviewing also can elicit information about subjects that are unobservable, such as behavior in private places or intrapsychic phenomena, such as beliefs and attitudes.

Taylor and Bogdan (1984) have described depth interviews as "face to face encounters . . . directed towards understanding informants' perspectives on their lives, experiences or situations as expressed in their own words" (p. 77). Douglas (1985) suggests that depth interviewing involves "the use of many strategies . . . of interaction, largely based on an understanding of friendly feelings and intimacy, to optimize cooperative, mutual disclosure and a creative search for mutual understanding" (pp. 25–26). Thus, this method can be especially appropriate in the collaborative service model that characterizes partnership approaches in human services.

Types of Depth Interviews

When interviewing is not preceded by observation, an *unstructured* approach is perhaps most appropriate. In this approach, conversation is informal, and no interview schedule is required. The purpose of a preliminary, unstructured interview in human services is to get to know the client and to gather information to help shape more structured interviewing or questionnaire development that will follow.

Once an observation or an unstructured interview has been completed, the practitioner should conduct either a *semistructured* or a *focused* interview. A semistructured interview is usually done early in the relationship between the service provider and service user and is often the most valuable means for identifying a client's resources, concerns, and priorities. Although the conversation is guided by an interview schedule developed by the provider, the structure is open to topics and issues raised by the client. Much of the rest of this chapter will focus on semistructured interviewing techniques.

Focused interviews are usually used later in the identification process, often as new concerns arise. In such a case, reviewing the client's history and opportunity structure usually is not necessary, and both client and practitioner usually are anxious to resolve the issue at hand. For example, a family that has been served by an early intervention program for several months may learn that their child needs surgery. This development may lead to concerns about transportation to the hospital, visiting rules for parents, and child care arrangements for siblings left at home. The professional thus may want to schedule a focused interview to determine what new information or other resources the family might now need. In such a case, the interview schedule would be a much abbreviated version of the kind of schedule developed for a semistructured interview.

Constructing an Interview Schedule

As in the case of observation, most of the interviewing techniques to be discussed here were originally developed for research purposes. These techniques are equally appropriate for use in the identification process in human services, because both research and identification require the elicitation of honest and complete responses. In discussing semistructured interviews for research purposes, Berg (1995) suggests a two-stage process: First, the interviewer develops an outline, listing all the broad categories that may be relevant; second, the interviewer writes questions relevant to each of the outlined categories. The same process is also appropriate in a human service situation. For example, a typical interview to help a new client identify his or her resources, priorities, and concerns might include the following categories:

- Demographic background information.
- General area(s) of concern (e.g., domestic violence; family member with a disability; drug/alcohol abuse; lack of food, clothing, or shelter, etc.).
- History of these concerns (previous experience with similar situations and events leading up to the current situation).
- Resources/description of client's opportunity structure (existing knowledge/research/self-advocacy skills; informal, formal, and material supports; strengths of other family members).
- Current definition of the situation/priorities (e.g., condition of family member with Alzheimer's disease has deteriorated, and the individual can no longer be left at home alone).
- Interest in available services

These categories would apply to intake or initial interviews in all kinds of human service situations. The following sections will address the development of questions in these areas.

Types of Questions

Primary, Broad-Range Questions

As suggested in Darling and Baxter (1996), these questions ask for general rather than specific information. Examples of questions of this type from the sample interview schedule included in this chapter (Fig. 7.1) include the following:

- Was your family large?
- How did you learn about this program?
- Are you and your child involved with any other agencies?
- Do you work?
- Does your family live nearby?

This interview schedule was designed for families of children with recently diagnosed disabilities who were entering an early intervention program. Although developed for a specific purpose, the schedule follows the topic outline suggested above and provides a model that can be easily adapted to other human service situations. For example, in a domestic violence situation, the question about whether the respondent knew any individuals with disabilities while growing up would be replaced with a question about childhood experiences with abuse both within and outside of the family. These primary questions provide the basis for secondary, narrow-range questions.

Secondary, Narrow-Range Questions

Secondary questions encourage people to talk further about an aspect of their experience. These questions enable the interviewer to clarify and expand on the information provided in response to the initial, primary question that introduced a topic. People may be unsure about how much information to provide in response to a primary question but may be happy to offer further information when encouraged to do so. Examples of secondary, narrow-range questions in Fig. 7.1 are marked with the designation, NRQ. For instance, the primary question, "Have you told other people about the diagnosis?" is followed by a secondary question, "How have they reacted to the news?"

Probes

In order to gain a complete understanding of an interviewee's situation, the interviewer will need to provide both verbal and nonverbal encouragement. Such expressions of encouragement are, unlike primary and secondary questions, not

Family Interview

I'd like to ask you some questions about your family to help us understand how we can best meet your needs and help you help your child. If I ask you anything you would rather not answer, just tell me and we will skip that question. Please tell me, too, if there is anything you would like to talk about that I may forget to ask.

First, it would help me to know a little about your background [asked of both parents; if one parent is absent, information is sought on both parents from the parent being interviewed].

What is your (your husband's/wife's) date of birth? ________________ (h) ________________ (w)

Where are you from originally? ____

Was your family large? ____

(family size)

While you were growing up, did you know any children or adults with any kind of disability?
______ (Yes) ______ (No)

Do you remember the kinds of things you were thinking before (__________________) was born?
child's name

[NRQ][1] Did you ever think he/she might have a problem of any kind? ____________________

____

____

Is ______________ your first child? (birth order position of child, etc.) ______________

____

When did you first learn that ______________________ had a problem? ______ (child's age)

[NRQ] How did you feel when you first heard (or suspected) this? ____________________

____

____

What kinds of things have you worried about since you first learned about __________________'s disability?

____

____

["Prompts"[2] until all worries have been expressed]

Who are the people who live here in this house with you? (list names and ages)

________________ ______ ________________ ______

________________ ______ ________________ ______

________________ ______ ________________ ______

[1]"NRQ" indicates narrow-range question.

[2]"Prompt" indicates either the verbal prompt specifically indicated in this interview schedule or any of the verbal or nonverbal prompts described in this chapter.

(Continued)

Have you told other people about the diagnosis?
[Prompts]

siblings ________, grandparents ________, friends _______,

minister/priest/rabbi ________, neighbors ________, co-workers ________?

[NRQ] How have they reacted to the news? ____

____

[NRQ] How have they reacted to the baby? ____

____

Do you know any other parents of children with special needs? ____________________________

____

[NRQ] Would you like to talk to other parents? _______ (Y) ________ (N)

How did you learn about this program? ____

____

Has it been hard to get information about available services? ____________________________

____

Have you been satisfied with your child's medical treatment so far? ________ (Y) ________ (N)

[NRQ If no] Have you done anything to try to get better treatment? ________________________

____

Are you and your child involved with any other agencies? ________ (Y) ________ (N)

[NRQ If yes] Which ones? ____

____

[NRQ] Have they been helpful to you? ________ (Y) ________ (N)

{NRQ if no] Have you done anything to try to make these services better?

____

How about your health—has it been good? ____

____

Has anyone else in the family had any medical problems? ____________________________

____

Have there been any other family problems lately? ________________________________

____

Do you work? ________ (Y) ________ (N) (If no) Have you worked in the past? ______________

____ (husband/wife both asked)

[NRQ] Do (did) you like your job? ________ (Y) ________ (N) (If not working)

(Continued)

Would you like to work if you had someone to take care of ________________________________?

________ (Y) ________ (N)

____

(If married) How long have you been married? ________ (number of years)

Who helps with child care? ____

____

Does your family live nearby? ________ (Y) ________ (N) Do they help you with anything?

____

What about friends and neighbors, have they been helpful? __________________________

____

Do any of your other children have any special needs? ______________________________

____

In general, how have your other children been doing? _______________________________

____

Do you have anyone who can take care of the baby so that you can get out once in a while?

____

____

Have you had any problems with the baby with sleeping? ______ feeding? ______ handling? _______ [prompts—for other areas of care?]

____

Is there anything you need for the baby? ____

Do you need anything for anyone else in the family? ________________________________

____

Do you have a car or any other means of transportaton? ________ (Y) ________ (N)

In general would you say you are satisfied with the way your life has been going lately? ____________

____

Would you say that you have been coping pretty well with your problems right now, or would you like some help with the things that are bothering you?

________ (Y) ________ (N) [If yes, prompts as appropriate] ____________________________

____

As part of this program, you will be asked to work on some activities with your baby at home. Do you think you will have any difficulty finding enough time to work on these activities? Do you like the idea of being your baby's teacher? ____

____

(Continued)

Do you think you might have any special experience, skills, or feelings that will make you a good teacher for your baby? ____________________

____

____

Can you think of anything right now that our program might be able to help you with? ____________________

____

____

Figure 7.1. Example of an interview schedule (From Darling & Baxter, 1996, pp. 133–137.) Reprinted with permission.

included in the interview schedule; rather, they are interjected by the interviewer in an ad lib fashion when appropriate. Verbal encouragement commonly takes the form of probes, or questions or comments that suggest an interest in knowing more about a particular feeling or event. Several probes have been identified by Minichiello, Aron, Timewell, and Alexander (1990, p. 125); these are adapted below:

- Please tell me more about that.
- Oh really?
- Please go on.
- And then . . . ?
- I see.
- Is that so?
- Please continue.
- Yes.
- Hmm . . .
- What happened then?
- Is that the way you feel now?
- What about his sister?

Other useful phrases, adapted from Darling and Baxter (1996, p. 149), include:

- Tell me a little more about . . .
- Why do you think you felt that way?
- What did you have in mind when you said . . . ?
- I'm not sure whether I understand what you mean by that.
- Anything else?
- What about other members of the family?

Gordon (1992) cautions against probing too much, because probing tends to interrupt the respondent's free-association pattern. He writes, "The only way to be sure you are not interrupting the respondent with a probe is to wait until the respondent has indicated, verbally or nonverbally, that he or she is expecting the interviewer to speak" (pp. 146–147). He also notes that probing that is too directive can remove topic control from the interviewee. Although the interviewer needs to keep the interview on track, probes that change the subject may be premature when a respondent has more to say about a topic.

Reflection

Another way of encouraging people to continue talking is to show that you are listening. In addition to the probes above, the interviewer should occasionally repeat parts of what a respondent has said. For example, after a mother I was interviewing described her son's hospitalization and discharge, I said, "And so you brought him home from the hospital . . ." This reflective comment provided a topic transition in this case, and the mother then proceeded to describe the post-hospitalization experience. In other cases, simply paraphrasing what a client has said can encourage him or her to continue a story. Kadushin and Kadushin (1997) suggest that "a good paraphrase is a condensation and crystallization of the client's communication" (p.141). They offer the following example:

> Interviewee: You make out applications one after the other, and you go out for interviews one after the other, and they take one look at you, and because you're African American you don't get any consideration for the job.
>
> Interviewer: You make every effort to find work, but you feel discrimination prevents you from getting a job. (Kadushin & Kadushin, 1997, pp.141–142)

Some phrases useful in paraphrasing are:

- In other words . . .
- So, you're saying that . . .
- It seems to me you're saying that . . .
- Am I understanding you correctly? . . .
- You mean . . . , don't you?
- You were talking about . . . , weren't you?
- Am I correct in assuming that . . . ?

In the status inequality model, practitioners sometimes use the term "reflection" to suggest an interpretation of feelings, rather than a simple restatement of what a client has said (see, for example, Samantrai, 1996). In the partnership approach being advocated here, however, reflection and paraphrasing are more or less synonymous.

Nonverbal Reactions

Egan (reported in Kadushin & Kadushin, 1997) suggests the acronym, SOLER—straight, open, leaning, eye contact, relaxed—as a way to remember the postures that indicate involvement. In general, interviewers should simply act as they would in any conversational situation; they should appear interested in what the other person is saying.

Another technique often useful in encouraging clients to talk is, paradoxically, silence. Most people are uncomfortable with lapses in verbal communication and have a tendency to keep talking in such situations. Thus, the interviewer should not rush to the next question on the schedule during a pause in a response. Samantrai (1996) suggests that an interviewer's silence can mean, "I'm with you, go on . . . I'm waiting, sensing that you have not finished . . . take your time, I am not going to rush you . . ." (p. 142). As discussed in Chapter 5, however, some cultural groups are able to tolerate long periods of silence, making this technique less useful in interviews with members of those groups.

Asking Good Questions

Questions can be constructed in a number of different ways. In general, the vocabulary used in any question should match the conversational style of the respondent. Thus, the schedule in Fig. 7.1 includes such conversational wording as, "Was your family large?" (rather than, "What was the size of your family?") and "Does your family live nearby?" (rather than, "What is your family's county of residence?"). Professional jargon also should be avoided.

Good questions are also *relevant.* Gorden (1992) suggests that, prior to developing questions, the interviewer should clarify the objectives of the interview. Interviewers should ask themselves what they are hoping to learn from the interview and how they will use this information to help the client. A long, life history format may not be necessary to address client concerns about a specific, time-limited issue, such as the closing of a treatment center in the client's neighborhood. If the client's only concern is where to obtain treatment in the future, the interviewer's questions should be limited to the availability of transportation or other material resourcs. (See Gorden, 1992, for some practice exercises in relevance determination).

Varying the structure of questions is sometimes a good way to obtain information and to help the client conceptualize responses. The following sections describe some types of question format (Darling & Baxter, 1996).

Descriptive Questions

These questions ask for descriptions of places, events, people, or experiences and are often asked early in an interview. Some examples follow:

- What happened when you took Michael to Children's Hospital?
- How many people work in your office?
- Who are the people who live in this house with you?
- How long has Jim been using cocaine?

Structural Questions

These questions allow interviewees to organize their knowledge about a particular event or experience. For example, to learn about a person's support network, the interviewer might ask, "Do you get together often with relatives, friends, or neighbors?" Structural questions commonly ask people to think in categorical terms. Some other examples follow:

- Of all the services you have received, which would you say have been the most helpful?
- Would you say that you get along well with the other residents on your floor?
- Did you know any other women who had been abused before you came to the shelter?

Contrast Questions

These questions ask interviewees to make comparisons between situations, events, or experiences. Such questions are especially useful in evaluating service options. Some examples follow:

- How would you say your life has changed since you entered this program?
- Which would you prefer, coming down to the agency to meet with me, or having me come out to your home?
- Were the services you received at Agency X more helpful than those you received at Agency Y?

Opinion/Value Questions

These questions, which are particularly useful in program evaluation, ask people to make judgments about situations or services. For example, the interviewer might ask, "Are you satisfied with the services you have received from this agency so far?"

Questions that Pose an Ideal

Schatzman and Strauss (1973) suggest that interviewees be asked to describe the most ideal situation they can imagine in relation to their current life situation. For example, an interviewer might ask the parents of an adult child with mental retardation to describe the best living situation they could imagine for their child. Alternatively, the interviewer might describe such a situation and ask the parents how that situation sounds to them. Such questions are helpful in learning about clients' goals and dreams.

Hypothetical Questions

In these questions, a number of plausible scenarios, options, or occurrences are presented, and the interviewee is asked to react to these. For example, the interviewer might describe several service options and ask which the client would prefer. These questions provide information to clients to help them make decisions. The following question might be asked by a professional at a hospital discharge interview:

> You have several options. You may want to enter a short-term care facility where you would still have assistance with dressing and eating until you felt strong enough to care for yourself. Or, you may want to have a nurse or a housekeeper come to your home to help you with these things. Or, perhaps you have a family member or friend you can rely on for assistance. Do you have a preference for a particular kind of help?

Devil's Advocate Questions

These questions begin with phrases like, "Some people think . . ." and enable people to express their attitudes and opinions about service options. The following example is illustrative:

> Some people think that parents of very young infants should receive services at home; other people think that services at a child care center are better. What do you think?

Mirror or Summary Questions

These questions are similar to the reflective questions described earlier in that they paraphrase what the interviewee has said. In this case, however, the questions are used at the end of a topic or interview to summarize what has transpired and to help bring closure to the situation. The following are examples:

- Let me see if I have this right . . .
- So, to summarize your situation, you began by telling me that . . .
- My understanding, then, of your situation is that . . . Is that right?

Halley, Kopp, and Austin (1992, p.291) suggest that summary questions/statements can serve the following purposes: (1) to begin an interview (summarizing past material); (2) to close an interview; and (3) to help the client focus during an interview.

Avoiding "Loaded" and "Double-Barreled" Questions

When formulating all questions, interviewers need to be mindful of not influencing their interviewees to respond in certain ways. "Loaded" questions imply that the interviewer is looking for a particular answer. For example, the question, "You won't have a need for child care, will you?" could encourage a parent to deny a need that may in fact exist. The more neutral, "Will you need child care?" would be preferable. Similarly, interviewers should avoid questions that could be interpreted as judgmental. A caseworker for a children's protective services agency is unlikely to receive a "yes" answer to the question, "Do you ever leave your [young] child alone in the house?" because the parent is likely to know that such behavior is regarded as a form of neglect that could result in the removal of the child. Instead, the worker might want to question the parent about child care arrangements and the parent's concerns relating to these arrangements.

Another type of question that is likely to evoke an inaccurate response is a "double-barreled" question, or one that includes two possibilities but only one response choice. For example, the question, "Have your family and friends accepted your choice of lifestyle?" forces the interviewee to consider family and friends together, when, in fact, friends may be accepting while family members are not. In this case, two separate questions could be asked: "Has your family accepted your choice of lifestyle?" and "Have your friends accepted your choice of lifestyle?"

Sometimes, loaded and double-barreled questions are not obvious to the person constructing the interview schedule, especially in cases of cross-cultural interviewing or in unfamiliar client situations. For this reason, pretesting the schedule with a few select clients, or at least with more experienced professionals, is always a good idea. This precaution is also important in questionnaire construction, which will be addressed in Chapter 8.

Question Sequence

In general, an interview should begin with nonthreatening questions that are easy to answer. Usually these are questions that provide background, demographic information about the interviewee, such as age, occupation, length of time at current residence, household composition, marital and parental status, and size of family of origin. Such questions usually help to establish rapport between the interviewer and the interviewee.

As the interview proceeds, more difficult and sensitive questions may be included. Topics that are known to be especially sensitive should not be introduced until the end of the interview. Such topics often include the following:

- Drug or alcohol use.
- Sexual preferences and behavior.
- Financial status [especially in the case of upper-socioeconomic status (SES) clients, who are sometimes reluctant to reveal their income or assets].
- Religion (especially in the case of members of some minority religious groups).
- Potentially stigmatizing medical conditions (such as sexually transmitted diseases, AIDS, some genetic conditions, mental illnesses, and diseases caused by stigmatized behaviors, such as liver disease resulting from alcoholism).
- Abortion history and, in some cases, pregnancy history.
- In some cases, previous involvement with human service agencies.
- Criminal history.

In general, questions that are likely to embarrass the client should not be asked at all, unless they are essential to provide the help that the client desires.

Normally, the question sequence will follow the topic outline described earlier in this chapter. A chronologically ordered sequence is usually also desirable in interviews designed to understand the context of a client's present situation. The interview schedule in Fig. 7.1 follows such a sequence, beginning with childhood experiences and ending with current concerns. As the interviewer moves from one topic to another, he or she should include transitional statements, such as: "What you've told me so far is really helpful. Now I'd like to ask you some questions about . . ." At the end of the interview, the interviewer should be sure to thank the interviewee for sharing valuable information and to let the interviewee know what to expect next in the helping process.

In research, interview schedules always should be pretested to determine their validity and reliability before being standardized. Because interview schedules used in human services are likely to vary as they are individualized for different clients, pretesting is not always possible. For this reason, interviewers need to be aware that clients' responses may reflect misunderstandings about question meaning or misrepresentation of actual beliefs and attitudes. Such misunderstandings and misrepresentations can usually be minimized by establishing good rapport with an interviewee and by careful reflection and probing. Methods for establishing rapport and facilitating the interview experience are discussed in the next section.

The Interview Process

The Interview Situation

Preparation for an interview involves a number of decisions. The professional needs to decide first where the interview is to be conducted. Whenever possible, the location should be determined by the client. Often, the client will be most comfortable at home or in other familiar surroundings. Sometimes, however, the client may prefer a more private location that would prevent intrusion or eavesdropping by other family members. In the agency I directed, one client who was living at a homeless shelter asked the caseworker to conduct the interview on a park bench rather than at the shelter; she was concerned about other shelter residents knowing about "her private business." Thus, the professional generally should ask the client about preferred locations.

A second decision involves the professional's presentation of self (see Chapter 4 for a further discussion of this concept). The interviewer must decide how to dress and whether to use a formal or informal communication style, among other options. In general, the goal is to establish rapport by making the client feel as comfortable as possible. Thus, the professional should probably adapt his or her approach to the client. Lower-SES clients may feel more comfortable with an interviewer who wears casual clothes and avoids professional jargon; upper-SES clients, on the other hand, may prefer a more "professional" approach.

Berg (1995) analyzes the interview situation in research from a dramaturgical perspective. He suggests that interviewees are likely to have a preexisting definition of the situation that changes over the course of an interview. Thus, the interviewer can shape an interviewee's definition through role-playing and self-presentation. From a dramaturgical perspective, the interviewer is an actor engaging in a self-conscious performance (Berg, 1995, p. 49), in which the "script" is continually readjusted to promote rapport, interest, and cooperation on the part of the interviewee. In order to encourage the person being interviewed to provide useful information, the interviewer needs to remain in control of the situation by keeping the conversation on track while not discouraging the interviewee from participating. Thus, the interviewer plays the role of director, as well as actor. This analogy probably applies equally well to human service situations, although in a partnership relationship, the professional should not be attempting to manipulate the client in any way.

Taylor and Bogdan (1984) note that, like observation, interviewing "requires an ability to relate to others on their own terms" (p. 94). Establishing such a relationship involves four related skills: Being nonjudgmental; letting people talk; paying attention; and being sensitive. Each applies to both research and human service practice and will be discussed in turn.

Being Nonjudgmental

In the course of an interview, a client may express opinions or beliefs that violate the interviewer's own values or knowledge. For example, I once interviewed a young mother about her living situation and inquired about her relationship with her landlord. She responded, "[The landlord] is Jewish, you know. She's a real [expletive]. She can't understand why we can't pay the rent." These remarks certainly affected me negatively, not only because they were antisemitic (this client no doubt did not realize that I was Jewish), but also because they involved a factual error (I happened to know that the landlord in question was Christian). However, I did not want to jeopardize the rapport I had managed to establish with this client after several weeks of providing services to her family. Thus, I did not attempt to correct her attitudes or beliefs, but rather focused on the concern she had raised by asking further questions about the nature of her interactions with the landlord and about the availability of alternative living arrangements. Taylor and Bogdan (1984) suggest that, in cases when interviewers feel morally compelled to state their own positions, they should do so, "but gently and without condemning the person as a whole" (p. 94).

The interviewer may need to work hard to make the client feel comfortable. When a client reveals something embarrassing or discrediting, the interviewer may wish to offer a reassuring comment, such as, "I've had the same experience with my own children" or "I know what you mean." Because human service interviewing often involves interactions with clients whose lifestyles and beliefs are different from the professional's, preservice practice in cross-cultural communication can be invaluable (see Chapter 5 for some suggested activities of this kind).

Letting People Talk

A general rule in depth interviewing is that the client always should do more talking than the professional. The role of the professional is to encourage the client to talk by using the techniques discussed throughout this chapter and to listen carefully.

Although some clients are reserved and reluctant to share personal information, others may seem too talkative. In general, the interviewer should not be too quick to interrupt in an attempt to get the interview back on track. Even though a client's remarks may not be relevant to the current situation, by interrupting, the interviewer suggests that he or she is not interested in what the client is saying. When clients share information, they are defining the information as important. The interviewer should listen politely but gently change the subject by asking a redirecting question during a break in the conversation. For example, when a woman I interviewed described at length all the minor details of her son's hospitalization (in response to a question about how she learned of his diagnosis), I waited until she paused and then said, "That was quite an ordeal. When did you finally see the doctor again?"

Paying Attention

Depth interviewing requires patience and perseverance. Not everything a client says will be of interest to the interviewer, and over the course of a long interview, interviewers' minds are likely to wander. Clients, on the other hand, need to believe that what they say is important. Thus, interviewers must work on concentrating on what their clients say and on communicating their interest. What Cottle (reported in Taylor and Bogdan, 1984, p. 95) has written about research is equally applicable to interviewing in the human service situation: "If there is a rule about this form of research it might be reduced to something as simple as pay attention."

Being Sensitive

Closely related to the qualities of being nonjudgmental and paying attention is the quality of being sensitive. Interviewers need to know when to probe and when to change the subject. To do this well, they must be good role takers (see Chapter 4), that is, they must be aware of their clients' thoughts and feelings. Good interviewers pay close attention to verbal and nonverbal cues; as a result, they are able to avoid prying into concerns that a client would rather not discuss and to encourage clients to provide more information about those concerns they do want to share. When interviewers sense that their clients are becoming bored with answering questions, they may want to terminate the interview and schedule another time to discuss issues that have not yet been addressed. The next section will provide some specific suggestions for obtaining information in a sensitive and appropriate way.

Interviewing Techniques

Beginning the Interview

An interviewer should never launch right into a prepared interview schedule without some preliminary small talk. The topic of such small talk will vary according to the situation. If the interview is to be conducted in a client's home, for example, the interviewer might comment on the surroundings ("What a beautiful Christmas tree!"), the circumstances of arrival ("Your directions were great! I had no trouble finding your house"), or that old standby, the weather ("It's really snowing hard out there"). In general, such small talk should follow normal social conventions and should be modeled after the kinds of conversations one typically has with new acquaintances.

The transition from this initial small talk to the interview should include some introductory remarks about the purposes of the interview. For example, the professional might say,

> I had a chance to get to know your family a little bit during my observation visit last week. Today, I'm hoping to learn a little more about your concerns by talking with you in some detail. Our conversation will give me some background information that will be valuable in helping you decide which services might be best for your family.

Establishing a Relationship

Kadushin and Kadushin (1997, p. 103) suggest some adjectives that characterize an interviewer who is likely to develop a positive relationship with a client: respectful, attentive, interested, caring, trustworthy, friendly, genuine, unpretentious, sympathetic, warm, concerned, empathetic, accepting, compassionate, understanding, supportive, reassuring, patient, comforting, solicitous. They suggest that the following interviewer characteristics are *not* likely to lead to a positive relationship: critical, impatient, aloof, uninterested, controlling, dogmatic, detached, judgmental, insensitive, egotistical, opinionated, uncaring, businesslike, mechanical, punitive, authoritarian, condescending, rude, patronizing, unresponsive.

Positive relationships sometimes take time to develop. At first, a client may have no basis for trusting a professional, especially in cases in which the service is court ordered or involuntary. Certainly, the professional should begin the interview with assurances about confidentiality, but such assurances may not be believed. With time, however, if a professional displays the positive characteristics listed above, the client is likely to accept the professional's interest in providing useful services. Such acceptance is important if the client is to try to answer the interviewer's questions honestly.

With patience, the professional can hope to become a significant other (see Chapter 4) for the client, as suggested by the following account by the mother of a child in an early intervention program:

> When I placed Matthew into a strange woman's arms on the first day in the infant program, I didn't know what she hoped to accomplish with my 4-week-old baby. . . . As the weeks and months passed, I sensed my baby's growing attachment to his teacher and his response to her obvious delight whenever he accomplished a new feat. I, too, unconsciously formed my attachment to her. . . . Professionals who work with families in the early months of the child's life can have a profound influence on parents. A mother may hear the first hopeful words about her child from a teacher or therapist. And those words and assurances can become the basis of strong attachments, acknowledged or unrealized, between parents and program staff. (Moeller, 1986, pp. 151–152)

The "Ten Commandments of Interviewing"

Berg (1995, pp. 57–58) summarizes some of the points made in the preceding sections with these "ten commandments of interviewing":

1. Never begin an interview cold.
2. Remember your purpose.
3. Present a natural front.
4. Demonstrate aware hearing.
5. Think about appearance.
6. Interview in a comfortable place.
7. Don't be satisfied with monosyllabic answers.
8. Be respectful.
9. Practice, practice, and practice some more.
10. Be cordial and appreciative.

Some Difficult Situations

Sometimes, even when an interviewer follows all the rules listed above, the interview process breaks down, and additional, useful information cannot be obtained by this method. The most common situations of this kind involve clients who cry or otherwise lose control of their emotions and clients who never seem to move beyond one-word answers.

Crying is not at all uncommon when clients are revealing sad or stressful events in their lives. Sometimes clients are embarrassed about losing control of their emotions, and acknowledgment by the interviewer can make the situation worse. No absolute rules apply here, because different clients react in different ways. Thus, good role-taking by the interviewer is important. Certainly, keeping tissues handy is always appropriate. Other appropriate responses may include any of the following:

- Sympathetic silence. The interviewer appears sympathetic but simply waits until the client has regained emotional control before proceeding with the interview.
- Appropriate questioning. The interviewer asks whether the client wants to continue talking about the current topic or prefers to move on to a different subject. In rare instances, the interviewer may want to ask the client if he or she would prefer to terminate and/or reschedule the interview. Sometimes, the client is just having a "bad day" for reasons unrelated to the interview and may be emotionally volatile as a result. Rescheduling the interview may be best in such circumstances.

- Appropriate reflection. The interviewer says, "It must be hard for you to talk about . . ." or , "I can understand how talking about this would make you feel bad" (can be used in conjunction with appropriate questioning).
- Changing the subject. Sometimes the best response is to subtly change the subject after waiting a short amount of time for the client to regain some emotional control.
- Proceeding with the interview. If the client seems unduly embarrassed about losing control, the interviewer may want to pay as little attention as possible to the crying and proceed as normally as possible. In such situations, the client often regains control without assistance. The methods above can be implemented if the situation deteriorates further.

A different kind of difficult situation involves clients who are especially nonverbal and either do not respond to questions or respond with only a word or a phrase. This situation is most likely to arise in the following instances:

- Involuntary or court-ordered clients.
- Clients who feel intimidated, commonly those of low SES or considerably less education than the interviewer.
- Culturally different clients.
- Clients who have difficulty understanding because of disability or lack of proficiency in language.

Some of the techniques discussed earlier in this and previous chapters, such as "dressing down," using lay language, engaging in small talk before beginning the interview, and using an interpreter, can be useful here.

Sometimes, however, clients may simply be shy or unfamiliar with the interviewer's expectations. The appropriate use of silence, probes, and follow-up questions is important. In addition, the interviewer may wish to remind the client that his or her views are important and that the interviewer needs as much information as possible to provide the kinds of help the client may want. In general, more experienced interviewers have the least difficulty with reticent clients. Novice interviewers will find that, with practice, their patience and comfort increases. Clients can sense when an interviewer is uncomfortable and are less likely to be open with an interviewer who is not relaxed. However, with some clients, an interview may not be the best method to use. When interviewing does not seem to be culturally appropriate or clients have great difficulty with verbal communication, professionals may need to rely on other methods, such as observation and written questionnaires.

Recording Methods

Although recording during the process of observation may be unnecessarily obtrusive, recording during interviewing is usually a good idea. An interview may cover many topics, and the interviewer needs to remember accurately and not misrepresent the client's responses. However, the recording method should still be as unobtrusive as possible and should not detract inordinately from the flow of conversation. The most common methods for recording interviews are taking notes, tape recording, and video recording. Each will be discussed in turn.

Taking Notes

Most clients will expect the interviewer to record what they say and will want to be sure that what they say is accurately recorded. In the collaborative partnership model being advocated here, the interviewer should never try to hide what is written; rather, note taking should be done openly, so that the client can see the notes.

In a conversational, depth interview, the interviewer should not try to record everything the client says verbatim. Doing so, even if it were possible, would detract from the flow of conversation and result in a stilted question-and-answer session. Instead, the interviewer should write only key words and phrases, just enough to help in remembering later when the interview report is written in narrative form. The interviewer may wish to record *a few* phrases or short sentences verbatim to capture the client's style of communication.

One way to reduce the amount of writing during the interview is to take notes using a topic outline rather than a blank piece of paper. This outline would list the major topics and questions to be used, leaving enough space between topics to allow the interviewer to write. Typically, an agency serves enough clients of a given type to make it feasible to develop a standardized interview form that can be used repeatedly with different clients.

Note taking may be the most natural way to record an interview. Most clients feel relatively comfortable with this method and seem to speak freely when it is used. However, the professional should always ask the client in advance whether he or she minds whether the interviewer takes notes "to be sure to get it right." Occasionally, a client may ask a professional not to write during a particular portion of the interview, and the professional should respect those wishes.

Tape Recording

For most human service purposes, note taking is appropriate and sufficient as a recording method during interviews. However, accuracy can be improved with audiotaping, and tape recording is less obtrusive than writing. Also, the interviewer can concentrate more on the interviewee's words, gestures, and facial expressions if he or she does not have to periodically stop and write.

The main reason for not tape recording is that it tends to make people uncomfortable. As a result, they may censor what they say and not provide truthful or useful information. In addition, time to transcribe long tapes is typically not available in human service work.

If a tape recorder is used, the interviewer always should ask the client's permission in advance. If the client agrees, the following suggestions from Taylor and Bogdan (1984, p. 103) should be heeded:

- Use a small recorder and place it out of sight if possible.
- The microphone should be unobtrusive and sensitive enough to pick up voices without having to speak into it.
- Use long-playing tapes, so the conversation will not be interrupted so often.

When complete accuracy is important, videotaping may be superior to audiotaping. A video recorder can capture facial expressions and "body language" that audio recording will miss. In group interviews, videotaping can be especially useful in capturing the reactions of participants while others are speaking. However, videotaping usually requires an additional person to operate the camera, and extra staff commonly are not available for such purposes in human service agencies. In addition, video cameras tend to be even more intimidating than tape recorders. Many people will refuse to be videotaped, and those who agree to the taping still are likely to be uncomfortable and act unnaturally as a result. Thus, this recording method is not practical in most human service situations.

Writing the Report

Regardless of the recording method used, a narrative report should be written as soon as possible after the interview is completed. If the report will not be written until several days after the interview, the interviewer should at least review his or her notes immediately, completing unfinished thoughts and adding a few words about the interviewee's presentation of self, apparent receptivity to the experience, and communication style. This information will be useful in helping the interviewer remember the context of the interview when the report is written.

Different agencies use different forms and/or expect different formats for reporting the outcomes of interviews and other communications with clients. The format to be suggested here may need to be modified in accordance with agency guidelines but will be valuable as a general framework for reporting interview results. The interview report should include the following information:

1. Identifying information. This section should include the name of the interviewee(s), along with any other identifying information required by an agency, such as social security number, address, or date of birth.
2. Location of the interview. The report should indicate where the interview was conducted; whether in the professional's office, the client's home or place of business, or elsewhere.
3. Time, date, and duration of the interview. In addition to information about when the interview was conducted and how long it lasted, the report also should indicate whether it was completed in a single session or extended over several sessions. Interruptions also might be noted.
4. Description of the setting. The report should include information about the physical surroundings, such as furniture and room arrangement, as well as the number and identity of all of the people who were present.
5. Summary of responses. The report should not be a list of questions and answers. Rather, the interviewee's responses should be summarized in narrative form, under headings to indicate the topics discussed. Both direct quotes and paraphrased statements may be included. A copy of the original interview schedule may be attached to illustrate the nature of the questions that were asked.
6. Analysis. In this section, the reporter attempts to draw conclusions about the interviewee's resources, priorities, and concerns, as revealed in the interview. These should be summarized under the headings previously discussed: information and formal, informal, and material support. In addition, the reporter should provide information relating to the likely reliability and validity of these conclusions. This information is usually derived from observed cues, such as the interviewee's presentation of self, the presence of other people in the room (perhaps causing responses to be censored), and from the circumstances surrounding the interview (Was it voluntary or court ordered? Was the interviewee reacting to other, unrelated life events that recently occurred?).
7. Service recommendations. The interviewer might wish to speculate about potential referrals or possible services that would assist the client in addressing concerns raised during the interview. Additional recommendations might involve additional identification activities, such as questionnaire administration, that could be used to further clarify the respondent's resources, concerns, and priorities.

An example of an interview report follows:

> Susan Doe was referred to this agency by the guidance counselor at her son's school. Bobby, age 12, has been absent from school 20 of the last 40 days. His teachers report that he seems distracted and that his grades are falling. During a previous home visit to observe the family, I learned that Mr. and Mrs. Doe have recently separated and

that Bobby cares for his younger siblings and performs other household chores while Mrs. Doe works. She works variable shifts.

The interview was conducted on November 6, 1999, in the Does' home (described in the observation report). The interview began at 4:00 PM and lasted until 5:15 PM. I was seated at the kitchen table, across from Mrs. Doe, who had just returned from work. Bobby was in the living room watching television. The other children, 3-year-old Katie, 5-year-old Nikki, and 9-year-old, Steven, entered and left the kitchen several times during the interview. Katie sat on her mother's lap for short periods of time, and the other children took food and drinks from the refrigerator.

Summary of Responses. Mrs. Doe expressed her love and concern for her children at several points during the interview. She said that things had been difficult since her husband moved out of the house two months ago and that she was concerned about the effect of the separation on the children, who "miss their father." She said she was proud of Bobby, who had become "the man of the house." She said he had been very helpful to her. She did express concern, though, about his school grades. When asked directly about his absences, she said that he had been "sick a lot." She reluctantly admitted that on a few occasions, Bobby had stayed home to take care of Katie and Nikki, because her "shift changed at the last minute" and she could not get a babysitter.

When I asked about her usual child care arrangements, Mrs. Doe said that, prior to the separation, her husband usually watched the children, because he worked different shifts. Mrs. Doe also had relied on her sister, but this sister had recently gotten a job and could no longer help. Also, a neighbor recently had been watching the children when their mother worked day shift but this neighbor was not always reliable.

Mrs. Doe said that she had no other friends or relatives who could help and that money was tight. She said her mother lived nearby but "has her own life" and "doesn't come over much." She reported that Mr. Doe had not given her any money since he left. She said that "in some ways" she was glad her husband had left, because he "had a drinking problem" and they "didn't get along real well." On the other hand, she was concerned about managing alone. She did not express any other concerns about herself or her children. Her main concern involves finding reliable child care.

Analysis. This interview seemed to accurately reflect Mrs. Doe's concerns. Although initially a little reticent, she seemed to relax as the interview progressed. She seemed to be close to tears when she talked about her children and her concerns. She seemed to want help with her concerns.

- Information. Mrs. Doe has talked to a lawyer recommended by a friend and plans to pursue getting child support payments from her husband. She does not think she needs any more information in this area. She would like more information about child care and other programs for the children.
- Material support. Mrs. Doe is working. As noted above, she is also pursuing child support payments from her husband. She is concerned about her financial situation.
- Informal support. Mrs. Doe receives some help from a neighbor. Bobby also has been helpful. She is concerned about the effect on Bobby. She also is concerned about the effect of the separation on her other children. She cannot depend on help from other family members or friends.
- Formal support. Mrs. Doe is familiar with legal services but has not used any other agency services. She is interested in knowing more about services that might be helpful. She is not interested in counseling for herself at this point but might be interested in talking with other mothers in her situation.

> *Recommendations.* I will explore subsidized child care arrangements that are available in this community. I also will look into latchkey programs for Nikki and Steven. I will provide Mrs. Doe with information about support groups for single parents. I also will provide information for Mrs. Doe to consider about counseling for the children. Our agency will need to work closely with Mrs. Doe to provide support and assistance to address her present concerns and to monitor any new concerns that may develop during this period of transition in her life.

Some Special Interviewing Situations

Face-to-face, one-on-one interviewing is the most frequently used method in human services to help clients identify their resources, concerns, and priorities. Sometimes, though, circumstances necessitate other formats, such as group interviews or telephone interviews. Some special adaptations for these formats are discussed below.

Conducting Group Interviews

Today in human services the "client" is often not an individual, but a couple, a family, or even a representative group of the members of an entire community. As Hedges (1985) and others have noted, interviews with more than one person provide an opportunity for group members to talk with one another, as well as with the interviewer. Group interviews also are an efficient way of gathering information from all the individuals who share a concern. In addition, this method allows all the members of a group to hear the definitions of the situation of other group members and may promote discussion and consensus when definitions differ.

Group interviews offer additional advantages in cases in which clients do not feel comfortable speaking for other members of their family or group (or are likely to be inaccurate reporters). For example, in one study (Briggs, 1986; Foddy, 1993), the investigators almost misinterpreted their subjects' interest in receiving services. The Navajo interviewees had answered, "No, I don't think so," when asked about the interest of other members of their families. The investigators later learned that, in contrast to other ethnic groups, the Navajo believed speculation about the beliefs of others to be highly inappropriate. For this group, then, either separate individual interviews or a group interview would be necessary.

On the other hand, group interviews also involve some disadvantages, such as those noted by Darling and Baxter (1996, p. 138):

- There is less time for an in-depth exploration of individual perspectives . . .
- Social pressure within the group, along with the influence of the more dominant and articulate members, can present problems. Individuals may

feel socially exposed and less inclined to express views they believe will not be acceptable within that group context.

- People sometimes feel compelled to present themselves in the best possible light when other members of their family or peer group are present.
- It is often logistically difficult to get all relevant members of a family or [other group] together at one time.
- Some individuals are simply intimidated by groups.
- In some cultural contexts group conversation is normal and expected; in others it is not (see Chapter 5).

The skills required for group interviewing are similar to those involved in individual interviewing. However, skills for controlling side conversations and arguments between group members also are important. In general, the interviewer should try to let members work out their disputes themselves. After all, the interviewer's role is to gather information, not to provide intervention. However, if the discussion becomes too heated, the interviewer may want to refocus it with a comment such as, "You two certainly don't seem to agree about this. We have a number of topics to cover today. Do you want to continue this discussion now, or should we save it for later and move on to something else?" Even in less heated discussions, the interviewer should acknowledge differences in definition or opinion with a comment like the following: "I'm hearing two different things here. That's OK; I don't necessarily expect you to agree about this. I just want to be sure that I'm hearing you correctly." An understanding of such intragroup differences may be important in the development of a service plan that meets the needs and addresses the wishes of all members of a group.

One specialized kind of group interview that is commonly used in human services is the focus group interview, involving approximately ten individuals and an interviewer–moderator. Although not designed for use in identifying the resources and concerns of clients, focus groups can be useful in program evaluation and needs assessment (see Chapters 10 and 11). They often are used in preliminary attempts to learn about attitudes toward and interest in the development of new services.

Designing an interview schedule for a focus group is similar to designing an unstructured or semistructured schedule for the identification of resources, concerns, and priorities. Usually, the questions are open-ended and are limited to a specific topic or topics. Stewart and Shamdasani (1998) note that a typical interview guide for a 90-minute discussion usually does not include more than 12 to 15 questions. The discussion begins with more general questions and becomes narrower as the group focuses on more specific issues.

As in the case of other group interviews, the focus group moderator may be more or less directive, depending on the nature of the topic and the nature of the group. The moderator generally would not want to interrupt discussion and would not intervene unless the group became unduly argumentative or strayed too far from the desired agenda. Because the members of a focus group were commonly unacquainted with one another prior to the group's establishment, they are not as likely as family groups to engage in conflict unrelated to the group's purpose. Thus, the moderator usually only needs to keep the discussion on track with occasional reminders about the topic being discussed or with transitional questions that introduce new topics.

Conducting Telephone Interviews

In general, face-to-face interviewing is superior to telephone interviewing for most human service purposes. Interviewing by telephone usually results in a less personal relationship between the interviewer and the interviewee. In addition, the interviewer will miss nonverbal cues issued by the client. Further, the interviewer cannot use such cues as eye contact and head nodding to encourage the interviewee to say more. For these and other reasons, telephone conversations tend to be briefer than in-person interviews.

However, on some occasions, clients prefer the convenience and lack of intrusiveness of telephone interviews. Such interviews also are useful in contacting family members who were not able to be present during the face-to-face interview conducted with other members of the family. In the early intervention program that I directed, work schedules often required that mothers be interviewed in person during the day, whereas fathers were interviewed by telephone in the evening. Telephone interviews also are useful as follow-ups to in-person interviews, whenever information needs to be clarified or additional questions need to be asked.

Some evidence (see, for example, Bradburn & Sudman, 1979; Weiss, 1986) exists to suggest that people are willing to talk on the telephone about sensitive issues. For example, in one study, participants talked on average for nearly an hour about issues such as racism (Kluegel & Smith, 1982) and women's opportunities (Smith & Kluegel, 1984). Clients who already know an interviewer well (usually after they have been receiving services for some time) are especially likely to feel comfortable talking about personal matters on the telephone.

Telephone interviews, like face-to-face interviews, should be scheduled in advance. The time should be convenient for the client and when distractions can be minimized. Parents of young children almost always should be interviewed after their children are in bed or when another caregiver is present in the house. Meal times and times when favorite television shows are on the air also should be avoided. The interviewer should inform clients in advance of the approximate duration of the interview and suggest that they make themselves comfortable.

Group interviews also can be conducted by telephone with the aid of features such as three-way calling or speakerphones. However, unless necessary, such adaptations tend to limit free participation and spontaneity even more than the telephone itself. Group interviews conducted in this way also can be confusing for the interviewer, who may not always be able to identify the speaker or to hear what is being said when several people are talking at once.

The Advantages and Disadvantages of Interviews

Although interviewing is usually the best method for identifying clients' resources, concerns, and priorities, it is not appropriate for all clients and in all situations, and the resulting information is subject to limitations in reliability and validity. The advantages of interviewing are clear: Like other qualitative methods, it allows the interviewer to establish the context of a client's concerns, and, unlike observation, it can assist the professional and the client in focusing and clarifying information.

The value of interviewing, however, depends on the skill of the interviewer in asking the right questions and asking them well and on the interviewer's ability to establish rapport. These skills may not be enough when clients are not very verbal or are not fluent in English. In such cases, observation may be the only qualitative method that can be used. In other cases, for cultural or personal reasons, the client may perceive the interview process as overly intrusive. Certainly, interviewing is more intrusive than observation. Such clients sometimes prefer questionnaires, which do not require face-to-face contact and which allow respondents to skip questions more easily (see Chapter 8).

Regardless of the client's comfort with the interview format, any information obtained through this method is subject to the biases, both intentional and unintentional, of the person being interviewed. In observation, the observer's biases can distort perceptions. In interviewing, the biases of the interviewee become important as well. Responses may be censored or otherwise altered to reflect what the client thinks the professional wants to hear. The client's recall of past events also may be inaccurate. As Darling and Baxter (1996) have written,

> Professionals and family members alike do not necessarily mean what they say or say what they mean. Nor do people necessarily have insight into their beliefs, resources, and concerns, let alone the capacity to articulate these in an interview. Moreover, one person's perception of an experience will not necessarily be the same as that of someone else who shared the experience. We all distort and exaggerate our experiences on occasion. What is said in a depth interview may surprise even the utterer and only later will it be possible for the informant to consider whether the statement is a true reflection of what he or she believes. (p. 157)

However, absolute validity may not be as important when interviewing is used as part of the identification process in human services as it is when interviewing is used in research. Within a partnership perspective, the service user's perception of his or her concerns and priorities is what matters. When the client's definition of the situation is the operative one, professionals need to be more concerned with whether or not they have succeeded in getting their clients to tell the truth as they see it than with whether their clients' accounts match some objective standard. Using interviewing in combination with other methods may be the best way to ensure that these accounts remain relatively consistent throughout the identification process. Questionnaires, the final identification technique to be presented in this volume, will be discussed in the next chapter.

Chapter Summary

This chapter continued the discussion of the identification process by presenting the method of interviewing. Like observation, interviewing is a qualitative method that promotes a deeper understanding of a client's situation. The chapter focused on the technique of semistructured depth interviewing and provided guidance on developing questions and conducting interviews of this type. Examples were used to illustrate appropriate interviewer behavior in both ordinary and difficult interview situations. Finally, the special cases of group and telephone interviews were addressed.

Suggested Exercises

In a classroom situation, students can practice the skills of designing an interview schedule, conducting an interview, and writing a report through the following exercise.

1. You will be interviewing a fellow student to learn how he or she arrived at the decision to attend this university. Your interview will follow a modified life history format, so you will want to know when your interviewee first started thinking about attending college. Who were the people who influenced this thinking? Did his or her thinking change over time? You will need to ask questions that trace your interviewee's "career path" (see Chapter 4), beginning with early life experiences relating to higher education and continuing with later experiences in chronological order, culminating with the decision to attend this particular university.

   You will need to do three things to complete this exercise:

   - Design an interview schedule.
   - Interview a fellow student using your schedule. (Ideally, your interviewee should not be a close friend.)
   - Write a narrative description of your interviewee's career path.

6:00 AM	
6:30 AM	
7:00 AM	
7:30 AM	
8:00 AM	
8:30 AM	
9:00 AM	
9:30 AM	
10:00 AM	
10:30 AM	
11:00 AM	
11:30 AM	
NOON	
12:30 PM	
1:00 PM	
1:30 PM	
2:00 PM	
2:30 PM	
3:00 PM	
3:30 PM	
4:00 PM	
4:30 PM	
5:00 PM	
5:30 PM	
6:00 PM	
6:30 PM	
7:00 PM	
7:30 PM	
8:00 PM	
8:30 PM	
9:00 PM	
9:30 PM	
10:00 PM	
10:30 PM	
11:00 PM	
11:30 PM	

Figure 7.2. Interview record form.

2. A second exercise involves interviewing a fellow student about what he or she did yesterday. To facilitate recording the interview, the student should use paper ruled to show times, as in Fig. 7.2. The interview should include probes in order to obtain as much information as possible. After the interview is completed, students can reverse roles, so that each has a chance to be both interviewer and interviewee.

After both exercises, students can discuss what worked well and what did not seem to work. Interviewees can discuss how they felt about being interviewed. Was it easy or difficult to be truthful?

Suggestions for Further Reading

Kadushin, A. & Kadushin, G. (1997). *The social work interview: A guide for human service professionals*. New York: Columbia University Press.

Taylor, S.J., & Bogdan, R. (1984). *Introduction to qualitative research methods: The search for meanings*. New York: John Wiley & Sons.

8

Identification Techniques III

Questionnaires

The techniques discussed in the two previous chapters were qualitative. Both observation and depth interviewing are subject to the actions and interpretations of the professional. Even when the same interview schedule is used, the process will vary depending on each client's responses and the interviewer's decisions based on those responses. Written questionnaires, on the other hand, can be standardized, so that many clients complete the same instrument in the same way. Data obtained from the questionnaire responses of many clients usually can be readily quantified and used for research purposes, such as program evaluation.

Questionnaires also can be valuable in the identification of clients' resources, priorities, and concerns. Clients are not necessarily aware of the resources available to meet their needs, and questionnaires incorporating checklists and scales can provide useful information in this regard. In addition, checklists can serve as an aid to memory by including concerns that might not be recalled when other formats are used. Questionnaires are also particularly useful for collecting factual and attitudinal information and for ascertaining clients' preferences in relation to a range of alternatives.

This chapter will discuss the uses of questionnaires as part of the identification process in human services. Good questionnaire design will be presented and illustrated with examples. Finally, the advantages and disadvantages of questionnaires in relation to other identification methods will be addressed.

Because questionnaires are relatively easy to administer, some human service professionals have a tendency to overuse them. Those who use a status inequality approach, especially, will find many standardized tests and assessment instruments available. Sometimes, these can be valuable in determining a client's need for services. Most, however, were designed from a professional's (rather than a client's) point of view (see Chapter 2), and therefore have limited usefulness in a partnership approach. Before administering any questionnaire, professionals should ask themselves whether it is really necessary in order to provide the services that the client might choose. In general, the fewest possible measures should be used, in order to minimize intrusiveness.

When Are Questionnaires Useful in Human Services?

Written questionnaires can be used in addition to or in place of other identification methods. Normally, because of the importance of qualitative information for most human service purposes, questionnaires should supplement other methods, such as observation and depth interviewing. However, given the administrative constraints of practice today, methods that are quick and easy sometimes must take precedence over those that might yield more valuable information. In general, written questionnaires are especially valuable in the following situations:

- At intake. Funder policies or client needs may dictate a short intake process, in which client concerns are identified in a fixed amount of time. Written questionnaires provide a way to obtain information quickly and easily. In addition, questionnaire administration is not necessarily dependent on the development of rapport between the professional and the client, and therefore may be more appropriate than other methods early in a relationship.
- Later in the client–professional relationship, when qualitative methods are no longer necessary. Usually, observation and depth interviewing occur during or shortly after intake, because qualitative information is important in determining service requirements and preferences. In a long-term client–professional relationship, the professional is likely to already know much about the context of the client's life. Life history questions need only be asked once, and home observations need not be repeated unless the client has moved or the living situation has changed significantly. In these cases, a questionnaire can serve as a quick update on the client's priorities and an indication of any new resources and concerns with less intrusiveness than other methods.
- For clients who prefer this format. Some clients find written instruments to be less intrusive than methods involving personal interaction. Depending on cultural and personal preferences, home observations or depth interviews may be regarded as unnecessary invasions of privacy. In my experience, such attitudes have been more common among middle-class clients than among those of lower socioeconomic status (SES), perhaps because of different values placed on individual and family privacy or differing amounts of past experience with human service agencies. In any case, all clients should be asked about their preferred methods, and qualitative techniques should be avoided when clients indicate that they their use would make them uncomfortable.
- As a follow-up to other methods. After observation and interviewing have been completed, some areas may need further clarification. For example, a client may have expressed a desire for assistance with child care but may

not have indicated a preference for in-home care versus family day care versus a child care center. A questionnaire could be useful in this case to assist the client in choosing among available services. Questionnaires also provide a way of checking on information obtained by other means. For example, observation and interviewing may have produced contradictory information, as in a case in which a home observation suggested a need for furniture or other material resources, but the client indicated no such concern during an interview. A checklist of concerns would provide a way to be surer that the client did not desire assistance in this area. Questionnaires also can be used to obtain information about subjects not included in an interview. Sometimes, clients prefer the less personal written format when discussing especially sensitive areas, such as illegal or sexual behavior. In addition, interview time can be saved by using questionnaires to obtain information about straightforward matters that do not require a qualitative context (e.g., demographic information).

- When information is already available regarding clients of this type. Certainly all clients are individuals, and no client should be assumed to possess any given characteristic. However, professionals may know a considerable amount about certain populations from the research literature and from past experience. When interviews repeatedly reveal the same concerns in a given population, written checklists may save time. For example, the Parent Needs Survey included here (Fig. 8.1) was developed from the research literature on parents of young children with disabilities, as well as from the concerns that had been expressed over time by numerous parents in an early intervention program.
- To determine service preferences when choices are limited. Some human service programs are not designed to address all the concerns that a client might have. A transportation service, for example, may only be interested in knowing the days and times when clients might need a ride. Programs of this type probably do not need to use qualitative methods in order to provide appropriate services.
- In research. Questionnaires are especially useful in needs assessment and program evaluation, when the identity of individual clients is not important. Written questionnaires can be administered anonymously, promoting honesty in responses. These uses will be explored more fully in Chapters 10 and 11.
- To measure progress. The same questionnaire can be administered at program entry and at various intervals throughout the course of service delivery. Responses can then be compared. For example, when the Parent Needs Survey was given to clients every six months, both the number and intensity of concerns decreased over time (Darling & Baxter, 1996). Thus, the program seemed to be successful in addressing these concerns.

Parent Needs Survey

Date: ____________________________

Name of Person Completing Form: ____________________________

Relationship to Child: ____________________________

Parents of young children have many different needs. Not all parents need the same kinds of help. For each of the needs listed below, please check (✓) the space that best describes your need or desire for help in that area. Although we may not be able to help you with all your needs, your answers will help us improve our program.

	I really need some help in this area.	I would like some help, but my need is not that great.	I don't need any help in this area.
1. More information about my child's disability.			
2. Someone who can help me feel better about myself.			
3. Help with child care.			
4. More money/financial help.			
5. Someone who can baby sit for a day or evening so I can get away			
6. Better medical care for my child.			
7. More information about child development.			
8. More information about behavior problems.			
9. More information about programs that can help my child.			
10. Counseling to help me cope with my situation.			
11. Better/more frequent teaching or therapy services for my child.			
12. Day care so I can get a job.			
13. A bigger or better house or apartment.			
14. More information about how I can help my child.			
15. More information about nutrition or feeding.			
16. Learning how to handle my other children's jealousy of their brother or sister.			

(Continued)

	I really need some help in this area.	I would like some help, but my need is not that great.	I don't need any help in this area.
17. Problems with in-laws or other relatives.			
18. Problems with friends or neighbors.			
19. Special equipment to meet my child's needs.			
20. More friends who have a child like mine.			
21. Someone to talk to about my problems.			
22. Problems with my husband (wife).			
23. A car or other form of transportation.			
24. Medical care for myself.			
25. More time for myself.			
26. More time to be with my child.			
Please list any needs we have forgotten:			
27.			
28.			
29.			
30.			
31.			
32.			
33.			
34.			
35.			

Figure 8.1. Example of a checklist-type instrument.

Developing Questionnaires

Characteristics of a Good Instrument

A good questionnaire will provide information that is useful to both the professional and the client. Certain characteristics are required to ensure usefulness:

- Appropriateness. Sometimes in human services, a questionnaire may need to be individualized for a given client or family. For example, if a client has expressed numerous concerns during a depth interview, the professional may wish to develop a questionnaire that lists all these concerns, along with a scale that assists the client in prioritizing them. When standardized (nonindividualized) instruments are used, the professional always should be careful to be sure that all the items are appropriate to the literacy level, cultural values, and known preferences of the client.
- Lay language. Questionnaires should be free of professional jargon and ideology. The professional should be sure that the instrument used is understandable to the client and not biased in any way.
- Promotion of problem-solving skills. Questionnaires should be useful to clients, as well as to professionals (Turnbull & Turnbull, 1990, p. 367). The process of completing a questionnaire should provide clients with the opportunity to think about their resources, concerns, and priorities.
- Necessity. Before administering any instrument, the professional should be sure that it will provide necessary and valuable information. Too often in human services professionals automatically use the same battery of written instruments for all clients. Sometimes, qualitative methods such as depth interviewing and observation are sufficient to identify all a client's resources, concerns, and priorities, and the use of questionnaires is both redundant and an unnecessary additional imposition on a client's time and privacy.

Designing an Instrument

Because standardized instruments developed from a partnership perspective are not readily available in all areas of human services, professionals need to have the skills to design their own. These skills include formatting, developing instructions, developing questions, and organizing. Each will be discussed in turn.

Format

The format of a questionnaire should assist the client in responding accurately and completely. To this end, the developer needs to consider length, language, and layout, as follows:

- Length. When questionnaires are too long, respondents tend to lose interest, and their responses to later questions are not as likely as their earlier responses to be accurate and complete. In general, clients with more education and better reading ability can complete a longer instrument than those who are less literate. Because most programs serve clients with a variety of literacy levels, shorter questionnaires are usually better than longer ones. No one length is right for all purposes, but as a general guideline, questionnaires longer than three pages are probably too long.
- Language. As noted above, written instruments must be understandable to those who are completing them. Simple, everyday language is usually best, because it can be understood by clients of all education levels. Computer programs that provide literacy-level checks are useful.
- Layout. The font should be large and clear enough to be read easily, especially for older clients. In addition, instructions and headings should be written in a different font from questions (or at least italicized or bolded). Open-ended questions should include enough space for long answers, and closed-ended questions should include response choices that are clear and easily marked. Questions that require answers of different kinds (e.g., checklists vs. scales of agreement) generally should not be included, and if included should not be in the same section. Respondents who are not highly literate may have difficulty with questions that offer too many choices; scales should probably be limited to three–five response choices at most, and these choices should be presented clearly.

Instructions

Instructions should be written in a way that promotes accurate completion of the questionnaire. If all questions use the same response format, one set of instructions may be sufficient. When different formats are used, questions should be grouped by response type and separate instructions provided for each group. When questions addressing widely divergent topics are included, grouping is also appropriate, even if the response format does not change. In this case, transitional statements should be included (e.g., "The following questions are about concerns relating to school.")

The instructions at the beginning of the questionnaire always should include the following elements:

- Assurances. The respondent should be assured that no "right" or "wrong" answers exist and that all responses are "normal." For example, the Parent Needs Survey includes the following statements: "Parents of young children have many different needs. Not all parents need the same kinds of help." Such statements help to counteract the tendency to try to respond in ways that are perceived to be normative or socially appropriate.

- Response method. The instructions should clearly state whether the respondent is to check, circle, make an "X", or otherwise respond to questions. If the response method is at all likely to be unfamiliar, an example should be provided. The Parent Needs Survey, which uses a simple checklist format, includes this statement: "For each of the needs listed below, please check (√) the space that best describes your need or desire for help in that area."
- Rationale. The instructions should help the respondent answer the questions, "Why am I doing this?" or "What's in it for me?" When questions are included that do not relate directly to some benefit that the agency might be able to provide, an explanation should be offered. The Parent Needs Survey states, "Although we may not be able to help you with all your needs, your answers will help us improve our program."

Question Type

Question wording and type are important in obtaining useful information. Two broad question type options are available: open-ended and closed-ended. Open-ended questions do not provide a range of response choices. For example, the question, "Are you satisfied with the services you have received from the agency?" is open-ended. If the same question were asked in the following way, it would be closed-ended:

> Please indicate your level of satisfaction with the services you have received from the agency. Are you
> [ ] Very satisfied
> [ ] Satisfied
> [ ] Not sure
> [ ] Not satisfied
> [ ] Very dissatisfied?

Closed-ended questions can help respondents organize their thinking and are generally easier to answer, especially for respondents with low literacy levels. These questions also can be informative, by suggesting a range of alternative responses. When used in program evaluation, closed-ended questions facilitate the quantification of results. When the same closed-ended questions are used with a single client over time, they provide for a ready comparison of results.

On the other hand, when professionals develop such questions, they may not be able to think of all possible responses, and as a result clients might not find a response choice that fits their thinking or preference. When only closed-ended questions are used, respondents have no way to explain their answers, and professionals may misinterpret responses. For example if in response to the question above a client checks "Very dissatisfied," is the client indicating dissatisfaction with all services, or with a few services, and which services does he or she have in mind? One way of addressing this problem is to include an open-ended option following the closed-ended one, for example,

Please explain your answer ______________________________.

Another way to address the limitations of closed-ended questions is to include the response choice, "other." This choice allows respondents to select an alternative that the professional may have missed in designing the question. Normally, an "other" choice should be accompanied by space for an open-ended response, along with directions such as "Please explain" or "Please specify."

Open-ended questions may also provide advantages for some respondents. Monette et al. (1998) note that well-educated respondents may prefer such questions, because they allow greater flexibility of expression and therefore are more satisfying. Generally, for human service purposes, including some open-ended questions, along with closed-ended ones, satisfies the needs of most clients.

Closed-ended questions can be presented using a variety of formats. In human services, formats that are commonly used include checklists, questions followed by response choices, and rank ordering. The Parent Needs Survey (Fig. 8.1) is a checklist. One advantage of checklists is that they generally are easy for respondents to complete. In addition, they tend to remind respondents about options they may have forgotten and to educate respondents about options with which they were previously unfamiliar. In human services, checklists are especially valuable in identifying client concerns (as in the case of the Parent Needs Survey) and resources and in facilitating choices among service options.

Another commonly used format lists response choices immediately after each question, as in the question about satisfaction with agency services above. Response choices may be listed either horizontally or vertically (as above). The horizontal option is often used in connection with attitude and opinion scales, which will be discussed later in the chapter.

Rank ordering is especially useful in identifying client priorities. This format is similar to checklists in that alternative responses are listed on one side of the form. However, rather than checking preferred alternatives, the client numbers alternatives in preferential order. As part of the identification process, all of a client's previously identified concerns can be listed, and the client can be instructed to number them in order of importance. For example, if a client had checked the "I really need some help in this area" column on the Parent Needs Survey for five items, the following form could be used to determine priorities:

Some of your concerns may be more important to you than others. Please write a number from 1 to 5 in the space next to each of the items listed below. Write a "1" next to those items with which you would like some help right away, a "2" next to those that are

next in importance, and so on. Write a "5" next to the items that are the least important to you. You may use a number more than once for items that are equally important:

Item	Number
More information about my child's disability	____
More money/financial help	____
More information about programs that can help my child	____
More information about nutrition or feeding	____
Problems with in-laws or other relatives	____

Rank ordering is sometimes confusing for clients with low levels of education or literacy. With such clients, priorities may be better addressed verbally.

Another use of rank ordering involves the prioritizing of service choices, as in the following example (Darling & Baxter, 1996, p. 187):

Please rank from 1 (most desirable) to 3 (least desirable):

Someone to look after my child in my own home ____
Someone to look after my child in his or her home ____
Someone to look after my child in a child care center ____

Question Wording

Unclear question wording can result in inaccurate or biased answers. All questions therefore should be pretested with respondents whose backgrounds are similar to those of the clients with whom the questions will be used. In general, the development of good questions should be guided by the following principles:

- Avoid vagueness. Questions generally should require respondents to speak for themselves rather than for people in general. For example, "Are you satisfied with the information you have received from the agency?" is less vague than "Is the agency information satisfactory?"
- Avoid "reinventing the wheel." If an established instrument is available, use it. Devising a new instrument is time consuming and requires pretesting.
- Avoid biased wording and "loaded" questions. Bias can arise from "strong" words as well as from questions posed in positive or negative ways. Words such as love, prejudice, or hate, for example, may result in responses that clients believe to be socially appropriate but that do not reflect their true feelings. Similarly, the question, "Are you satisfied with the program?" is more likely to produce a positive response than the question, "Are you satisfied or dissatisfied with the program?" Question wording should suggest that negative or critical responses are acceptable. Questions that suggest an answer also are likely to produce inaccurate information. For example, the

question, "You won't be needing our transportation services, will you?" implies that a "No" response is expected. A client who does need transportation might be inclined to deny his or her need when the question is asked in this way.

- Avoid complex questions. Questions should be as short and simple as possible and should address only one issue at a time. One human service agency with which I am familiar uses the following question in its intake questionnaire: "Generally, do you express your feelings, opinions, and wishes to others in an open, appropriate manner?" This question could confuse a respondent who believes that his expression is open but not "appropriate." Another respondent may express wishes openly but not feelings and opinions, and so forth.

  Darling and Baxter (1996) further note that

  > . . . the key idea in the question should come last and any conditional clauses first. For example, if the key idea is transportation to and from preschool, it is better to ask: "If [name of child] is accepted by the preschool, what arrangements could you make to get her there?" rather than "What arrangements could you make to get her there if [name of child] is accepted by the preschool?" In the latter case, the notion of whether the child will be accepted may be given more attention than the issue of transportation, which is intended to be the major focus of the question. (p. 171)

- Devise questions at an appropriate literacy level. Questions should usually use simple vocabulary and avoid professional jargon. A questionnaire used by one state to evaluate its early intervention programs included the following statement (followed by a seven-point agreement scale): "Intervention practices promote mutually beneficial exchanges between my family and other informal and formal community members." In the program I directed, parents with less than a high school education had difficulty understanding some of the words in the statement. Even highly educated parents did not understand the terms, informal and formal community members. These terms come from the language of human service professionals and are likely to be misunderstood by lay clients.
- Avoid assumptions. Several writers (Judd, Smith, & Kidder, 1991; Neuman,1991) have noted that unwarranted assumptions in research questions can produce invalid data. Similarly, in human services, professionals should not assume anything about their clients. For example, the question, "What are your major concerns about John?" assumes that the client has concerns, and major ones. A better question might be, "Do you have any concerns about John?"

  Double-barreled questions (see Chapter 7) also make an assumption, namely, that a connection exists between two separate ideas. For example, as part of a program evaluation, a "Meals-on-Wheels" program asked their clients "Are you satisfied with the quality and quantity of the meals you receive?" This question does not allow for the possibility that the quantity is sufficient but the quality is poor or that the quality is good but the portions are too small.

- Use tense consistently. Monette et al. (1998) note the importance of not mixing tenses in a questionnaire. If a question about the past is inserted between two questions on the present, the respondent may have difficulty shifting from one time frame to another. Thus, questions about a particular period of time should be grouped together, and shifts in time should be marked by a transitional statement such as the following: "The following questions are about your experiences during the past month."

Response Categories and Scales

In closed-ended questions, the number of response choices will depend on the type of information that is needed. In some cases, a simple yes/no response may be all that is required. For example, a question such as "Do you wish to receive more information about transportation services?" requires only an affirmative or negative response when the degree of the respondent's desire is not important.

On the other hand, in both the identification and evaluation processes, knowing about such matters as the magnitude of a particular need or the degree of satisfaction with program services may be important. In these cases, response categories can take the form of scales. Various scaling formats are used for research purposes. For the human service purposes being discussed here, the most common format is the Likert scale (Likert, 1932). Some scales of this type are the following (Darling & Baxter, 1996, p. 178):

- Strongly agree, agree, no opinion, disagree, strongly disagree
- Always, most of the time, some of the time, rarely, never
- Excellent, good, fair, poor
- More likely, less likely, no difference
- Much better, slightly better, about the same, slightly worse, much worse
- Very satisfied, satisfied, unable to judge, dissatisfied, very dissatisfied.

Likert-type scales always should be properly balanced, with an equal number of positive and negative choices. Usually, too, a neutral choice such as "no opinion" or "unable to judge" should be provided to reduce the likelihood of invalid responses. The Parent Needs Survey (Fig. 8.1) presented earlier uses a three-point scale in checklist format. The most commonly used Likert scale includes five response categories: two positive categories, two negative ones, and one neutral one. Generally in human services, five-category scales are sufficient for measuring degrees of concern or agreement, and additional categories could be unnecessarily confusing. For example, one evaluation instrument with which I am familiar used the following categories: strongly disagree, mildly disagree, disagree just a little, neither agree nor disagree, agree just a little, mildly agree, strongly agree. Many clients had difficulty distinguishing between "mildly disagree" and "disagree just a little" when completing this form.

Likert scales can be especially useful when used as part of the resource identification process to measure the level of assistance that is available from various formal and informal supports. Fig. 8.2, which is part of a questionnaire entitled, Personal Network Matrix (Dunst et al., 1987), illustrates such a scale designed for use in an early intervention program. Figure 8.3 illustrates a scale developed for a similar purpose for use with a general population sample.

Whenever a person needs help or assistance, he or she generally can depend upon certain persons or groups more than others. Listed below are different individuals, groups, and agencies that you might ask for help or assistance. For each source listed, please indicate to what extent you could depend upon each person or group if you needed any type of help.

To what extent can you depend upon any of the following for help or assistance when you need it:	Not at all	Sometimes	Occasionally	Most of the Time	All of the Time
1. Spouse or Partner	1	2	3	4	5
2. My Children	1	2	3	4	5
3. My Parents	1	2	3	4	5
4. Spouse or Partner's Parents	1	2	3	4	5
5. My Sister/Brother	1	2	3	4	5
6. My Spouse or Partner's Sister/Brother	1	2	3	4	5
7. Other Relatives	1	2	3	4	5
8. Friends	1	2	3	4	5
9. Neighbors	1	2	3	4	5
10. Church Members	1	2	3	4	5
11. Minister, Priest, Rabbi	1	2	3	4	5
12. Co-Workers	1	2	3	4	5
13. Babysitter	1	2	3	4	5
14. Daycare or School	1	2	3	4	5
15. Private Therapist for Child	1	2	3	4	5
16. Child/Family Doctors	1	2	3	4	5
17. Early Childhood Intervention Program	1	2	3	4	5
18. Hospital/Special Clinics	1	2	3	4	5
19. Health Departments	1	2	3	4	5
20. Social Service Department	1	2	3	4	5
21. Other Agencies	1	2	3	4	5
22. ____________________	1	2	3	4	5
23. ____________________	1	2	3	4	5

Source: C. J. Dunst, C. M. Trivette, and A. G. Deal (1987). *Enabling and Empowering Families: Principles and Guidelines for Practice.* Cambridge, MA: Brookline Books. May be reproduced.

Figure 8.2. Example of a questionnaire that uses a Likert scale designed for an early intervention program.

SECTION G. PERSONAL NETWORKS

THE NEXT QUESTIONS ARE ABOUT YOUR SITUATION AT THE PRESENT TIME. THEY ARE ABOUT YOUR "PERSONAL NETWORK"

G1. Please list, by first name or initials, the people in each of the categories below who are important to you or to whom you are important. The categories are SPOUSE/PARTNER, FAMILY/RELATIVE, CO-WORKER, SUPERVISOR PROFESSIONAL (E.G., CLERGY, DOCTOR, PSYCHOLOGIST PSYCHIATRIST, SOCIAL WORKER, ETC.) FRIEND. If no people in a category are important to you, leave it blank.

(For each person whose name or initials you list, answer the questions in columns A through E)

	A	B	C			D					E				
	Age	Sex	Was This Person In Your Network Last Year? (check one)			How Important Is This Person To You? (check one)					How Important Do You Think You Are To This Person? (check one)				
	in years	M or F	Yes	No	Don't know	Very important		Important		Not very important	Very important		Important		Not very important
			1	2	3	1	2	3	4	5	1	2	3	4	5
a.. SPOUSE/PARTNER															
1.															
b. FAMILY/RELATIVE															
1.															
2.															
3.															
4.															
5.															
c. CO-WORKERS (Includes friends who are co-workers here)															
1.															
2.															

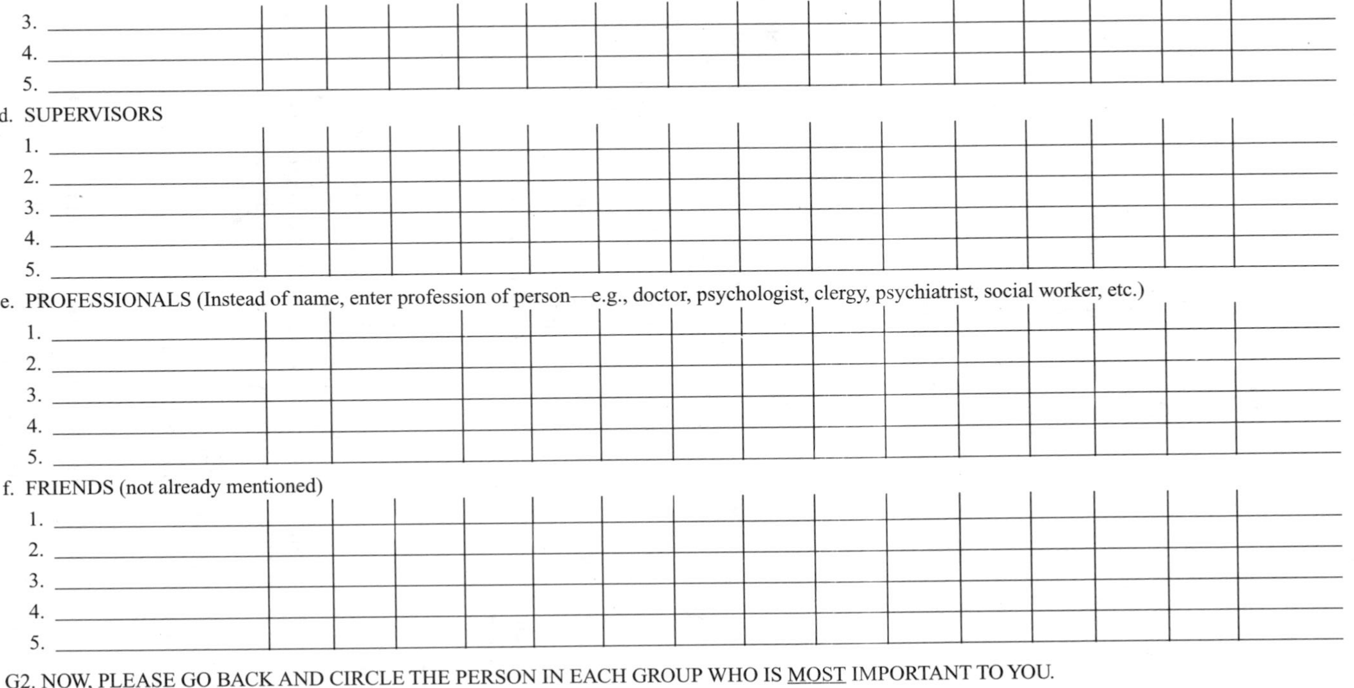

3.
4.
5.

d. SUPERVISORS
1.
2.
3.
4.
5.

e. PROFESSIONALS (Instead of name, enter profession of person—e.g., doctor, psychologist, clergy, psychiatrist, social worker, etc.)
1.
2.
3.
4.
5.

f. FRIENDS (not already mentioned)
1.
2.
3.
4.
5.

G2. NOW, PLEASE GO BACK AND CIRCLE THE PERSON IN EACH GROUP WHO IS MOST IMPORTANT TO YOU.

From: Antonucci, T.C. & Depner, C.E. (1982) Social support and informal helping relationships. In T.A. Wills (Ed.) Basic process in helping relationships (pp. 233–254). New York: Academic Press.

Figure 8.3. Example of a questionnaire that uses a Likert scale designed for a college-educated population. (From Antonucci & Depner, 1982. Reprinted with permission)

Similarly, scales have commonly been used to measure degree of need or concern. The Parent Needs Survey (Fig. 8.1) is a scale that measures need across a range of areas. More specific scales could be developed to measure need for assistance in a particular area. For example, in the field of mental retardation services, staff may want to know whether caregivers want help in teaching a family member various life skills. Figure 8.4 (Darling & Baxter, 1996, p. 185) presents such a scale developed for use in an early intervention program.

Another scaling format that could be useful in the identification and evaluation processes is the *semantic differential* (Osgood, Suci, & Tannenbaum, 1957). A semantic differential scale presents adjectives that are polar opposites at either end, with numbered points in between. Respondents select a numbered point to represent their attitude toward a particular person, event, or service. For example, in program evaluation, a scale such as the following might be used:

In my opinion, program staff were:

Helpful	1	2	3	4	5	6	7	Unhelpful
Caring	1	2	3	4	5	6	7	Uncaring
Competent	1	2	3	4	5	6	7	Incompetent
Efficient	1	2	3	4	5	6	7	Inefficient
Friendly	1	2	3	4	5	6	7	Unfriendly

A semantic differential scale also might be useful in the identification process for the purpose of clarifying the nature of resources or supports. For example, a client could be asked to rate each of the supports listed in the Personal Network Matrix above (Fig. 8.2) in terms of characteristics such as dependable (undependable), helpful (unhelpful), available (unavailable), caring (uncaring), and concerned (unconcerned).

Organization: Question Order

As noted in Chapter 7, the order in which questions are asked can influence the quality of the information that is obtained. In general, in both interviews and questionnaires, easier, less threatening questions should be asked first. Monette et al. (1998) suggest some other considerations in decisions about question order:

- Earlier questions can bias responses to later ones.
- Interesting questions should be asked first in order to capture the respondent's attention.

Questions generally should be grouped by topic, with transitional statements or subtitles separating the topics. Such grouping is especially important in the case of long questionnaires that cover a variety of subject areas.

Would you have liked more assistance regarding how to teach your child new skills like:

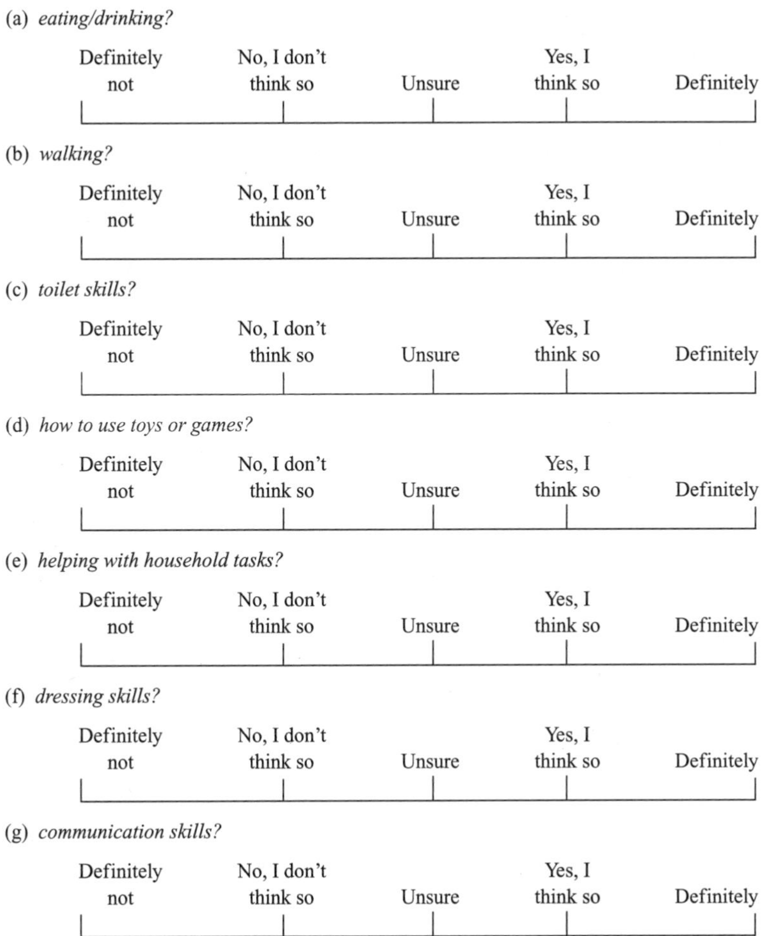

(a) *eating/drinking?*

Definitely not	No, I don't think so	Unsure	Yes, I think so	Definitely

(b) *walking?*

Definitely not	No, I don't think so	Unsure	Yes, I think so	Definitely

(c) *toilet skills?*

Definitely not	No, I don't think so	Unsure	Yes, I think so	Definitely

(d) *how to use toys or games?*

Definitely not	No, I don't think so	Unsure	Yes, I think so	Definitely

(e) *helping with household tasks?*

Definitely not	No, I don't think so	Unsure	Yes, I think so	Definitely

(f) *dressing skills?*

Definitely not	No, I don't think so	Unsure	Yes, I think so	Definitely

(g) *communication skills?*

Definitely not	No, I don't think so	Unsure	Yes, I think so	Definitely

Figure 8.4. Questionnaire to measure need for assistance in teaching skills. (From Darling & Baxter, 1996, p. 185. Reprinted with permission.)

Evaluation Exercise

The following questionnaires, to be completed by clients of various educational levels, have been designed by actual human service agencies for the purpose of program evaluation. Based on the principles of good questionnaire design discussed above, evaluate each of the questionnaires below in terms of length, language, layout, and question type. Do you think that these agencies will get the kinds of information they need from these instruments? Why or why not?

The following questions are specific to each of these instruments:

1. Senior Center Participant Questionnaire (Fig. 8.5):
   - Are any scales used in this questionnaire?
   - Should a "Please explain your answer" item follow any of the questions?
   - Are open- and closed-ended questions used appropriately?
2. Client Evaluation Form (Fig. 8.6):
   - Are any of the questions double-barreled? Which ones?
   - Do you think clients will provide honest answers? Why or why not?
3. Consumer Survey (Fig. 8.7):
   - Would the language be clear to most laypersons?
   - Does the format allow sufficient space for client responses?
   - Should a "Please explain your answer" item be added after any of the questions?
   - Is the question sequence logical?
4. Family Survey of Early Intervention Services (Fig. 8.8)
   - Is the length appropriate?

Senior Center Participant Questionnaire

---

1 Which Center do you attend?______________________________

2. How often do you receive a meal provided by Services, Inc.?

   _____ Almost every day   _____ About once a week   _____ A few times a month

3. Are you satisfied with the *quality* of meals you receive?   _____ yes   _____ no

4. Are you satisfied with the *quantity* of food you receive?   _____ yes   _____ No

5. What meal do you enjoy the most?______________________________

6. What meal do you enjoy the least?______________________________

7. Please list below any comments or suggestions you have regarding our meal service.

____

____

8. Are you satisfied with the programs that are presented in your center?   _____ yes   _____ no

9. What type of program would you like presented in your center?______________________________

____

Thank you for your time and cooperation.

Figure 8.5. Senior center participant questionnaire.

Client Evaluation Form

In evaluating our agency and its services, we need your help! Please answer the questions below. We would appreciate your signature but it is not necessary.

1. Did you receive the service, information and referrals that you needed? yes ______ no ______
2. Briefly identify the service(s) you received.

____

____

____

3. How would you rate the service(s) you received from our agency?

   Good ______ Fair ______ Poor ______

4. Was the person with whom you had contact considerate, polite, and knowledgeable?

   yes ______ no ______

5. Comments and suggestions: How could we better serve you?

____

____

____

____

____

____

____

____

____

____

______________________________ ______________________

Signature Date

Figure 8.6. Client evaluation form from an agency serving families in poverty.

- Are the scale choices clearly different from one another?
- Is lay language used? If not, cite examples of professional jargon that might not be understood by clients.
- Is the use of a variety of scales appropriate?
- Are the instructions clear?

If you found any problems in these instruments, rewrite the questions/redesign the surveys as appropriate to correct these problems.

Consumer Survey

1. Was your training as a supervisor of an attendant adequate? ____ yes ____ no

   If NO which areas do you feel could be improved?

   ____ Attendant Recruitment ____ Form completion ____ Interview/Selection

   ____ Termination/Firing Attendant ____ Interpersonal Relations

   ____ Attendant Supervision

2. In what areas could the attendant training be improved, if any?

   ____ Efficient use of time ____ Adaptability to your needs ____ Call off procedure

   ____ Dress Code ____ Transfers ____ Confidentiality

   ____ Other, please state ____________________

3. How has attendant care affected your life? ____________________

4. Do you receive the amount of service hours that you need? ____ yes ____ no

   Please explain ____________________

5. Do you feel that Agency support is adequate? ____yes ____no

   Please explain ____________________

6. Is Agency supervisory staff available to listen to your concerns? ____ yes ____ no.

   Please explain ____________________

7. Are you visited or called by Agency staff on a regular basis? ____ yes ____ no

8. Were the different service options adequately explained to you? (i.e. "Agency/Employer Option", "Consumer/Employer Option") ____ yes ____ no

9. Was the Waiver Program explained to you? ____ yes ____ no

10. Does the Agency encourage you to be independent? ____ yes ____ no

11. Has the service given family caregivers relief? ____ yes ____ no

12. In what areas are you satisfied with the service? ____________________

    ____

13. In what areas are you dissatisfied with the service? ____________________

    ____

14. What would you suggest to improve the service? ____________________

    ____

15. Does your attendant permit you to accomplish tasks that you yourself can do?

    ____ yes ____ no If NO, why not? ____________________

    ____

____________________ ____________________

Date Signature of Consumer

Figure 8.7. Consumer survey form from an agency serving adults with disabilities.

Family Survey of Early Intervention Services

INSTRUCTIONS

This survey is being conducted to learn more about the ways early intervention services are provided to children and their families. The information you provide will help us learn how families feel about these services. Please complete each section and return the survey in the stamped envelope we have enclosed. Your participation in this project is very much appreciated.

FAMILY-ORIENTED PRACTICES

This section of the survey asks you to indicate the extent to which different program components, methods, and approaches are part of the family-oriented early intervention pratices adopted or endorsed by YOUR CHILD'S PROGRAM. Please indicate whether or not you agree or disagree that each statement reflects the official position of YOUR CHILD'S PROGRAM with respect to the adoption or endorsement of the different types of practices listed.

To what extent do each of the following statements reflect the official position of YOUR CHILD'S PROGRAM?	Strongly Disagree	Mildly Disagree	Disagree Just A Little	Neither Agree Nor Disagree	Agree Just A Little	Mildly Agree	Strongly Agree
1. Nothing is written on the IFSP without my family's explicit permission	1	2	3	4	5	6	7
2. My family's involvement in implementing IFSPs is determined by my family's level of interest	1	2	3	4	5	6	7
3. Case managers mobilize resources to meet my child's needs so my family doesn't have to be bothered with doing this themselves	1	2	3	4	5	6	7
4. My family is encouraged to follow what is professionally prescribed to meet my child's needs	1	2	3	4	5	6	7
5. Early intervention assessment practices focus on my child's need for services and resources provided by the early intervention program	1	2	3	4	5	6	7
6. Intervention practices promote mutually beneficial exchanges between my family and other informal and formal comunity members	1	2	3	4	5	6	7

To what extent do each of the following statements reflect the official position of <u>YOUR CHILD'S PROGRAM</u>?	Strongly Disagree	Mildly Disagree	Disagree Just A Little	Neither Agree Nor Disagree	Agree Just A Little	Mildly Agree	Strongly Agree
7. Early intervention program staff encourage professionals from other agencies to inform my family about their decisions during transitions between settings	1	2	3	4	5	6	7
8. My family's input is routinely obtained as a basis for making changes in my child's early intervention program	1	2	3	4	5	6	7
9. Early intervention staff have autonomy in developing and implementing child-level interventions	1	2	3	4	5	6	7
10. Early intervention program staff are primarily responsible for determining appropriate IFSP services and resources for my child and family	1	2	3	4	5	6	7
11. IFSP goals/needs are changed as often as my family desires even if it means making a completely new plan	1	2	3	4	5	6	7
12. Case management practices teach my family how to establish linkages with informal and formal community resources	1	2	3	4	5	6	7
13. My family determines when and how we receive services from early intervention programs	1	2	3	4	5	6	7
14. Intervention practices primarily enhance my child's development rather than other areas of family functioning	1	2	3	4	5	6	7
15. IFSP goals/needs are jointly identified by early intervention program staff and my family	1	2	3	4	5	6	7
16. Early intervention staff roles in implementing IFSPs are restricted to professional areas of expertise related to my child's development	1	2	3	4	5	6	7
17. My family's needs and lifestyle determine the roles of our case managers	1	2	3	4	5	6	7

18. My family and professionals are equally responsible for mobilizing resources to meet my family's needs	1	2	3	4	5	6	7
19. My family's concerns and needs determine the assessment methods and practices used by my child's early intervention program	1	2	3	4	5	6	7
20. My child's behavior and development is the focus of all or most of my parental involvement in my child's early intervention programs	1	2	3	4	5	6	7
21. My family is the "sole owner" of the IFSP	1	2	3	4	5	6	7
22. Implementing IFSPs centers around services aimed at effecting changes in my child's behavior and development	1	2	3	4	5	6	7
23. Intervention practices are flexible so they fit into my family's lifestyle	1	2	3	4	5	6	7
24. Early intervention assessment practices emphasize the assessment of my child development skills	1	2	3	4	5	6	7
25. My family participates in a parent-training program as part of our involvement in early intervention programs	1	2	3	4	5	6	7
26. Early intervention staff can seek assistance or advice from other multidisciplinary team members without my consent	1	2	3	4	5	6	7
27. The IFSP is written in words understood by my family	1	2	3	4	5	6	7
28. The IFSP process "fits" my family's unique lifestyle even if child-level needs are not addressed	1	2	3	4	5	6	7
29. My family determines which areas of child functioning and family concerns are the focus of early intervention assessment practices	1	2	3	4	5	6	7
30. The "bottom line" is that my child is the focus of all intervention practices	1	2	3	4	5	6	7

(Continued)

Please indicate to what extent <u>you</u> agree or disagree with whether the following principles have been adopted or endorsed by <u>YOUR CHILD'S PROGRAM</u>			Strongly Disagree	Mildly Disagree	Neither Agree Nor Disagree	Agree	Strongly Agree
31. The case manager who works with my family is selected at the convenience of the early intervention program	1	2	3	4	5	6	7
32. It's important for early intervention staff to identify and "stick to" long-range IFSP goals	1	2	3	4	5	6	7
33. Prevention or remediation of family dysfunctional patterns is the focus of the IFSP process	1	2	3	4	5	6	7
34. Case management practices emphasize the transfer of knowledge and skills from professionals to my family	1	2	3	4	5	6	7
35. Intervention practices place primary emphasis on early intervention program staff promoting my child's development	1	2	3	4	5	6	7
36. Assessment practices are restricted to my family's needs only as they relate to my child's development	1	2	3	4	5	6	7
37. All information that early intervention staff know about my family's situation is shared in an unbiased and complete manner with my family	1	2	3	4	5	6	7
38. Early intervention program staff are primarily responsible for deciding the appropriate placement for my child as part of planning transitions	1	2	3	4	5	6	7
39. My family has complete and immediate access to all forms of documentation maintained on my child and family	1	2	3	4	5	6	7
40. Interventions are begun prior to obtaining my consent or approval	1	2	3	4	5	6	7

GUIDING PRINCIPLES

This section of the survey asks you to indicate the extent to which certain principles have been adopted or endorsed by YOUR CHILD'S PROGRAM regarding ways in which resources and services ought to be made available to infants and toddlers with special needs and their families. Please circle the response that you feel best describes whether or not the principles listed have been adopted or endorsed by YOUR CHILD'S PROGRAM.

Please indicate to what extent you agree or disagree with whether the following principles have been adopted or endorsed by YOUR CHILD'S PROGRAM	Strongly Disagree	Mildly Disagree	Neither Agree Nor Disagree	Agree	Strongly Agree
1. Interventions build upon family's strengths rather than correct weaknesses or deficits	1	2	3	4	5
2. Resources and supports are made available to my family in ways that are flexible, individualized, and responsive to the needs of the entire family unit	1	2	3	4	5
3. Interventions are needs-based and family-driven rather than professionally prescribed	1	2	3	4	5
4. Resource and support mobilization for families of infants and toddlers with special needs occur in the same ways as those for all families of very young children in our community	1	2	3	4	5
5. Interventions use partnerships between parents and professionals, rather than traditional client-professional relationships, to strengthen family functioning	1	2	3	4	5
6. Resource and support mobilization interactions between my family and professionals are based upon mutual sharing of information and expertise	1	2	3	4	5
7. Interventions focus on building and strengthening informal support networks for my family rather than developing new professional service systems	1	2	3	4	5
8. Resources and supports are provided in ways that encourage, develop, and maintain healthy, stable relationships among all our family members	1	2	3	4	5

(Continued)

Please indicate to what extent you agree or disagree with whether the following principles have been adopted or endorsed by YOUR CHILD'S PROGRAM	Strongly Disagree	Mildly Disagree	Neither Agree Nor Disagree	Agree	Strongly Agree
9. Interventions focus on the integration of my family and our child with developmental delays or disabilities into the mainstream of all normalized community activities	1	2	3	4	5
10. Resources and supports are made available to my family in ways that maximize our control over and decision-making power regarding the services we receive	1	2	3	4	5
11. Interventions focus on promotion of healthy family functioning rather than prevention or treatment of dysfunctional behavior	1	2	3	4	5
12. Interventions minimize "professional" intrusion upon my family and our personal and cultural values and beliefs	1	2	3	4	5

This section of the survey asks you a number of questions about your child's development and the services you and your child receive from the early intervention program.

1. Since your child has been involved in the early intervention program, would you say he or she has made more or less progress in each of the following areas:

How much progress, has your child made?

AREAS OF DEVELOPMENT	Much Less than Expected			About What Was Expected			Much More Than Expected
Communication Skills	1	2	3	4	5	6	7
Gross Motor Skills	1	2	3	4	5	6	7
Self-help Skills	1	2	3	4	5	6	7
Playing with Toys	1	2	3	4	5	6	7
Interacting with People	1	2	3	4	5	6	7

2. Since you have been involved in the early intervention program, how much help has the staff provided you in the following areas:

	None At All	A Little	Some	Generally	A Lot
Teaching you how to work with your child	1	2	3	4	5
Providing you information about your child's development	1	2	3	4	5
Improving your child's ability to learn new things	1	2	3	4	5
Improving your child's ability to do things for him/herself	1	2	3	4	5
Helping you see that family and friends might be able to help you with a problem	1	2	3	4	5
Helping you find child care or respite care	1	2	3	4	5
Learning about other agencies that could help your child and family	1	2	3	4	5
Finding community opportunities (for example, recreational) for your child	1	2	3	4	5
Working through the "paperwork" that had to be done for other agencies	1	2	3	4	5
Helping you and your child during the transition from early intervention to preschool, or preschool to school	1	2	3	4	5
Helping you identify public school services for your child	1	2	3	4	5

This section of the survey asks for your opinion and feelings about the early intervention program and yourself.

1. Please indicate which of the following ratings best describes how the early intervention staff interact with you and your family.

   A. Which rating best describes whether the early intervention staff believe you know your <u>needs and strengths</u>?
   __ Rarely treats me as if I know my needs and strengths.
   __ Seldom treats me as if I know my needs and strengths.

(Continued)

__ Sometimes treats me as if I know my needs and strengths.
__ Generally treats me as if I know my needs and strengths.
__ Almost always treats me as if I know my needs and strenghts.

B. Which rating best describes whether the early interventions staff view you in a <u>negative or positive way</u>?
__ Almost always views me in a negative way.
__ Sometimes views me in a negative way.
__ Views me neither positively or negatively.
__ Sometimes views me in a positive way.
__ Almost always views me in a positive way.

C. Which rating best describes how the early intervention staff <u>support</u> you when <u>you make a decision</u> about your child?
__ Rarely supports my decisions about my child.
__ Seldom supports my decisions about my child.
__ Sometimes supports my decisions about my child.
__ Generally supports my decisions about my child.
__ Almost always supports my decisions about my child.

D. Which rating best describes how the early intervention staff <u>try to understand</u> your concerns by putting themselves in your situations?
__ Rarely tries to understand my concerns.
__ Seldom tries to understand my concerns.
__ Sometimes tries to understand my concerns.
__ Generally tries to understand my concerns.
__ Almost always tries to understand my concerns.

E. Which rating best describes how well the early intervention staff <u>listen</u> to what you have to say about your child and family?
__ Rarely listens to what I have to say.
__ Seldom listens to what I have to say.
__ Sometimes listens to what I have to say.
__ Generally listens to what I have to say.
__ Almost always listens to what I have to say.

2. Please circle the response that indicates approximately the number of hours a month that you have contact with the staff from the early intervention program. This can be any type of contact: phone calls, home visits, or group meetings.

Less than 1 hour a month
1 hour a month
2 hours a month
3 hours a month
4 hours a month
5 hours a month

3. How pleased are you with the services you and your family receive from the early intervention program?

__ Not at all pleased
__ A little pleased
__ Somewhat pleased
__ Generally pleased
__ Almost always pleased

4. At this moment in your life, to what extent do you feel you have control over the help you receive from the early intervention program staff working with your child and family? Please indicate on the scale below the sense of control you feel you have.

1	2	3	4	5	6	7	8	9	10
Very Little Control									A Great Deal of Control

5. This series of questions asks you to describe your own well-being. These questions are being asked because we often find that people's responses to the items differ depending on what they do on a regular basis.

How often did you feel this way DURING THE PAST WEEK?	Not at All	Once or Twice	Several Times	Often
1. On top of the world?	1	2	3	4
2. So restless you couldn't sit long in a chair?	1	2	3	4
3. Relaxed and calm?	1	2	3	4

(Continued)

4. Bored?	1	2	3	4
5. Particularly excited or interested in something?	1	2	3	4
6. Uneasy about something without knowing why?	1	2	3	4
7. Well-rested?	1	2	3	4
8. That you couldn't do something because you just couldn't get along?	1	2	3	4
9. That you had more things to do than you could get done?	1	2	3	4
10. Proud because someone complimented you on something you had done?	1	2	3	4
11. Depressed or very unhappy?	1	2	3	4
12. Content with just the way things are?	1	2	3	4
13. Upset because someone criticized you?	1	2	3	4
14. Pleased about accomplishing something?	1	2	3	4
15. Very lonely or remote from other people?	1	2	3	4
16. Angry at something that usually wouldn't bother you?	1	2	3	4
17. Calm, cool, and collected?	1	2	3	4
18. That things were going your way?	1	2	3	4

Figure 8.8. Family survey of early intervention services.

Reliability and Validity

As noted in Chapters 6 and 7, concerns about reliability and validity are generally more important in research than in the identification process in human services. In a client-driven partnership approach, an understanding of the client's subjective reality takes precedence over the accuracy or consistency of a client's actions, statements, or questionnaire responses. However, designers of questionnaires to be used for either identification or evaluation still need to be concerned about whether their instruments are eliciting information that is relevant and useful.

Face validity is established by ensuring that an instrument does indeed measure all aspects of what one is attempting to measure. One way to increase validity is to read all the available literature on the subject in question. A questionnaire designed to address treatment options for new clients who abuse drugs, for example, should be based on first-person accounts by abusers and their families, as well as on studies by professionals. A draft of the questionnaire then should be pretested with similar population groups, perhaps those who are on a waiting list for services or who are already participating in other agency programs. The draft then can be revised to include items that emerge from the pretest.

Validity also is suggested by pretest responses that seem to appropriately address the questions that are asked. If certain questions are consistently left unanswered or are answered inappropriately, the designer may want to interview pretest respondents in an attempt to improve the instrument. The Parent Needs Survey presented earlier in the chapter was initially presented in conjunction with the Family Interview in Chapter 7. When answers to the questionnaire were consistent with the in-depth information provided in the interview, the validity of the instrument was supported:

> A series of 100 PNS forms was compared with information obtained from the same parents during the Family Interview. This comparison revealed that for 96% of the items checked by parents on the PNS, the parents' indication of need (or lack of need) was supported by the interview data. Of the 26 items on the PNS, an average of 24.95 items per person were confirmed by the interview data. (Darling & Baxter, 1996, p. 195)

In addition, the Parent Needs Survey was field tested in early intervention programs in five states, and parents in all of the states responded in similar ways. Such large-scale testing may not be feasible for all questionnaires developed by human service agencies to meet agency-specific needs, but at least some pretesting is clearly advisable.

Reliability—whether the responses of any given respondent are consistent from one administration of the instrument to the next—is more difficult to determine in a human service context. New clients are usually eager to begin receiving services and may not respond favorably to being asked to complete the same form twice. Research with such a vulnerable population also may be ethically questionable.

However, when the administration of a questionnaire is immediately followed by an interview, professionals often can determine whether questionnaire responses accurately reflect a client's intentions. In the agency I directed, for example, the social worker reviewed the Parent Needs Survey with the client after it was completed; this follow-up interview usually confirmed the written responses but sometimes revealed that a survey item had been misunderstood.

One technique for assessing reliability without administering a form twice involves the use of "split halves." When an instrument is designed to measure only one variable, the responses to the first half of the instrument's items should be correlated with the responses to the items in the second half. Typically in the identification process in human services, however, instruments are designed to identify a variety of resources and concerns. The Parent Needs Survey, for example, assumes that parents have a variety of distinct needs; a parent who indicates a need for help with child care would not necessarily be expected to also have a need for counseling. The split-half technique might be more useful in program evaluation research, at least in the case of a unidimensional study concerned only with general levels of satisfaction with services.

The Relative Advantages and Disadvantages of Questionnaires

In summary, then, questionnaires, when used carefully, can be very useful in human services, both in identifying client concerns, resources, and priorities and in evaluating program services. The following lists of the advantages and disadvantages of questionnaires in relation to other methods will serve as a review of the material that has been covered in this chapter.

Advantages

- Unlike qualitative techniques, questionnaires are relatively easy to validate and check for reliability; identical forms can be used for many clients.
- Questionnaires generally can be administered more quickly than interviews and can be administered by people without high levels of skill and training.
- Clients often find questionnaires to be less intrusive than interviews.
- Questionnaires with closed-ended response choices help respondents to organize their thoughts.
- Questionnaires can be administered to people who are not physically present.
- Questionnaires are especially valuable with nonverbal clients or those with culturally based prohibitions against talking about sensitive issues.
- Questionnaires are more efficient for identifying changes in resources, concerns, and priorities in clients who have been receiving services for a long time and are well known to the service provider.

- Questionnaires eliminate the possibility for bias that can occur in interviews when a respondent is influenced by the way a question is asked.

Disadvantages

- Unlike qualitative techniques, questionnaires do not provide a context for a respondent's answers, which may result in misinterpretation by the professional.
- Questionnaires require literacy and writing skills, making them less useful with clients who are poorly educated, who do not speak English, or who have certain disabilities.
- Questionnaires may not be perceived as culturally appropriate in some groups.
- Unlike interviews, questionnaires do not allow for as many probes or follow-up questions (although questionnaire responses can be clarified through follow-up interviews).
- Questionnaires limit serendipity. In observation and interviewing, professionals may discover resources and concerns that had not previously occurred to them. In questionnaires, on the other hand, all areas to be explored will be those that the designer thought about in advance.

Chapter Summary

This chapter presented the quantitative method of questionnaire development and administration. Questionnaires have certain advantages over other methods; in essence, they are easier and quicker to administer than more qualitative techniques. However, unlike observation and interviewing, questionnaires may not provide an in-depth understanding of a client's situation. The elements of good questionnaire construction were presented, and examples of both well-designed and poorly designed instruments were provided. Questionnaires are useful in human services both in the identification of clients' resources, concerns, and priorities and in the evaluation of services. Evaluation will be discussed further in Chapter 11.

Suggested Exercise

Students can practice their questionnaire construction skills by developing a questionnaire to identify the resources and/or concerns of a segment of the student population, for example, sociology majors at their university. They may wish to determine whether the services these students are receiving (classes, advising, etc.) are in fact meeting their needs. Students then can exchange and evaluate each other's questionnaires.

Suggestion for Further Reading

Monette, D.R., Sullivan, T.J., & DeJong, C.R. (1998). *Applied Social Research: Tool for the Human Services*. Fort Worth: Harcourt Brace.

III

Models of Intervention and Evaluation

9

Linking Identification and Intervention

Developing and Implementing Service Plans

The previous three chapters have presented techniques for identifying service users' resources, concerns, and priorities. The next step in service provision is the development of a plan for addressing concerns. This chapter will illustrate the process of translating the data obtained through the identification process into a plan for intervention. Several case examples will be used to illustrate this process. The chapter will focus on intervention at the microlevel, that is, intervention to change the client's immediate opportunity structure.

Selecting Methods[1]

The first step in working with clients is the identification process. As already noted, the three primary methods for identifying client resources, concerns, and priorities are observation (Chapter 6), interviewing (Chapter 7), and questionnaires (Chapter 8). Ideally, all three methods make valuable contributions when used in combination. However, certain limitations are suggested by the context within which services occur. These limitations include client choice, cultural appropriateness, and time constraints.

Client Choice

Some service users prefer answering questions verbally, whereas others prefer paper-and-pencil instruments. Some would find either method too intrusive. In

[1] Some of the material in this and the following sections is taken from Darling and Baxter (1996, pp. 201–252), with permission.

keeping with a partnership approach, before using any method for the identification of client resources, concerns, or priorities, the professional should ask clients what they would prefer.

Observation, of course, occurs regardless of client preference. However, the professional can choose not to include information obtained in this way in the development of the intervention plan. For example, an early intervention professional might say to a parent, "I notice that Suzie [sister of child receiving services] seems to want all of your attention when we work with the baby. If it's a problem for you, we can address it in the plan. If not, that's fine, too." If the parent indicates that Suzie's behavior is not a concern, the interventionist would not include it on the written document.

When using more formal methods such as interviews and questionnaires, the professional should always discuss the method with the client first. An explanation such as the following might be helpful:

> Many people who have used our services have told us they find it helpful to have a checklist of possible needs to help them remember any concerns they want to share with us. This is the checklist we usually use. (Show the checklist to the client.) Do you think it would be helpful to you to fill it out?

Client choices may reflect privacy concerns but also may indicate literacy limitations. Sometimes service users are more receptive to having a questionnaire left at the home to be returned at the next session than to completing it in the presence of the professional.

For most clients, offering a choice among methods is appropriate. The professional can explain the pros and cons of all three methods, being careful not to overwhelm the client with great methodological detail, and even suggest that using several methods in combination is usually helpful. With informed consent, service users can select the methods with which they are comfortable.

Cultural Appropriateness

As indicated in Chapter 5, subcultural groups differ considerably in communication styles. Some Italian Americans, for example, may be highly verbal and comfortable with an interview format, whereas others, like Native Americans or Asian Americans, may be reluctant to share personal information in this way. Similarly, complex written questionnaires may be intimidating to some groups of low educational status. The use of indigenous professionals may make any method more acceptable to clients of different cultural backgrounds.

The language used in any written or verbal instrument should be that with which the service user feels most comfortable. Bilingual clients should be asked which language they prefer. As indicated in Chapter 5, native-speaking interviewers are preferable to interpreters, and bicultural interpreters are preferable to those who are only bilingual.

Time Constraints

Bureaucratic requirements typically limit the time allowed for the identification process. When I was working in the field of early intervention, for example, professionals had 45 days from the date a family entered a program to complete a service plan. Regardless of requirements, clients of all human service programs are usually anxious to begin receiving services as soon as possible, making a protracted identification process impractical or even unethical.

Such time limitations may dictate which identification methods are used. As noted in previous chapters, questionnaires are generally quicker and easier to administer than more qualitative methods like observation and interviewing. On the other hand, valuable understanding can be lost when qualitative methods are eliminated. Thus, a multimethod approach should always be regarded as the ideal or best practice.

Developing Action Statements

Determining Resources, Concerns, and Priorities

In research, observers, interviewers, and questionnaire administrators do not also provide intervention to change their subjects' life situations. In human services, however, both information gathering and intervention are usually part of the same practitioner's job. Thus, the professional who conducts the identification process is likely to be the one to write the service plan. After the identification process has been completed, the service user and the service provider together should select activities for inclusion in the intervention plan. First, though, they should review any written instruments verbally to be sure that the service user's meanings and intentions are clearly understood by the provider. Sometimes, written responses reflect misunderstandings or misinterpretations of a question. For example, on the Parent Needs Survey discussed in Chapter 8, the checklist item, "more friends [for myself] with a child like mine" was occasionally read by parents to mean, "more friends for my child." Obviously, the intervention would differ depending on whether friends were being sought for the parent or for the child.

After all observations and responses have been clarified, the user and professional should develop a list of resources and concerns in each of the areas discussed in Chapter 5: information, informal support, formal support, and material support. Concerns can then be prioritized. Priorities may be determined on the basis of interviews and questionnaires already administered. For example, an item checked in the "I really need help in this area" column on the Parent Needs Survey would be assumed to be more of a priority than one checked in the "I could use some help with this, but my need is not that great" column. If the identification instruments used did not provide a good indication of the client's priorities, the professional could simply ask, "Which of these concerns is most important to you?" or "Which of these things would you like us to work on first?" Table 9.1 is an example of a list of resources and concerns for a woman seeking help at a domestic violence shelter.

Writing Action Statements

The list of resources, concerns, and priorities can be used as the basis for a written intervention plan. Most human service agencies use written plans as contractual arrangements between the provider and the client specifying the specific obligations of each in bringing about desired outcomes. In agencies using a status inequality approach, the treatment plan typically is written by the professional, who sets a series of goals for the client. A statement from such a plan might read, "John will attend a support group meeting each week" or "Mary will wash the dishes every day."

Table 9.1. **Sample List of Resources and Concerns**

Area	Resources	Concerns
Information	Knows about the shelter and its policies Some knowledge of laws relating to domestic violence	No concerns in this area
Informal support	Mother lives nearby Children are doing well in School Has some close friends who provide emotional support	In-laws are not supportive Husband has threatened harm if children are taken from the home
Formal support	Familiar with some service agencies in the community	Did not complete high school Needs help with child care in order to work Needs assistance in obtaining a protection from abuse (PFA) order
Material support	Mother can provide some short-term financial assistance	Needs income Needs job skills Needs housing

Priorities: (1) a safe place to live; (2) additional short-term financial assistance; (3) education and job training; (4) information about child care; (5) counseling relating to long-term relationship with in-laws.

In the partnership model being advocated in this volume, actions are based on the wishes of the client rather than on professional preference. Further, in this model, professionals do not presume to be able to dictate the actions of their clients. Thus, action statements specify only what the professional will provide to enable the client to make useful choices. Rather than stating that John will attend a support group meeting, for example, the plan might suggest, "The service coordinator will provide information to John about support group meetings." Practitioners trained in a status inequality model might argue that some clients are not able or willing to act on their own. Such clients are often labeled "noncompliant," regardless of the language used in the service plan. Although some clients may in fact do better with status inequality approaches, most are more likely to act in self-beneficial ways when goals are based on their expressed concerns and priorities and when their ability to act in their self-interest is respected.

VanDenBerg and Grealish (1997) further suggest that action statements need to be strengths based. They advocate using informal supports chosen by the family rather than formal supports such as professional services. For example, in the case of parents looking for assistance in dealing with a rebellious teenager, they recommend using a relative "who knows them and who they and the family services worker both agree is a good parent" (p. 5), rather than a parent training course or a professional family preservation worker. They also note that low-priority concerns may not need to be addressed at all if high-priority concerns are satisfied. For example, they describe a couple whose marriage is in jeopardy, because of the stress created by having a child in a group home and by the father's unemployment. The parents tell their service provider that if the family is reunited and the father finds work, they will not need any help in keeping their marriage together. Thus, an action statement related to marriage counseling would be inappropriate.

Based on a partnership model, a plan for the woman whose resources and concerns were listed in Table 9.1 might include the following action statements:

1. Within 1 week, the caseworker will provide information about obtaining a PFA [Protection From Abuse] order.
2. Within 2 weeks, the caseworker will provide information about relocation opportunities in other communities and /or information about low-cost housing in this community.
3. Within 2 weeks, the caseworker will provide information about applying for TANF [Temporary Assistance for Needy Families].
4. Within 3 weeks, if the client decides to remain in this community, the caseworker will provide information about GED courses and job training programs.
5. When the client is ready to look for a job, the caseworker will provide a list of subsidized child care providers.

6. After an arrangement for secure, independent living has been established, the caseworker will provide a list of counselors with experience in family situations involving domestic violence.

The specific format to be used in writing action statements may vary depending on agency or regulatory requirements in different localities.

The Process of Plan Development: Case Illustrations

To further illustrate the process of plan development, this section will present the cases of three clients, based on actual situations in human services. All names, identifying information, and some details have been changed, and some descriptions represent a composite of several clients.

The Jones Family: Addressing Family Concerns in Early Intervention

This family consists of Amy Jones, a 2-year-old child with blindness, her 17-year-old father, Bill, and her grandparents, Mary and Pete, with whom they live. Amy's mother, who has chosen not to be involved in Amy's life, decided to give custody of Amy to Bill and his parents when she learned about Amy's blindness. Amy was 2 months old at the time. Amy has been receiving early intervention services since she was 3 months old. These services have included home visits by a vision specialist (Ann) and a social worker (Barbara).

Now, at 2 years of age, Amy is scheduled for a developmental reassessment, after which a new Individualized Family Service Plan will be developed. Ann, Barbara, Bill, and Mary will be involved in this process. Pete was invited to participate but declined the invitation. The family has requested that Ann, the professional they know best, serve as their service coordinator.

OBSERVATION. Ann and Barbara know the Jones family well after almost 2 years of home visits. Through informal observation, they know that Mary cares for Amy during the day while Bill is at school. They know from some evening visits that Bill is very much involved in Amy's care when he is at home. However, he also has a part-time job after school in a convenience store. Both Bill and Mary obviously care a great deal about Amy and try to do the best they can for her. Pete is not home much. He works long hours at a restaurant and comes home late at night. Bill and Mary report that he is fond of Amy but does not have much time to spend with her. The family lives in a house in a working-class neighborhood. The furnishings are modest but comfortable, and Amy appears to have many toys.

QUESTIONNAIRES. Barbara has chosen to use the Parent Needs Survey (see Chapter 8) with this family. She has used it with them several times before, and the

Parent Needs Survey

Date: 8/26/93

Name of Person Completing Form: Bill Jones

Relationship to Child: father

Parents of young children have many different needs. Not all parents need the same kinds of help. For each of the needs listed below, please check (✓) the space that best describes your need or desire for help in that area. Although we may not be able to help you with all your needs, your answers will help us improve our program.

	I really need some help in this area.	I would like some help, but my need is not that great.	I don't need any help in this area.
1. More information about my child's disability		✓	
2. Someone who can help me feel better about myself			✓
3. Help with child care			✓
4. More money/financial help			✓
5. Someone who can babysit for a day or evening so I can get away			✓
6. Better medical care for my child			✓
7. More information about child development		✓	
8. More information about behavior problems			✓
9. More information about programs that can help my child		✓	
10. Counseling to help me cope with my situation			✓
11. Better/more frequent teaching or therapy services for my child			✓
12. Day care so I can get a job			✓
13. A bigger or better house or apartment			✓
14. More information about how I can help my child	✓		

Figure 9.1. PNS for Bill Jones. From Darling and Baxter (1996, pp. 209–211).

	I really need some help in this area.	I would like some help, but my need is not that great.	I don't need any help in this area.
15. More information about nutrition or feeding			✓
16. Learning how to handle my other children's jealousy of their brother or sister			✓
17. Problems with in-laws or other relatives			✓
18. Problems with friends or neighbors			✓
19. Special equipment to meet my child's needs		✓	
20. More friends who have a child like mine	✓		
21. Someone to talk to about my problems			✓
22. Problems with my husband (wife)			✓
23. A car or other form of transportation			✓
24. Medical care for myself			✓
25. More time for myself			✓
26. More time to be with my child		✓	

Please list any needs we have forgotten:

27. ______________________________

____

28. ______________________________

____

29. ______________________________

____

30. ______________________________

____

Figure 9.1. (*continued*)

Parent Needs Survey

Date: 8/26/93

Name of Person Completing Form: Mary Jones

Relationship to Child: grandmother

Parents of young children have many different needs. Not all parents need the same kinds of help. For each of the needs listed below, please check (✓) the space that best describes your need or desire for help in that area. Although we may not be able to help you with all your needs, your answers will help us improve our program.

	I really need some help in this area.	I would like some help, but my need is not that great.	I don't need any help in this area.
1. More information about my child's disability		✓	
2. Someone who can help me feel better about myself			✓
3. Help with child care			✓
4. More money/financial help			✓
5. Someone who can babysit for a day or evening so I can get away		✓	
6. Better medical care for my child			✓
7. More information about child development			✓
8. More information about behavior problems		✓	
9. More information about programs that can help my child		✓	
10. Counseling to help me cope with my situation			✓
11. Better/more frequent teaching or therapy services for my child			✓
12. Day care so I can get a job			✓
13. A bigger or better house or apartment			✓
14. More information about how I can help my child			✓

Figure 9.2. PNS for Mary Jones. From Darling and Baxter (1996, pp. 212–213). Reprinted with permission.

	I really need some help in this area.	I would like some help, but my need is not that great.	I don't need any help in this area.
15. More information about nutrition or feeding			✓
16. Learning how to handle my other children's jealousy of their brother or sister			✓
17. Problems with in-laws or other relatives			✓
18. Problems with friends or neighbors			✓
19. Special equipment to meet my child's needs			✓
20. More friends who have a child like mine			✓
21. Someone to talk to about my problems			✓
22. Problems with my husband (wife)			✓
23. A car or other form of transportation			✓
24. Medical care for myself			✓
25. More time for myself		✓	
26. More time to be with my child			✓

Please list any needs we have forgotten:

27. ________________

28. ________________

29. ________________

30. ________________

Figure 9.2.

family has found it useful. Both Bill and Mary complete the survey forms. Their completed forms are included as Fig. 9.1 and 9.2.

These forms suggest the following concerns:

Bill:
- More information about Amy's disability
- More information about child development
- More information about programs that can help Amy
- More information about how he can help Amy (strong concern)
- Special equipment to meet Amy's needs
- More friends with a child like Amy (strong concern)
- More time to be with Amy

Mary:
- More information about Amy's disability
- Someone who can babysit for a day or evening so she can get away
- More information about behavior problems
- More information about programs that can help Amy
- More time for herself.

Ann uses other questionnaires to obtain Bill's and Mary's input into desired outcomes for Amy (such as toilet training and feeding herself). These outcomes involving technical support will be included in a separate part of the intervention plan.

INTERVIEW. Because the family has been receiving services for almost 2 years, Barbara already has interviewed the family members several times. She already knows about Amy's birth history. She knows that Bill is a senior in high school and is studying drafting. She knows that, although they cannot afford many luxuries, Pete is able to provide comfortably for the family. At this interview, then, she does not repeat any of her earlier questions; she simply asks if anything has changed in the family's life situation. Bill explains that he is looking forward to graduating and hopes to find a day job so he can help support his daughter and spend more time with her.

Barbara reviews the Parent Needs Survey with both Mary and Bill to clarify their responses. She talks with each of them separately. Bill confirms that he wants to know as much as possible about Amy's disability and about any programs of which he might not be aware. He also wants more information about the development of children in general and children with blindness in particular. He feels strongly about doing everything he can for Amy. He also would like Amy to have her own adapted toys. She seems to do well with the special sound ball and lighted toys that Ann brings and would like to have access to similar toys that they can borrow for an extended period of time. He also says that none of Amy's cousins or the other children in the neighborhood is blind. He would like to see other children like Amy and talk with their parents. Finally, he believes that his concern about not having enough time to spend with Amy will be alleviated once he graduates and finds a full-time job.

Barbara does not bring up some concerns that are not expressed by Bill on the Parent Needs Survey. For example, Bill has not checked the item "More time for myself." She suspects that any 17-year-old who goes to school all day, works all evening, and plays with his daughter at night would like some time for himself or some time to be with his friends. In the traditional status inequality approach, Bill would have been asked about such concerns. In the less intrusive partnership approach, however, Bill defines the topics for discussion, and the social worker accepts his definition. She is guided only by the items indicated by Bill as those with which he wants help. However, she does try to establish a comfortable, open relationship with Bill, one in which he would not be embarrassed to reveal his true feelings, even if he thought those feelings were not appropriate.

In her interview with Mary, Barbara learns that she, too, would like as much information as possible about Amy's disability. In addition, she sometimes feels "tied down" by Amy, because she does not have any babysitters who are available during the day to provide some respite for her. She also mentions that caring for Amy has become more difficult lately, because Amy is "into everything" and "doesn't seem to understand 'No.'" Like Bill, she also wants to be sure that she is aware of any programs that can help Amy.

Developing Action Statements. Ann and Barbara meet with Bill and Mary to develop activities for their plan. They talk about Amy first, and Ann shares the results of her developmental assessment. Based on these results and on the family's priorities for Amy, they develop some child-centered activities relating to Amy's self-help development, vision skills, and behavior.

Barbara then leads the discussion on activities related to the family. They agree that Ann will provide additional information to the family about child development in general and the development of children with vision disabilities. Several informational booklets from the agency library will be useful in this process and are listed in the plan (see Fig. 9.3). Some of these materials also address Mary's concern about Amy's behavior. Some of Amy's behavior is typical of 2-year-olds in general and unrelated to her disability, and Barbara thinks that Mary will be reassured by reading some general literature on child development.

In addition, Barbara informs Mary of the availability of a series of early childhood behavior management classes offered by the agency. Mary says that she would like to try the suggestions in the written materials first and would not like to include the classes on the plan at this time.

Ann explains to the family that she already has given them all the materials she has about Amy's disability. Bill and Mary agree that they have enough information but would like Ann to keep them in mind if she encounters any additional information in the future. Ann assures them that she will.

Ann tells the family that she can call the library at the Bureau of Blindness and Vision Services to see if it has any of the adapted toys that the family would like to borrow. Bill offers to call the library, and Ann says that she will give him the long-distance telephone number and the name of a contact person there.

Barbara tells Bill that in previous inquiries she has been unable to locate another child in the area with the same diagnosis as Amy. She suggests that the family contact the National Organization for Rare Disorders or send a letter to *Exceptional Parent* magazine. She also offers to post a notice on an electronic mailing list, as the family does not own a computer. Bill says that, although he would like to meet parents of children with the same diagnosis, he would not mind meeting any parents of children with blindness. Barbara offers to call local school districts to see if they would provide names. She notes that the only other children with blindness currently enrolled in the early intervention program also have major disabilities in other areas as well. She offers to check the agency's records for the names of other children with only vision disabilities and to check with early intervention programs in neighboring counties. She asks Bill if he is interested in the agency's support group, which includes parents of children with various disabilities. He responds negatively, saying he is interested only in talking with parents of children whose only disability is blindness.

Barbara talks with Mary about her need for babysitting. She tells her about a family aid program sponsored by another agency. This program provides free babysitting services for families of children with disabilities. Mary is very interested in learning more about the program, and Barbara promises to provide her with additional information. The action statements that result from this discussion are included in the service plan (Fig. 9.3).

The Velez Family: Preventing Neglect

This family consists of 3-month-old Amanda, who was just discharged from a neonatal intensive care unit; her 2-year-old brother, Raymond; her 4-year-old sister, Jessica; and her 21-year-old mother, Elena. Amanda was born prematurely and experienced a number of medical complications shortly after her birth. The social worker at the hospital was concerned, because Elena missed several appointments for the cardiopulmonary resuscitation (CPR) classes that were required prior to the baby's discharge and did not visit regularly while Amanda was in the hospital. As a result, the social worker referred the family to a family support program associated with the local child protective services agency.

OBSERVATION. Kate, the caseworker from the program, makes a home visit. She sees that the family lives in a cramped, sparsely furnished, two-bedroom apartment in a run-down building. She does not see any toys. The paint on the baby's crib is peeling. The older children are sitting at a kitchen table eating their break-

Family Section

Summary of Family Resources in Areas in Which Family Has No Concerns at Present

Area: Material Support	Resources: Mrs. Jones feels that she and her family are able to provide for Amy's needs. Bill is employed and contributes toward Amy's care.
Area:	Resources:
Area:	Resources:
Area:	Resources:

Area: Information

Family Resources: Mrs. Jones and Bill feel that they have a good understanding of Amy's developmental needs. They are always interested in learning ways to help her.

Family Concerns: Mrs. Jones and Bill would like information on child development and behavior of children with visual impairment.

Action Statements (steps to address concerns):

PROGRAM (WHO)	ACTION (WHAT)	FAMILY SATISFACTION (Initial)	COMMUNITY/PROGRAM RESOURCES	ANTICIPATED DATE	ACTUAL DATE
Ann will	Provide information on the development and behavior of children with visual impairments		Discussion Hand-Outs —Learning Together Chapter 5 —Guiding the Development of the Young Child with Visual Impairments —Ready, Set, Go —Daily Living Skills —Overbrook Series —Listening and Moving —Enhancing Orientation and Mobility —Developing Social Skills —Communication —Eating Skills —Learning to Move Around —Suggested Activities 24–36 months	10/93	

—Managing Behavior
24–36 months
—Managing Behavior

Area: Formal Support

Family Resources: Mrs. Jones and Bill have been satisfied with Amy's medical care and with the services provided by Beginnings. They are familiar with comunnity agencies and services and use these as needed.

Family Concerns: Bill would like to be kept informed of any special equiment that might be helpful to Amy. Mrs. Jones would like information on babysitting services.

Action statements (steps to address concerns):

PROGRAM (WHO)	ACTION (WHAT)	FAMILY SATISFACTION (Initial)	COMMUNITY/PROGRAM RESOURCES	ANTICIPATED DATE	ACTUAL DATE
Ann will	Continue to work with B.V.S. concerning Amy's special equipment needs.		B.V.S. contact: Sue Adams Phone: 555-2222	10/93 and ongoing	
Barbara will	Discuss options for babysitting services		Discussion A.R.C. Family Aide Program Contact: Kathy Galosi, A.R.C. Service Coordinator phone: 555-1511/ 555-6548 fees: none	10/93	

Area: Informal Support

Family Resources: Mrs. Jones and Bill feel that they have a supportive network of family members and friends. Bill and Mrs. Jones feel that things are going well for them and their family. Bill expects to have more time to spend with Amy after he graduates.

Family Concerns: Bill would like to have more contact with other parents of children with visual impairments.

Action statements (steps to address concerns):

PROGRAM (WHO)	ACTION (WHAT)	FAMILY SATISFACTION (Initial)	COMMUNITY/PROGRAM RESOURCES	ANTICIPATED DATE	ACTUAL DATE
Barbara will	Put Bill in contact with other parents		Discussion —United City-School District —Willowbrook School District —Regional School for the Blind	11/93	

Figure 9.3. Service plan for the Jones family. Revised from Darling & Baxter (1996) pp. 224–229. Reprinted with permission.

fast—cereal and milk. It is one o'clock in the afternoon, and they have just awakened. The baby is asleep. Elena looks as though she has been crying.

INTERVIEW. Kate asks Elena how the baby has been doing since she has been home. Elena says she is concerned because the baby cries for long periods of time and does not sleep very much. Kate asks Elena for some additional information about the family, including household composition and who cares for the baby. She learns that Elena lives alone with the children; Elena is the only caregiver.

Kate also asks other questions based on the Family Interview presented in Chapter 7 and learns that Elena comes from a large family. One of her sisters lives a few blocks away from her, but the rest of the family lives in another state.

Elena dropped out of high school in her senior year while she was pregnant with Jessica. She lived with Jessica's father, Joe, for a while and planned to marry him, but while she was pregnant with Raymond, Joe started seeing other women. They had arguments, which were sometimes violent. Elena says that her mother was not supportive, because "they didn't want me to live with Joe in the first place." As a result, Elena reports that she moved to the state where she currently resides to be near her sister, who paid her moving expenses.

Elena met Amanda's father, Mike, shortly after moving here. He was very nice to her at first and brought presents for her and the children. However, while she was pregnant with Amanda, her history started to repeat itself. Elena and Mike argued often. He would drink and become abusive. Elena says that she does not see Mike very often anymore and that he has no interest in Amanda; however, he made one of his infrequent visits the previous night.

Kate asks Elena about her resources. She learns that the family receives public assistance, and Elena's sister, who has a clerical job, helps them some, but "we still don't have enough to pay the bills." Elena's sister, Maria, also helps a little with babysitting, but she works full-time and has two school-aged children of her own, including one who is "hyperactive." Elena says she has no close friends. Her neighbors are "nice but have enough of their own problems." Elena does not have a car and relies on public transportation, although the nearest bus line is located almost a mile from her house.

Elena reports that Raymond and Jessica are healthy. Jessica goes to Head Start and really likes it. She says that Mike has never hurt the children but that they are scared when he hits her. She does not think they are in danger.

As for her own needs, Elena notes that she has some concerns relating to her health and to her ability to find a job when her public assistance payments end. She says that she has had intermittent bleeding since Amanda was born and that she always feels tired. When asked, she says she has no regular doctor for herself but has recently found a pediatrician she likes for the children, and he accepts the medical card. Kate asks whether she has any difficulty getting to medical appointments. Elena says she usually takes the bus, but that walking to the bus with three young children is not easy. Her concerns about finding a job relate to her lack of education and job experience and to finding child care.

Kate asks whether Elena needs anything for herself or the children. Elena says she could use a new crib; the one she got from a neighbor is not in good condition. She says she gets food stamps and help from WIC [Women, Infants, and Children Program] and usually has enough food in the house, "but we can't afford anything extra that the kids want." She says she does not need clothes for the baby—she has "hand-me-downs" from Jessica and her sister's children. She says she does not have enough money to buy the children toys. Elena says often throughout the interview that she wants the best for her children.

QUESTIONNAIRES. Kate asks Elena whether she would like to complete a checklist of concerns designed for parents of young children "in case there's something I forgot to ask you about," but Elena declines. The intake worker has told Kate that Elena seemed to have difficulty with the intake forms and did not seem to be able to read very well. Kate does not try to get Elena to complete the form.

Because she hopes to help Elena acquire some toys for the children, Kate would like to use the toy checklist section of the HOME Screening Questionnaire (JFK Child Development Center, 1981) to determine the kinds of age-appropriate toys that are needed. She offers to read the checklist to Elena and Elena accepts her offer. The results confirm that the family does not have most of the items on the list. The only appropriate toys that Elena has for Amanda are a few rattles.

DEVELOPING ACTION STATEMENTS. After reviewing all the information that has been gathered, Elena and Kate list the family's resources, concerns, and priorities. Their list is included here as Table 9.2.

Based on this list, the following action statements are included in a written plan for the family:

1. Kate will immediately make a referral to the public health nurse, who will make home visits to provide information and support to Elena regarding Amanda's care and development. (formal support)

Because of Elena's apparent difficulty with printed material, modeling and discussion appear to be better in this case than booklets, handouts, and library references.

2. Kate will make a referral to the free babysitting program provided by the family center. (formal support)

This program provides up to 10 hours of free babysitting each week to families believed to be at-risk for child abuse or neglect. Elena could use this service while she attended to her own medical needs or could use it for one or more of the children while attending to the needs of the others.

3. Kate will give Elena a list of family doctors and OB-GYN specialists who accept the medical card and are easily accessible with public transportation. (information, formal support)
4. Kate will give Elena information about the support group for abused women and the children's counseling services offered by the Women's Help Center. (formal support)

During their discussion, Elena indicated to Kate that she did not want her to make a referral; she wanted the information so she could call and get help "when she needed it." If the children *were being abused, Kate would have*

Table 9.2. The Velez Family's Resources, Concerns, and Priorities in Various Areas

Area	Resources	Concerns
Information	Elena knows about child development in general, because she has two older children Elena knows the rules relating to the receipt of public assistance and some other services	Elena would like more information about the development of premature babies
Informal support	Elena's sister helps with babysitting when she can Jessica and Raymond are healthy Elena wants the best for her children	Elena is concerned about the effect of Mike's violence on the children
Formal support	Elena is satisfied with the children's medical care Jessica is enrolled in Head Start Elena is interested in learning more about agencies that can help the family	Elena would like medical care for herself Elena would like more help with child care Elena would like to find a program that would help improve her job skills
Material support	The family receives support through public assistance and WIC and some help from her sister and neighbors The children have enough clothes and have some toys The family has limited access to public transportation	Elena would like a new crib and more toys for the children Elena is concerned because her public assistance benefits will be ending in a few years

Priority: Help in caring for Amanda.

an ethical (and probably legal) obligation to report the situation to children's protective services. In the current circumstances, however, a partnership approach would dictate that she respect Elena's decision. She will continue to work closely with Elena and encourage her to seek help for the children if necessary. Such situations always involve a delicate balance between respecting a family's privacy and doing what the professional considers to be best for the children.

5. Kate will assist Elena in locating a crib at the Salvation Army store or another thrift shop. (material support)
6. Kate will review the family center's toy lending library list with Elena and will bring to the home the toys that Elena selects. (material support)
7. Kate will provide Elena with information about GED and job skills training programs. (information)

Michael King: Creating a Future for a Young Offender

Michael King is a 17-year-old who recently was released from a juvenile correctional facility, where he had been sent at the age of 15 as a result of participating in an armed robbery. John, his probation officer, makes a home visit.

OBSERVATION. Michael's home is located in a city housing project. The family, which consists of Michael, his mother Linda, his brother George, age 14, and his sister Tonya, age 8, occupies a three-bedroom apartment. The apartment is clean and well furnished. At the time of the early evening visit, Linda has just returned from work, and the children are watching television. John talks with Linda in the kitchen for awhile; then he and Michael have a private conversation in a bedroom. Both Linda and Michael are polite and seem receptive to any assistance that John may be able to provide.

INTERVIEW. Because Michael's life situation involves his family, John interviews Linda as well as Michael, his client. These interviews cover the time period from before Michael's arrest to the present. John asks questions about Michael's plans for the future and about resources and concerns relating to those plans.

Linda reports that she works as a nurse's aide in a hospital. She has been taking college courses and expects to graduate in a year. She is divorced from the children's father, who, she says, does not see the children very often and does not contribute to their support. She has relied on Michael and George to watch Tonya after school. Both boys were in day care until they were 12 and are no longer eligible for a subsidized child care program.

Linda reports that George and Tonya seem to be doing well. However, she is concerned that George may follow in his brother's footsteps. She says that she is unhappy about the children being alone after school. She often works late, and her college courses are in the evening. She says she needs the degree to be a better provider for her children. She also would like to be able to move out of the projects. She says that she has few friends there and that the environment is dangerous for the children. When John asks her whether she can count on anyone to help with the children, she says, "No."

Linda is very concerned about Michael. He was a good student when he was younger, but got involved with friends who were a "bad influence" when he was around 12 and started skipping school. She took him to a counselor for awhile, "but it didn't do any good." She says that she has no control over Michael and is afraid that he will get into trouble again.

Michael says that he wants to go back to school, but his school will not admit him because of his record. He says his mother does not want him to go to a special school for juvenile offenders, because she is afraid that the other students will be a bad influence on him. As a result, mostly he has been staying home watching television since his release from the correctional facility. He says he is trying to stay away from his old friends.

Michael reports that he started skipping school and stealing because "school was boring" and "I needed the money to buy things." He says he started carrying a gun after he was robbed by some older boys from his neighborhood. At first, he wanted the gun for protection, but then his friends convinced him to use it to steal. He says he had successfully robbed a pizza delivery man and a grocery store before he was caught. He has a girlfriend and says he spent most of the money he stole on her. He has seen her a few times since coming home but is concerned because he cannot afford to take her out or buy her anything.

Michael says he feels bad about disappointing his mother. He is proud of her for going to college and he wants her to be proud of him. He says he also wants to be a good model for his brother. Michael says he has no respect for his father and has no interest in seeing him. He says that no other adults are regularly involved in his life and that he might be interested in getting to know an adult with whom he could talk about his concerns.

John asks Michael what he likes to do for fun, and Michael says he likes to watch television and used to like to play basketball. When John asks about his favorite subjects at school, Michael says he likes math and was pretty good at it when he was younger. He says he had thought about becoming an accountant but is no longer sure about what he would like to do in the future.

QUESTIONNAIRES. John asks Michael to complete a checklist developed by the local family center, which includes a variety of activities and interests. This checklist will be useful in connecting Michael with programs that might interest him and allow Michael to choose activities of interest on his own.

According to Michael's completed form (Fig, 9.4), he is very interested in playing basketball, getting a part-time job, and learning about different jobs. He also may be interested in playing a musical instrument, helping other kids with their schoolwork, playing pool, learning about computers, and playing baseball.

Developing Action Statements. John works with both Michael and Linda to develop a written plan. The following action statements are written for Michael and the other children:

1. John will talk with the principal of Michael's old school about the possibility of placement in other city schools. (formal support)
2. John will talk with the Alternative Education Office at the city school district about the school placement possibilities for Michael. (formal support)
3. John will give Linda and Michael information about the Big Brothers/Big Sisters program. (formal support)
4. John will introduce Michael to the youth director at the Arlington Street Family Center and tell him about Michael's interests. (information, formal support, informal support, material support)
5. If the family center cannot help Michael find a part-time job, John will give him information about the job service at the City Employment Center. (information, material support)
6. John will provide information to Linda about after-school programs at the family center that may interest George and Tonya. (information, formal support, informal support)

Locating Resources and Creating Opportunities

As the above examples illustrate, writing a plan involves knowledge about community resources. In order to expand clients' opportunity structures, professionals need to be familiar with existing programs and services. In addition, they need to have the skills to create new resources when existing services are not sufficient to address their clients' concerns. Intervention, then, can take any of the following forms:

1. The professional can assist clients in *recognizing* resources and opportunities they already have. For example, an early intervention teacher can demonstrate how to make homemade toys from materials already in the home.
2. The professional can assist clients in *discovering* opportunities that already exist. For example, an eligible family can be made aware of government benefits such as food stamps or Supplemental Security Income (SSI).
3. The professional can assist clients in *creating* new opportunities. Commonly described as advocacy, this activity may involve calling

Arlington Street Family Center Interest Survey

The following list includes activities that sometimes interest people your age. You may be interested in most of the activities or only a few of them. Please indicate which ones interest you by checking (✓) the column next to each item that best describes your interest.

	I am definitely interested in this activity and would like to know more about doing it at the Center.	I might be interested in this activity. I'm not sure.	I am not interested this activity.
1. Playing basketball	✓		
2. Playing a musical instrument		✓	
3. Playing chess			✓
4. Getting help with my schoolwork			✓
5. Helping other kids with their schoolwork		✓	
6. Cooking			✓
7. Taking care of babies			✓
8. Getting a part-time job	✓		
9. Writing stories or poems			✓
10. Helping to take care of younger kids			✓
11. Playing pool		✓	
12. Drawing and painting			✓
13. Learning about different jobs	✓		
14. Playing baseball		✓	
15. Reading			✓
16. Learning about computers		✓	

17. Other things I like to do (Please list activities not included in the list above):

Figure 9.4. Instrument for the identification of interests.

legislators or organizing a demonstration at the State Capitol. Or it may simply involve talking with the director of a local agency about the need to create a new program.

In order to be a resource for clients, then, the professional needs to become as knowledgeable as possible about (1) opportunities that already exist and (2) methods for creating new opportunities.

Locating Existing Opportunities

Mobilizing Informal Supports

As noted in Chapter 5, most clients are embedded in networks of family, friends, neighbors, co-workers, and fellow church members. These relationships can be organized to provide assistance to clients in need, as the examples in the following paragraphs illustrate.

Halley et al. (1992) describe the Member-Organized Resource Exchange in St. Louis. This project, organized by a group of neighborhood centers, has compiled a computerized database of residents' skills, such as child care, carpentry, and other services. Co-ops also have been formed to meet the food and clothing needs of neighborhood residents. The project trains residents to operate the computers used to link people with needed services.

Similarly, O'Looney (1996) describes an information system tool that would maintain a database of community residents' skills, talents, interests, hobbies, willingness to volunteer, needs, pay requirements (e.g., in money or in "time dollars"), business and other experiences, and civic group associations that could be accessed by other members of the community and by human services staff who are in search of resources. In addition, the tool would maintain a database of civic associations and would match families with others who can provide desired goods or services.

Capossela and Warnock (1997) describe how a group of friends was organized by a professional to aid a woman who was dying of cancer. The friends took turns providing transportation and support for medical visits, keeping track of medications, and even arranging a wedding. Once organized, the group remained together to assist one another in times of need. Such a group can be especially important when clients live far from their families. Schwartz (1997) has described similar efforts to engage community members in helping one another.

Not all instances of informal support mobilization are as complex as these. Parents in many neighborhoods have gotten together to provide play groups or child care for each other's children, and churches have a long history of providing services and material assistance to their members. In my community, a group calling itself MOPs (mothers of preschool children) meets regularly for mutual support. Often such groups are organized without any assistance from professionals.

Sometimes, professionals need only make a suggestion to clients who are empowered to act on their own. Other times, professionals may want to suggest the inclusion of organizational assistance on a service plan.

Developing a Directory of Formal Supports

In addition to databases of informal supports such as those described above, directories and databases of formal supports should be included in agency resource libraries. Many communities maintain published directories of local agencies, including contact information and brief descriptions of the goods and/or services they provide. In addition to keeping a copy of such a directory on hand, agency staff should schedule visits to other agencies to learn firsthand what they provide and to meet staff who may serve as contacts for future referrals. Most communities have consortiums of human service agencies that meet on a regular basis. These meetings provide an opportunity for networking, learning about existing services, and forming partnerships for the creation of new resources.

Agencies also may want to include in their resource libraries information about services available in other geographic areas or through the Internet. For example, agencies serving individuals with disabilities may need to look outside their own communities to link their clients with others with similar disabilities. Services such as information and advocacy also may be available from state or national organizations.

A resource library can be organized in a variety of ways. One method that works well is to organize information according to categories taken from the instruments used by the agency for the identification of client concerns. For example, in the agency I directed, categories were based on the Parent Needs Survey discussed in Chapter 8, and files were established under headings such as information about childcare, information about specific disabilities, information about public transportation, and so forth.

Regardless of the categories selected, typical information that might be included in a resource library is suggested by the following list:

- Lists of medical/dental providers (including information about whether they accept Medical Assistance or other forms of insurance)
- Lists of landlords, shelters, and housing authority programs
- Bus schedules
- Lists of child care providers
- Lists of mental health counselors and family therapists
- Lists of summer camp programs and playgrounds
- Information about and catalogs from companies that produce special equipment for people with disabilities

- Lists of support groups
- Information about loan programs
- Lists of food banks
- Lists of thrift shops
- Lists of church programs
- Lists of neighborhood associations
- Information about government benefits, including WIC, SSI, energy assistance, Section 8 housing, TANF, social security, veterans' benefits, and so on
- Information about legal aid services
- Lists of advocacy organizations
- Contact information for state and federal legislators
- Lists of school guidance counselors and social workers
- Lists of nursery schools and preschool programs
- Lists of programs for older adults
- Lists of recreational programs, Scout troops, teen drop-in centers, and so on.
- Books written by and about individuals with conditions or in situations similar to those of clients served by the agency (e.g., books about children with disabilities)
- Subscriptions to periodicals for individuals like agency clients (e.g., *Exceptional Parent* magazine, *The Disability Rag*)
- Pamphlets and fact sheets about issues of client concern
- Subscriptions to newsletters from relevant organizations
- Information about Internet discussion and support lists and web pages
- Information from similar agencies in other communities and statewide associations.

Creating New Opportunities

Sometimes, existing resources are insufficient to address client concerns or existing opportunities are inequitably distributed, resulting in unequal access for clients. In such situations, practitioners have an obligation to expand their clients' opportunity structures by working to create new resources or to reallocate existing ones. Intervention by human service professionals can occur on two levels: individual or group *advocacy* or *social change*. Advocacy involves microlevel interventions in response to client concerns that are unique or community specific. Social change involves meso- or macrolevel interventions that address concerns that are shared by many individuals or groups. Advocacy will be discussed here, and social change will be addressed in Chapter 10.

Client advocacy can take two forms: (1) client empowerment techniques, including the provision of information about lobbying, and (2) acting on behalf of a client. Each will be discussed in turn.

Client Empowerment Techniques

As noted in previous chapters, human service clients often come from the segments of society with the least power, including the poor, people with disabilities, and members of racial and ethnic minority groups. As a result, they do not always have the skills or resources to get what they need from the "system." Professionals can provide a valuable service by educating them and facilitating their access to those in positions of authority.

Clients who have not had higher levels of education may need assistance with their letter-writing skills. In order to gain access to opportunities, they may need to write to the principal or teacher at their children's school, to the director of a local human service agency, or to their legislator. Instructing clients in the following pointers on writing effective letters (Pennsylvania Partnerships for Children, 1997) may be helpful:

- Be informed. Understand the pros and cons of the specific issue in question.
- Be positive and constructive. Thank the person to whom you are writing for any past assistance.
- Include favorable articles and editorials from local newspapers.
- Write legibly. Handwritten letters are fine.
- Make your letters personal. Include pictures when appropriate.
- Be brief and to the point. Limit the subject matter to a single issue.
- Be persistent. Write again if your first attempt is unsuccessful.

SUGGESTED EXERCISE. Your client, Mrs. Smith, is concerned because her child, John, is not doing well in school. John is in the fifth grade and until this year got all As and Bs. Mrs. Smith says that John doesn't like his teacher. He says that she likes the girls in the class but "picks on" the boys. Mrs. Smith tried calling the teacher, but the teacher, Mrs. Jones, just blamed John and said he was lazy. You suggest that Mrs. Smith write a letter to the principal, but she says she does not know what to say (she has only a tenth grade education herself). How would you help Mrs. Smith write a letter?

In addition to assistance with letter writing, clients may want advice regarding telephone calls or in-person visits to persons in positions of authority. With clients who have not been empowered, professionals first may need to convince them that they have the *right* to advocate for themselves. Sometimes providing contact information for consumer advocacy groups, such as the Alliance for the Mentally Ill or the National Union of the Homeless, is helpful. Representatives of these groups can provide success stories about people in similar circumstances who have gotten what they needed, along with information about techniques that have worked for others.

Acting as an Advocate

Because of their lack of status, power, and/or education, clients are not always successful when they act on their own behalf. Moreover, coping with the stresses of poverty, disability, or other personal problems may leave little time or energy for effective advocacy. In such situations, clients may want professionals to assist with their advocacy efforts or to advocate for them. As Biehal (reported in Bateman, 1995) has explained,

> Welfare users are not equivalent to consumers in the world of commerce. They include some of the most powerless and stigmatized members of society. For some, ill health, frailty or disability may further hamper their ability to "shop around" and make untrammelled choices in a marketplace of care services. (p. 21)

Thus, in some cases professionals may want to accompany their clients to legislators' offices, school conferences, hospital specialty clinics, or meetings with agency representatives. Such situations are typically intimidating for clients, especially when the client is outnumbered by a "team" of professionals or "outclassed" by a higher-status professional who appears to be more knowledgeable than the client. (Situations involving difficult client–professional interactions are discussed further in Chapters 3, 4, and 5.)

In order to be most helpful to clients, professionals will need to be familiar with the laws and regulations that apply in the situations their clients face. These might include laws relating to eviction, school attendance, domestic violence, or other areas. Certainly, human service practitioners cannot be expected to be legal experts. Although they should have basic familiarity with the laws that apply most commonly to their clients, they should maintain access to legal services provided by agency or Legal Aid attorneys and by advocacy organizations.

The following example of successful advocacy, based on an actual situation, is illustrative:

> Ellen was a 5-year-old child with spina bifida. In kindergarten she was in an inclusive classroom with children without disabilities and had been successful in that setting. At the end of the year, Ellen's mother attended a conference with the kindergarten teacher and school principal. They recommended that Ellen be placed in a segregated (for children with disabilities) classroom in the first grade. Ellen's mother wanted her daughter in an inclusive first-grade classroom and called a caseworker who knew the family to ask for help. The caseworker suggested they set up another meeting with school officials to try to understand the basis for the placement recommendation.
>
> At the meeting, the principal mentioned that all nonsegregated first-grade classrooms were on the second floor. The school building was old and did not have an elevator; Ellen used a wheelchair. Everyone agreed that Ellen would probably do well in a nonsegregated classroom.
>
> Following the meeting, the caseworker called the local chapter of the Spina Bifida Association of America to inquire about Ellen's legal rights. She learned that under the Individual with Disabilities Education Act Ellen was entitled to a "free, appropriate, public education" in the "least restrictive environment." The caseworker shared this

information with Ellen's mother, who said, "I know there's a law, but you can't ask the school to move their classrooms." "Why not?" the caseworker asked. Ellen's mother replied that she was afraid of being "too pushy," because the school might "take it out on Ellen." She asked the caseworker to call the school on her behalf.

The caseworker called the principal and told her what she had learned about the law. She also mentioned the law's provision for a due process hearing if the issue could not be resolved. The principal reluctantly agreed to move one of the inclusive first-grade classrooms to the first floor.

The goal of advocacy is to expand clients' opportunity structures. In the case cited above, a law already existed to protect Ellen's rights. The caseworker's advocacy efforts enabled Ellen to take advantage of the law by creating a change in her social structure (the school). The resulting change also may incidentally have benefited other children with disabilities. However, advocacy on an individual or microlevel does not necessarily help anyone other than the client in question. Chances are that the parent of a younger child with spina bifida entering the first grade in a few years might find that the inclusive classroom had been moved back to the second floor. Chapter 10 will address meso- and macrolevel initiatives that change social structures for larger groups.

Chapter Summary

This chapter addressed the next step in the provision of services after identification of a client's resources, concerns, and priorities. This step is usually called intervention. In human services, intervention at the individual or family (micro) level involves the development of a service plan. The chapter discussed the process of plan development and provided examples of action statements for clients in a variety of situations. Service plans may include activities of two types—those that help the client gain access to resources that already exist and those that create new resources. The creation of resources can involve advocacy on behalf of the client. Examples of advocacy activities, such as assistance with letter writing and talking to authority figures, were provided.

Suggestions for Further Reading

Bateman, N. (1995). *Advocacy skills: A handbook for human service professionals*. Brookfield, VT: Ashgate Publishing Company.

VanDenBerg, J, & Grealish, E.M. (1997). Finding families strengths: A multiple-choice test. *Reaching Today's Youth, The Community Circle of Caring Journal, 1(3) (http://www.air.org/cecp/wrap-around/articles.html).*

10

Social Change, Social Problems, and the Limits of Intervention

The last chapter explored intervention at the microlevel. Such intervention is appropriate when a client's concerns can be addressed with existing resources or with resources that can be created by changing the client's immediate opportunity structure. Sometimes, though, existing structures are inadequate to address a client's concerns. In some cases, changing a client's opportunity structure requires changing the opportunity structures of many individuals. In other cases, client concerns derive from problems in the structure of the larger society that require change on an even broader scale. This chapter will address both of these situations. First, the chapter will consider mesolevel intervention, or changing opportunities for groups of individuals with common concerns. Then, the case of changes that require the expansion of opportunities on a macrolevel—in society as a whole—will be addressed. Finally, the chapter will discuss the nature of social problems and its relation to the limits of human services.

Creating organizational change involves both internal and external activities. Before attempting to convince politicians, funders, and others with the power to change the service system of the need for change, activists need to be sure that others in their own agency, organization, or community are "on board." Erlich, Rothman, and Teresa (1999) note the importance of identifying key members of the organization, whose support will be needed. They also discuss strategies for gaining that support, including informal discussion and presentations at meetings. Generally, professionals who work for human service agencies will need to convince their supervisors and/or boards of directors of the value of their case before seeking support from external agents. Discussions with board members may either precede or follow a process of needs assessment, depending on the scope of the project.

Social Change I: Needs Assessment

When a client's localized or unique concerns cannot be addressed through existing resources, advocacy is an appropriate course of action. In some cases, however, concerns that cannot be addressed within existing systems are shared by many. In the example near the end of the last chapter, Ellen's needs could be met by moving a class to the first floor. In other cases, school officials have argued that the needs of children with disabilities could not be met at all within regular classrooms. During the 1970s, for example, many children with spina bifida were denied access to regular classrooms because of their need for clean intermittent catheterization, a relatively simple procedure that can be easily performed by a school nurse. As a result of action by several parents and their professional allies, the Supreme Court ruled that schools had to provide this service. Numerous children benefited from these actions.

In order to determine the appropriate course of action, then, professionals need to determine whether a client's concerns are shared by others. In other words, the professional needs to know whether the concern in question is a personal problem or a social problem. How can such a determination be made?

Sometimes, the professional is already aware of others with similar concerns. For example, when no adult day care services are available in a community, the professional may have a number of clients who are having difficulty caring for elderly family members. A few phone calls to other community agencies may confirm a widespread need.

In order to convince funders or legislators that such a need exists, however, professionals usually will need to gather supporting data. Various methods can be used to conduct a community needs assessment, including gathering and analyzing existing data, such as census reports, conducting surveys, convening focus groups, conducting interviews, and gathering anecdotal evidence.

Using Secondary Sources

Usually, existing demographic data are useful in demonstrating need. For example, an aging population can suggest a growing need for an adult day care center. Such data are available in government documents such as Census Bureau reports and vital statistics summaries. In addition, state and local departments of human services, health, welfare, and corrections usually maintain databases containing information about their clients. Various advocacy agencies, such as the Children's Defense Fund and its state-level equivalents, also publish reports containing information about child poverty rates, teen pregnancy rates, delinquency rates, and other statistics that can support a need for services in a given locality. Some universities also have research centers that support databases. In addition, local human service agencies and their state associations may collect information about past and current clients, including rates of service utilization and completion. As Porteous (1996, p. 40) notes, although existing data are readily available, they may "tell us little about [the] need beyond the fact that it appears to exist." Thus, some additional research is usually advisable.

Conducting Surveys

The principles of good questionnaire design in the identification of client concerns were discussed in Chapter 8. These principles also apply to large-scale surveys. For the purposes of community needs assessment, surveys are generally administered to a representative sample of the population. The population in question may be limited to the clients of one or more agencies or it may include everyone living in the target community. Using clients generally provides for a more manageable study but will not reveal the extent of need among people who are not already receiving services of any kind. Many research texts exist to instruct professionals in techniques for obtaining a random or probability sample of a given population (see, for example, Monette et al., 1998); these techniques will not be repeated here. Most surveys are conducted by mail or by telephone, although some are conducted in person. In-person surveys may be especially valuable in the case of potential human service clients who may not have telephone service or who are unable to read well. Because many localities already conduct community needs assessment surveys on a regular basis, professionals should contact their local human service departments before reinventing the wheel.

Convening Focus Groups

Focus group interviewing was discussed briefly in Chapter 7. Like other qualitative methods, focus group interviewing provides data in the participants' own words and can suggest a contextual basis for responses. In addition, as Porteous (1996, p. 37) notes, unlike interviews with individuals, focus group interviews "bring together different perspectives on issues and can generate new ideas and insights through the process of discussion and debate." This method has become increasingly popular in human services in recent years because of its relative ease and efficiency. Focus groups are generally based on *purposive* rather than probability sampling (Berkowitz, 1996) and involve fewer participants than surveys. For most human service purposes, groups of both service providers and service recipients or potential service recipients should be convened.

Conducting Interviews and Gathering Anecdotal Evidence

Although most funders like to see statistics to document a need for potential services, the inclusion of qualitative or anecdotal data serves to attach a "human face" to the numbers. Thus, most needs assessment studies can benefit from a small number of depth interviews (see Chapter 7) that will yield quotes from potential service users to supplement the tables and graphs produced from survey data.

The most common format for presenting the results of a needs assessment study designed to create social change is a grant application, although results often are presented in simple report form as well. Carter (1996) describes a commonly used format for such reports, which includes the following elements:

- Executive summary. A brief overview of the findings, usually less than five pages.
- Background. A description of the target population, the geographical area, and the reasons for the study.
- Methods. A description and rationale for the research and data analysis.
- Findings. A summary of the needs that were identified by the study.
- Recommendations. A discussion of services that could be developed to address the identified needs.

Further information on conducting needs assessments is available in many research methods texts.

Social Change II: Grant Proposals

After a need has been identified and its extent documented, funding for the establishment of a new service to address the need must be considered. The best way to begin a funding search usually is to contact the funders that currently support other agency services. Government funders and private donors and grantmakers who already provide support to an agency may be interested in extending their funding to a new service. If current funders are unable or unwilling to underwrite the cost, then new funding sources must be located.

Many books about grant writing are available (see, for example, Lauffer, 1997) and should be consulted by novice grant writers. Here, I will present only a brief overview of the process. The first step is to locate an appropriate request for proposals (RFP). The primary source for RFPs from the federal government is the *Catalog of Federal Domestic Assistance* (CFDA) (available from the Superintendent of Documents, Government Printing Office, Washington, DC 20402). Grant announcements also are published in the *Federal Register*. Although federal grants usually provide significant amounts of money, they tend to be highly competitive and to involve more paperwork than other grants. Smaller agencies are likely to have greater success in applying for grants from state and local governments and from private foundations.

The *Federal Register* has parallel, state-level publications (e.g., the *Pennsylvania Bulletin*). In addition, RFPs can be requested directly from the government agencies that issue them. Potential grant writers should make inquiries to appropriate officials. For example, practitioners in an agency seeking funding for a child abuse prevention program should get to know the people who develop proposals for the state office of children, youth, and families or its equivalent.

Private foundations also are a good source of potential funding for small agencies. Normally, foundations based in the same geographic area as the agency should be contacted first. Many locations have community foundations designed to support local programs. Local corporations and wealthy community residents also commonly sponsor services that are close to home. National foundation directories are available, but, as in the case of government grants, state-level directories (e.g., *Directory of Pennsylvania Foundations*) are sometimes more useful. These directories list funders by geographic location and provide information about funding interests and about projects that have recently been funded.

Hall (reported in Brody, 1991, p.47) suggests that those considering corporate support ask the following questions:

- Does the firm have significant business or employees in the community?
- Is the business related in any way to the type of project you are attempting?
- Does your organization deal with issues that are of unique importance to the firm?
- Would the firm gain a special benefit from being associated with the project, including publicity or visibility with key customers?
- Does the firm sell substantial products or services to your primary constituents?

Another important consideration in locating an RFP is the odds of success. Many federal RFPs generate hundreds of proposals but may fund fewer than ten. Because grant writing is labor intensive and time consuming, writers should concentrate their efforts on RFPs that offer a reasonable likelihood of success. Writers always should inquire about the number of proposals that are likely to be submitted, as well as the number likely to be funded.

Grantsmanship has been described as an art. Successful grant writers are not necessarily those who write the best proposals. Rather, grants are commonly the result of the cultivation of a relationship. Before responding to an RFP, a writer should make an appointment to talk with the funder, in person if possible. During their conversation, the writer should talk about identified needs and inquire about the funder's interests. Sometimes, the result will be a mismatch, and the writer will look elsewhere for funding. In other cases, though, the funder will express interest in the proposed project. At a grant-writing workshop I once attended, the presenter told us never to submit a proposal until we heard the "magic words" from the funder: "I am looking forward to seeing your proposal." Such conversations are usually most productive in the case of corporate and foundation funders. Government grantmakers may discourage or even prohibit personal contact.

Although RFPs vary from one funding source and grant to another, most proposals follow the same general format. Writers always should be careful to follow the format suggested by the RFP exactly; proposals may be disqualified for deviations, even minor deviations like exceeding the specified number of pages. The components of most proposals are as follows:

1. *Statement of the problem*. This section will be based on the needs assessment discussed earlier. Potential grant writers should maintain an updated file containing demographic data for their geographic area, newspaper clippings that document need, and the results of client satisfaction surveys, community needs assessment surveys, and focus group outcomes. In the grant proposal, information from this file will be used to demonstrate a need for funding. The problem statement should indicate both the extent of the identified need (that is, how many people might benefit from the proposed service) and the fact that current services available in the community are inadequate to meet the identified need. As noted earlier, both quantitative data (in the form of tables and graphs) and qualitative data (in the form of quotes from and anecdotes about potential service users) are important in documenting need.
2. *General goals*. This section should include outcome statements that make clear what the writer intends to accomplish with the grant money. Many funders prefer statements that include specific measures of accomplishment (e.g., "The child abuse rate in the county will be reduced by 50%," "At least 75% of program participants will be employed full-time by the end of the project"). In one funded proposal, this section was written as follows:

   The primary goal of this project is to prevent child abuse and neglect in families of at-risk infants and toddlers in Cambria County. This goal will be achieved through the following objectives:

   - To provide home-based education about normal infant and toddler development and parenting skills to the parents of 20 at-risk infants and toddlers each year.
   - To provide emotional support and referrals for other needed services to these parents.
   - To make developmentally appropriate toys available to all children in the program who need them.
   - To ensure that all children in the program receive ongoing medical care.

3. *Work plan*. In this section, the general goals are broken down into specific action steps. Usually, these steps are incorporated into a timetable. For example, the objectives above were broken down as follows:

   - Month 1: Hire and train child development specialist. Publicize the program in the community. Notify potential referral sources about the program and begin accepting referrals.
   - Months 2–12: Continue accepting referrals until 20 families have been enrolled in the program. Begin home visits (Child Development Specialist and Social Worker):

Identify family resources, concerns, and priorities; provide information; make referrals to cooperating pediatricians as needed; provide or make referrals for support.

- Months 2–36: Continue home visits according to the following schedule: (1) first 6 months after referral—once a week; (2) second 6 months to end of second year—twice a month; and (3) third year—once a month.

4. *Organization and personnel qualifications.* In this section, the writer must convince the funder that the organization sponsoring the proposed program is capable of carrying it out. The writer should provide information about the organization's history, including data on numbers of clients successfully served in the past. Funders also may want documentation of the organization's nonprofit status. In addition, the qualifications of the personnel who will be involved in the proposed project should be included. Usually, vitae or resumes are placed in the proposal's appendix rather than in the body of the document. For personnel who will be hired under the grant, job descriptions (including required qualifications) are included in the appendix in place of biographical information. Organizational charts help show the relationship of project personnel to one another and to others in the organization.
5. *Evaluation plan.* Normally, the proposal should include a discussion of a plan to evaluate the project. Program evaluation will be discussed in Chapter 11.
6. *Budget.* Writers should follow the format suggested by the RFP. Many grants require a local match, which should be reflected in the budget. Typically, the budget is accompanied by a narrative that explains and provides a rationale for the various items or categories.
7. *Appendix.* The appendix is sometimes the most important part of the proposal. In addition to the vitae and job descriptions noted above, the appendix usually also contains letters of support. Letters should be solicited from all collaborating agencies and possibly from referring agencies and government officials as well. For example, the child abuse prevention proposal quoted above included a letter from the pediatric social worker at the local hospital, who wrote about the need for a program where she could refer the many at-risk families she encountered in the neonatal intensive care nursery. The appendix also may contain agency licenses, certification of nonprofit status, or other required documents.

In addition to these required elements, good proposals usually

- Are written with the funder's priorities in mind.
- Do not include jargon or undefined acronyms.
- Are proofread and spell checked.
- Are well organized and easy to understand.

- Include references to the professional literature and bibliographic citations when appropriate.
- Propose projects that can be accomplished with assigned personnel only.
- Have budgets that correspond to their narratives.
- Have budgets sufficient to accomplish what is being proposed.
- Show collaboration among various community organizations when appropriate.

Social Change III: Community Organization and Political Action

The availability of RFPs to address client concerns implies that funders are already aware of those concerns or at least of the possibility of those concerns. Sometimes, though, identified concerns cannot be readily addressed by existing legislation or funding sources. In these cases, advocates may need to engage in political action or lobbying. Such action creates new, enabling legislation or increases funding based on existing legislation, which in turn can support services that address client concerns.

Because legislators are more likely to pay attention to large groups than to isolated individuals, lobbying sometimes initially takes the form of community organization. As Biklen (1974) has noted, service users may not be aware of others who share their concerns, or because of lack of resources, skills, or self-confidence they may not be able to readily contact others in similar situations. Thus, providers may need to facilitate bringing them together. Community organization has long been an important strand in sociological practice and in social work, and a number of instruction manuals in organizing techniques are available (see, for example, Kahn, 1982). The following case illustrates the value of organization in political action for social change.

Establishing A State-Level Entitlement for Early Intervention: The Case of Pennsylvania Act 212

In the mid-1980s, Congress passed PL 99-457, which provided for federal funding to states that established an entitlement for early intervention services for infants and toddlers with disabilities. At that time, some young children in Pennsylvania already received these services, but many more were on waiting lists. Legislators were reluctant to expand state funding for early intervention because of the cost involved.

In the mid-1980s, approximately 100 agencies were providing early intervention services in Pennsylvania, but most agency administrators knew only the administrators in surrounding counties. The families receiving these services and those on waiting lists were not organized at all. A few service providers recognized the need to get together and to begin talking to state legislators about the need for entitlement legislation.

With the help of information provided by some interested staff from the state Department of Public Welfare, a small group of service providers contacted all the other providers in the state. These providers held regional meetings, followed by a state meeting, at which the benefits of collaboration became clear. At the same time, other providers began talking with a sympathetic legislator, who agreed to write the enabling legislation.

After the bill was written, the service providers used their newly organized network to distribute information on talking to local legislators about supporting the bill. Families receiving services were urged to let their legislators know about the value of those services and those on waiting lists were encouraged to visit their legislators to share their concerns about insufficient funding for services. Every legislator in the state was contacted. Most received several visits from concerned parents, who brought their children or pictures of their children with them. Busloads of parents converged on the State Capitol to hold a rally for the bill. The local press and television stations were contacted, and the rally received good media coverage. The result of all this activity was that in 1990, during a time of fiscal restraint, the Pennsylvania legislature unanimously passed Act 212, which created a new entitlement program for infants and toddlers with disabilities.

Although a considerable amount of work was involved, organizing and empowering clients was relatively easy in the case just described, because the client population was essentially known. A large number of affected children were already receiving services, and many others were on waiting lists. Potential service users are not always so easy to locate. Many drug addicts and homeless people, for example, are not well known to community agencies. Organizers can work through existing organizations such as neighborhood associations, churches, unions, and grassroots groups and can hold community meetings, but potential service users are sometimes difficult to reach. Organizing is often a full-time job that is not included in the job descriptions of most human service practitioners.

The political action described in the case above also was relatively easy to implement because the legislator who wrote the bill was a strong ally. He was the chairperson of the state House Education Committee and was well respected by his colleagues in both parties. Political allies should be cultivated *before* specific legislation is needed. Local legislators should be invited to visit human service programs, and those who are sympathetic to various human service interests should be identified.

Although some policymakers may be predisposed toward a particular initiative, most initially lack at least some of the information they need to decide to support it. Richan (1991) suggests that the lobbying process is one of "modifying the audience's definition of the situation." He argues that the advocate needs to ask three questions:

1. What is the target's present focus of attention and what do I want it to be?
2. What are the target's presumptions about reality and how might I modify these?
3. What are the target's value preferences regarding this question and how can I connect my argument with those? (Richan, 1991, p. 95)

Moore (1991) notes a number of written and verbal formats that lobbyists can use, including testimony (before committees and special hearings), office visits to legislators, letters of support/opposition, press releases, and television and radio interviews. He suggests the following strategies:

- *Do not* inundate legislators and bureaucrats with too much information.
- *Do* synthesize technical information in an easily communicable fashion.
- *Do not* create sensationalism.
- *Do* include examples. Well-presented personal accounts humanize the rhetoric and the theoretical.
- *Do not* present supporting evidence that cannot be defended if its validity is questioned. *Credibility is essential to success* (Moore, 1991, pp. 84–85).

Additional strategies for meetings with policymakers include the following:

- Make an appointment.
- Go with a specific purpose.
- Prepare for the meeting.
- Always introduce yourself.
- Cover only one or two topics.
- Do not be argumentative.
- Expect questions.
- Leave a fact sheet.
- Thank the person for his or her time and courtesy.
- Follow up with a note later.
- Call or write with answers or information requested. (Guide to Citizen Education, 1995).

To some extent, then, human service practitioners can and should become involved in helping to bring about meso- and macrolevel change. In the Pennsylvania case cited above, the change involved the creation of additional services. Certainly, human service professionals have more expertise regarding the need for service expansion than most others in society; hence, their involvement in activities to expand services is both appropriate and necessary. (However, because of legal restrictons, professionals who work for publicly funded agencies may need to be careful about the sources of funds that support lobbying activities).

Another area in which such professionals should become involved in lobbying for change is in the redesign of service structures. Chapter 3 included an example of a child who was denied needed services because of the inflexibility of a bureaucratic system that judged her ineligible although she had genuine needs. Schorr (1997) cites numerous examples of human service agencies that have succeeded in creating alternative modes of service delivery that are more responsive to client needs. Redesigning national- and state-level service systems poses more of a challenge. Large, bureaucratic systems are well entrenched and are not readily amenable to change. However, some recent federal initiatives suggest that change is possible. Recent years have seen major initiatives in "reinventing government," that have included streamlining government bureaus and procedures and limiting the power of some federal agencies.

Chapter 2 presented many examples of service system reform. These included the development of new service models such as family centers and community policing. During the past decades, the human service system has been undergoing rapid changes in service delivery. Along with the movement toward a partnership approach, the organization of services has been moving toward more holistic and inclusive models that integrate diverse services within a single structure. In addition, services are becoming more universalistic and preventive, eliminating the need for eligibility determinations and labeling. These changes have occurred largely at the mesolevel, that is, in the organization of agencies and in statewide service systems.

The Limits of Human Services: Can Human Services Solve Social Problems?

The Relationship between Human Services and Social Problems

As the preceding sections have suggested, human service practitioners can intervene on various levels to help their clients. On a microlevel, they can assist in enhancing their clients' opportunity structures by helping their clients gain access to existing resources. When existing resources are insufficient to address identified concerns, practitioners may need to determine whether these concerns are shared by other clients or potential clients through a process of community needs assessment. When concerns are shared by many, intervention moves to a more mesolevel in the form of securing grants or shaping public policy. All these interventions, whether micro- or mesolevel, are based on an assumption that the concern in question is *well-defined, limited in scope*, and *able to be addressed through improved or expanded services.*

Unfortunately, many of the concerns facing human service clients today stem from social problems like poverty or racism that are broad in scope and not readily solved by traditional human service approaches. Kozol's (1995) description of an impoverished community in the South Bronx suggests the limits of human services as solutions to social problems:

> All the strategies and agencies and institutions needed to contain, control, and normalize a social plague—some of them severe, others exploitative, and some benign—are, it seems, being assembled: defensible stores, defensible parks, defensible entrances to housing projects, defensible schools where weapons-detectors are installed at the front doors and guards are posted, "drug-free zones" in front of the schools, "safety corridors" between the schools and nearby subway stations, "grieving rooms" in some of the schools where students have a place to mourn the friends who do not make it safely through the "safety corridors," a large and crowded criminal court and the enormous new court complex now under construction, an old reform school (Spofford) and the new, much larger juvenile prison being built on St. Ann's Avenue, an adult prison, a prison barge, a projected kitchen to prepackage prison meals, a projected high school to train kids to work in prisons and in other crime-related areas, the two symmetrical prostitute strolls, one to the east, one to the west, and counseling and condom distribution to protect the prostitutes from spreading or contracting AIDS, services for grown-ups who already have contracted AIDS, services for children who have AIDS, services for children who have seen their mothers die of AIDS, services for men and women coming out of prison, services for children of the men and women who are still in prison, a welfare office to determine who is eligible for checks and check-cashing stores where residents can cash the checks, food stamp distribution and bodegas that accept the stamps at discount to enable mothers to buy cigarettes or diapers, 13 shelters, 12 soup kitchens, 11 free food pantries, perhaps someday an "empowerment zone," or "enterprise zone," or some other kind of business zone to generate some jobs for a small fraction of the people who reside here: all the pieces of the perfectible ghetto. . . .
>
> All these strategies and services are needed—all these and hundreds more—if our society intends to keep on placing those it sees as unclean in the unclean places. (pp. 135–136)

In the same vein, the eminent American sociologist, C. Wright Mills (1959) distinguished between "private troubles" and "public issues":

> *Troubles* occur within the character of the individual and within the range of his immediate relations with others; they have to do with his self and with those limited areas of social life of which he is directly and personally aware. . . .
>
> *Issues* have to do with matters that transcend these local environments of the individual and the range of his inner life. They have to do with the organization of many such milieux into the institutions of an historical society as a whole, with the ways in which various milieux overlap and interpenetrate to form the larger structure of social and historical life. (p. 8)

Mills (1959) illustrates this distinction using a number of examples, including the following:

> In these terms, consider unemployment. When, in a city of 100,000, only one man is unemployed, that is his personal trouble, and for its relief we properly look to the character of the man, his skills, and his immediate opportunities. But when in a nation of 50 million employees, 15 million men are unemployed, that is an issue, and we may not hope to find its solution within the range of opportunities open to any one individual. The very structure of opportunities has collapsed. . . .
>
> In so far as an economy is so arranged that slumps occur, the problem of unemployment becomes incapable of personal solution. In so far as war is inherent in the nation–state system and in the uneven industrialization of the world, the ordinary individual in his restricted milieu will be powerless—with or without psychiatric aid—to solve the troubles this system or lack of system imposes on him. (pp. 9, 10)

Thus, social problems like widespread poverty derive from the structure of the larger society. Modern societies are characterized by an unequal distribution of political and economic power and unequal opportunities based on differences in class, race, and gender. Such inequalities can only be redressed by social change on a macrolevel that is beyond the scope of most human service work. Human services are structured to operate primarily at the microlevel and, to some extent, at the mesolevel. Human service practitioners usually cannot, at least within the confines of their agency positions, work to change the values and norms of the larger society.

The growing inequality between rich and poor in American society reflects a value system that favors individualism over communitarianism. Americans generally have been reluctant to pay higher taxes or to extend benefits to support those they perceive to be different from themselves (see, for example, Gans, 1995). On the other hand, in many European countries a high tax rate supports a variety of social programs that keep a large proportion of the population above the poverty level (see, for example, Bergmann, 1996). Thus, some macrolevel systems are more successful than others at reducing social problems.

Certainly, individuals *feel the effects* of these social problems and may seek assistance from human service agencies when public issues are manifested as private troubles. As Wood and Middleman (1989) have noted,

> The massive influence of poverty on human suffering, on social and health needs, can be appreciated by considering these figures from a report to the Joint Economic Committee of Congress: "for a 1% increase in umemployment over a period of one year, there are attributed 1,540 suicides, 5,320 state hospital admissions, 7,660 state prison admissions, 1,740 homicides, 870 deaths traced to cirrhosis of the liver, 26,440 deaths caused by cardiovascular and renal disease." (p. 5)

Thus, practitioners need to be skilled in locating the level of a problem's source. A background in sociology is essential to a complete understanding of human problems. Problems with microlevel causes can be addressed with traditional human service tools derived from both psychology and sociology and by the identification and intervention methods presented in this volume. However, these tools are insufficient to address problems whose macrolevel causes are not amenable to change through service-based intervention. Historically, large-scale social change has occurred as a result of social movements and revolutions, as well as in more evolutionary ways. Although the subject of broad social change is beyond the scope of this volume, it is addressed elsewhere in a large body of sociological literature. Of course, until large-scale change occurs, human service practitioners, especially those trained in counseling and psychology, can assist clients in coping with the effects of social inequality in their daily lives.

Human services, then, cannot compensate sufficiently for structural conditions that create or perpetuate macrolevel social problems. As Kozol (1995) suggested, no amount of services will change the nature of life in the South Bronx without fundamental changes in the way the residents of that community are viewed by others in society. On a microlevel, human service practitioners can help to expand the opportunity structures of individuals or even of entire communities. However, without major macrolevel changes in values and social structures, these practitioners cannot affect the overriding social conditions that limit the possibilities for opportunity expansion.

The problem of practitioner burnout, which has long plagued human service agencies, is caused by more than the low salaries in the field. Many caring practitioners become frustrated, because regardless of their best efforts many of their clients do not succeed. These practitioners are often idealistic individuals who unrealistically expect the provision of good services to solve social problems. Microlevel services cannot address macrolevel social problems. As a result, many clients remain in impoverished circumstances, even after years of receiving help. Similarly, many marriages fail, even after expert marriage counseling, because structural constraints (like public assistance policies that penalize couples, job markets that favor women, and gender-based expectations that create strains for women) make marriage undesirable as an institution. A better understanding of problem level might help burned out practitioners adapt more successfully to the limits of their work.

Although recognizing the limitations of human service practice is important, practitioners need to remember that many people are helped even by minor changes in their opportunity structures. Most agencies can cite a number of "success stories" of clients whose lives have changed as a result of services they received. One of my graduate students suggested the following analogy: The seas are filled with fog, rocks, and other dangers. Lighthouses do not eliminate those dangers, but they enable ships to steer safely through them. Human services, well provided, can help clients navigate the waters of their lives as successfully as possible.

The Process of Problem Analysis

In order to determine whether human services at any level can help a client, practitioners need to engage in a process of problem analysis. The components of this process and their relationships are presented in Fig. 10.1.

The process begins with the identification of a client's resources and concerns through the methods discussed in earlier chapters. After concerns have been identified, the practitioner needs to determine the level of causation. Microlevel concerns result from a lack of awareness of or lack of access to existing resources. Microlevel concerns can be addressed by providing information and referral, services, and advocacy. Mesolevel concerns are caused by gaps or problems in the service delivery system and are addressed by establishing new services or creating service system reform. Finally, macrolevel concerns are tied to socially structured inequalities in opportunity. These inequalities are not readily addressed through traditional human service means; rather, they require large-scale social change.

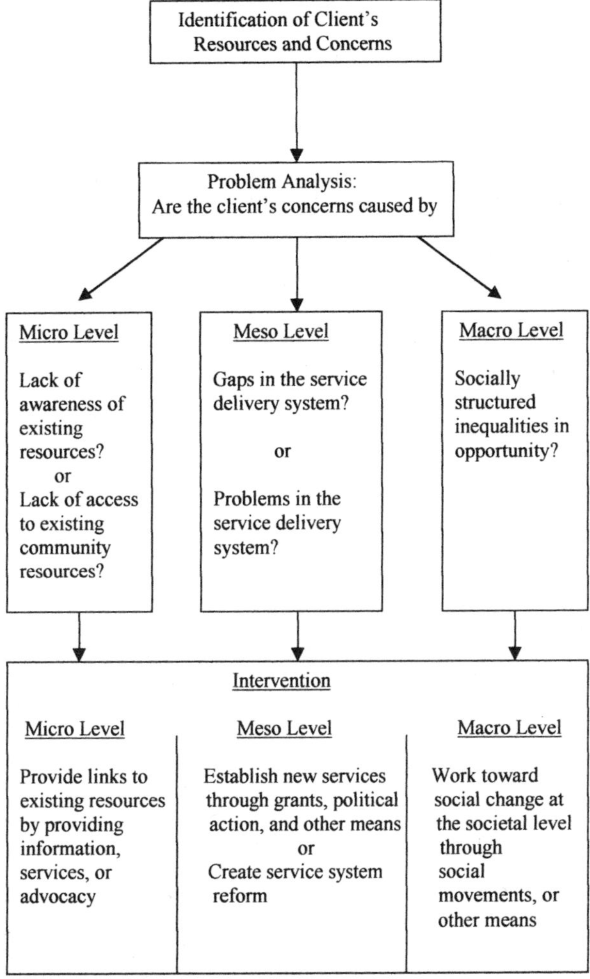

Figure 10.1. The process of problem analysis: Understanding levels of intervention.

Chapter Summary

This chapter shifted the focus of intervention in human services from the micro, or individual, to the meso- and macrolevels. First, the chapter addressed the situation in which many clients share a common concern and discussed using needs assessment techniques to determine the magnitude of the problem. Next, the chapter presented the process of grant writing as a means for addressing shared concerns. Political approaches based on community organization were suggested as strategies for increasing or improving services systemwide. Finally, the chapter explored the limits of human service practice using Mills's distinction between private troubles and public issues. Macrolevel public issues result from the differential allocation of opportunities in society, which has an impact on human service clients but is not amenable to change through traditional human service interventions.

Suggestions for Further Reading

Lauffer, A. (1997). *Grants, etc.* Thousand Oaks, CA: Sage.

Mills, C.W. (1959). *The sociological imagination.* New York: Oxford University Press.

Reviere, R., Berkowitz, S., Carter, C.C., & Ferguson, C.G. (Eds.). (1996). *Needs assessment: A creative and practical guide for social scientists.* Washington, DC: Taylor & Francis.

Richan, W.C. (1991). *Lobbying for social change.* New York: The Haworth Press.

11

Service Evaluation

The last two chapters presented intervention strategies based on the partnership approach that has been advocated throughout the volume. Regardless of the approach from which it derives, any intervention strategy should be continually evaluated to be sure that it is effective. "Effective" can have a variety of meanings. In much of the literature on program evaluation, effectiveness is professionally defined, and measures are based on change *in the client*, for example, increase in IQ score, having remained alcohol-free for a given period of time, or a lower stress score on a standardized instrument. Such measures may or may not be useful in a partnership approach.

In keeping with a partnership approach, evaluation measures must determine whether service outcomes reflect client-desired changes. In this chapter, I will review some of the literature on client-defined outcomes and will suggest some appropriate measures of these outcomes. In addition, I will discuss the relationship between service evaluation and program planning.

The Nature and Purposes of Evaluation Research

Definitions and Scope

Rossi and Freeman (1993, p.5) define evaluation as follows: "Evaluation research is the systematic application of social research procedures for assessing the conceptualization, design, implementation, and utility of social intervention programs." They suggest that *comprehensive* evaluations contain three components: (1) they relate to the conceptualization and design of the intervention, that is, they address the relationship between intervention outcomes and the needs assessment that prompted the intervention; (2) they monitor program implementation, that is, they determine whether the intervention occurred as intended; and (3) they assess program effectiveness and efficiency (benefits in relation to costs).

Rossi and Freeman (1993) use the term *impact* to describe the degree to which a program produces desired outcomes. They note the importance of having an impact model to explain how and why a program works; otherwise, outcomes may be the result of factors other than program interventions. Monitoring the process of service delivery is important for the same reason. Rossi and Freeman suggest that evaluation must be theory based. In other words, the evaluation process must relate to the intervention used in the program, which, in turn, is based on a theory of problem causation. Thus, evaluations of services based on a partnership model would need to look at variables like changes in clients' opportunity structures and definitions of the situation.

Rutman and Mowbray (1983) use the term *attribution* to describe impact. In addition, they suggest the importance of generalizability, or the extent to which the results of the evaluation are relevant for clients or situations other than those studied. Although generalizability is clearly important for research and replication purposes, it is probably less important in the partnership approach being advocated in this volume. Most partnership-centered practitioners would want to know whether or not their interventions have actually helped *their* clients.

Another distinction that is commonly made in evaluation research is that between *formative* and *summative* studies. Formative evaluation generally takes place relatively early in a program's implementation and helps to shape the process of service delivery. Monette et al. (1998) suggest that formative evaluation may include needs assessment as well as pretesting. Formative studies also can be conducted during the course of service delivery to determine whether intervention strategies are feasible or appropriate. For example, the implementation of a new service delivery procedure can be accompanied by a study to determine whether clients understand the procedure or find it acceptable. Summative evaluations, on the other hand, are intended to address impact, usually after services have been delivered for a given period of time. Summative evaluations are used to judge program success for purposes of funding or support.

Underlying Principles

Program evaluation has become a large and often profitable enterprise among researchers today. Funders concerned with effectiveness and efficiency have come to rely on evaluation studies to confirm the wisdom of their investments in programs. Some writers have expressed concern that the process of evaluation not be abstracted from the original purpose of human services, that is, helping clients. Shadish, Cook, and Leviton (1991) reiterate the importance of theory-based evaluation in this context:

> . . . the fundamental purpose of program evaluation theory is to specify feasible practices that evaluators can use to construct knowledge of the value of social programs that can be used to ameliorate the social problems to which programs are relevant. (p. 36)

They argue that evaluators should begin by asking the question, "What is the problem to which the intervention is a response?"

Patton (1997) also argues for a grounded approach, which he calls "utilization-focused evaluation." In this approach, the focus is on the evaluation's use by intended users, and evaluation becomes part of the service delivery process. Patton suggests the value of "participatory evaluation," in which the evaluator is a facilitator, collaborator, and resource, and the participants are the decision makers. Participants' perspectives and expertise are valued, much as they are in the partnership model of service delivery. Similarly, Stecher and Davis (1987) suggest that clients and staff are more likely to make use of findings if they have been involved in the evaluation process.

The *action research* perspective (Elden & Chisholm, 1993; Sussman, 1983) also promulgates a user-friendly approach to evaluation, based on the following principles (Darling & Baxter, 1996, pp. 257–258):

- The action evaluator rejects the idea that science can be "value neutral" and believes that the evaluation process is necessarily influenced by the evaluator's values and beliefs and conceptual framework.
- Problems are selected with a view to being resolved in accord with humanistic values, and these are openly stated at the outset. A concern for the perspective of less powerful groups, such as service users and lower-ranking workers in the service, is typically expressed by action evaluators.
- The aim is not only to extend knowledge, but also to solve problems.
- Evaluation using the action research method is change oriented, and its focus is on how organizations, agencies, and programs can function more responsibly and effectively in the interest of clients and workers.
- A basic assumption of program evaluation using the action research method is that ordinary participants in the operation of the program, including clients, can participate as partners in the evaluation using their own framework, language, categories, and other tools for understanding and explaining the work of the organization and their own attitudes toward it.
- Not only collaboration, but codetermination by groups within the organization, is required at all stages of the inquiry, including the analysis and interpretation of the data.
- While the major objective of action research is to identify and resolve problems, the major purpose of the participative process used is to educate and is designed to empower participants in this process.

The New Emphasis on Accountability

In these times of fiscal restraint, funders and other stakeholders have been demanding outcome measures that demonstrate that programs work (see, for example, Schorr, 1995). The terms *outcomes measurement* and *performance measurement* commonly have been used to describe the resulting processes (see, for example, Martin & Kettner, 1996; Mullen & Magnabosco, 1997). These processes derive, at least in part, from the "total quality management" (TQM) approach that has characterized business administration during past decades. This approach emphasizes improving the quality of outcomes while keeping costs down. A similar approach characterizes recent managed care initiatives in the health field.

Mullen and Magnabosco (1997) note, "Fundamental to the TQM . . . thinking is consumer/client/patient satisfaction" (p.xxxiv), and consumer satisfaction ratings are now typically required in health delivery systems. Similarly, Martin and Kettner (1996) note that the federal government increasingly has been using "service efforts and accomplishments" (SEA) reporting, with both quantity output measures, such as number of units of service and service completions, and quality measures, such as number of service completions with high consumer satisfaction.

Although the impetus for the recent interest in performance measurement may have been concerns about resource allocation, its implementation also can have positive consequences for service users. The emphases on client outcomes and client satisfaction can promote more client-centered service delivery approaches. On the other hand, the goal of cost containment may come into conflict with the principles of partnership-based practice. In managed care and similar approaches, services are typically standardized, so that all clients of a certain type receive similar treatments and are subject to the same expected outcomes. However, as earlier chapters have shown, clients' opportunity structures and definitions of the situation vary considerably, even though they may have been similarly labeled by the human service system. A "one-size-fits-all" approach cannot adequately address the diverse concerns of client populations. A challenge for human service administrators today is to maintain a balance between respecting their clients' autonomy and satisfying the efficiency concerns of their funding agencies.

Administrators who adopt a partnership approach need to be as accountable to their clients as they are to their funders. In some cases, client-desired outcomes may be the same as those required by funding agencies. For example, a drug treatment agency might be expected to produce low rates of relapse, and the voluntary clients of such an agency are also likely to want to remain drug free. In other cases, agencies may need to establish different sets of outcomes to address the concerns of both clients and funding agencies. The remainder of this chapter will be concerned with methods for the identification and measurement of outcomes from a partnership perspective.

Determining Outcomes

The Relation between Service Activities, Outputs, and Outcomes

Chapter 9 described the process of developing service plans. The purpose of such plans is to help clients achieve desired *outcomes*. Service plans include *action statements*, which are the activities that are intended to produce outcomes. The general outcome in partnership-based practice is an expanded opportunity structure or positive definition of the situation for the client. Some specific examples of outcome statements follow:

- John will be employed steadily for 1 year.
- The Jones family will obtain safe, affordable housing.
- Mary will be satisfied with the counseling services she receives.
- Tom and Sue will be satisfied with their child care arrangements.

Intermediate between activities and outcomes are *outputs*. These are the services that are actually received. For example, the following are some possible outputs that might lead to the outcomes listed above:

- John will be enrolled in a job training program.
- The Jones family will use the information provided by the homeless shelter to help them locate permanent housing.
- Mary will receive counseling services from the Family Guidance Center.
- With the help of the family center, Tom and Sue will organize a babysitting co-op in their neighborhood.

Thus, the relationship between action statements, outputs, and outcomes is as follows:

Action→Output→Outcome

If service plans are developed in accordance with the principles discussed in Chapter 9, they will include action statements based on goals and objectives proposed by clients rather than by professionals. The completion of these activities is an indicator of effective program functioning. Over time, programs should be able to demonstrate improvement in the percentage of plan activities that have been accomplished. Outcomes need to be measured in conjunction with a review of service plan activities; otherwise, their basis in the provision of services cannot be demonstrated. The purpose of action statements is to produce desired outcomes. Evaluation involves judgments about a cause–effect relationship between the actions of service providers and client outcomes. In order to evaluate program success, action statements on client service plans need to be translated into outputs and outcomes.

For example, Chapter 9 included a list of action statements for a woman using the services of a domestic violence shelter (see page 215). The following outputs might result from those actions:

1. The client obtains a Protection From Abuse (PFA) order.
2. The client finds an apartment.
3. The client is enrolled in the Temporary Assistance for Needy Families (TANF) program.

4. The client enrolls in a GED course and enters a job training program.

As a result of these actions and outputs, the following outcome may be achieved: *The client lives independently and no longer fears abuse from her husband.* This outcome is a status change, that is, an expanded opportunity structure. Status changes are indicators of program success. Intermediate outputs can be used as partial indicators of successful intervention but are not sufficient for demonstrating service effectiveness.

The outcomes chosen in any evaluation study are likely to reflect the point of view of one or more groups of stakeholders. In status inequality programs, the perspectives of the staff and administration may be different from that of the service users. However, as Mullen and Magnabosco (1997) have written, "The justification for human services must be found in their value to the actual and potential recipients of those services. Accordingly, community- and client-based outcomes measures should be the pivotal focus" (p. 318).

In keeping with the partnership focus of this volume, I will be concerned with outcomes that derive from the clients' definitions of the situation. Client-defined outcomes can take the form of satisfaction with services or status changes. The importance of client satisfaction relates directly to the centrality of the concept of definition of the situation. Status changes are important because of their relation to the concept of opportunity structure that has been stressed throughout the voume. These outcomes are discussed in greater depth in the following sections.

Satisfaction with Services

Today, human service agencies commonly conduct client satisfaction surveys at regular intervals, and client satisfaction is an important indicator of program success. Although they have limitations, these surveys can be used to demonstrate the appropriateness and value of human service programs. Martin and Kettner (1996, p. 42) suggest a number of dimensions of service quality that can be included in satisfaction measures:

- Accessibility—ease of access to services.
- Assurance—accessibility and knowledgeability of staff.
- Communication—ease of access to program information.
- Competency—technical ability of staff.
- Conformity—compliance of services with established standards.
- Courtesy—respectfulness toward clients.
- Deficiency—lack of some needed element.
- Durability—longevity of service results.
- Empathy—ability of staff to relate to and understand clients.
- Humaneness—protection of clients' dignity.

- Performance—accomplishment of intended purposes.
- Reliability—dependability of service provision.
- Responsiveness—timeliness of service provision.
- Security—safety of service setting.
- Tangibles—appropriateness of facilities and materials.

One study of service quality (Zeithaml, Parasuraman, & Berry, reported in Martin & Kettner, 1996) found that reliability, responsiveness, assurance, empathy, and tangibles were ranked in importance above other dimensions. Methods for constructing client satisfaction surveys based on these and other dimensions will be discussed later in this chapter.

Status Changes

Status changes represent expansions of a client's opportunity structure and can be measured in terms of decreases in concerns and increases in resources. Some indicators of change in resources for each of the areas discussed in Chapter 5 are presented below:

Area	**Indicators**
Information	Increased knowledge about services and access to resources; improved research skills
Material support	Increased family income; higher education level; improved housing type and stability; improved nutrition status; better access to transportation; improved access to food/clothing/employment opportunities
Informal support	Greater satisfaction with relationships; increased proximity to family; improved well-being of other family members; more relationships with friends and neighbors
Formal support	Greater use of services; improvement in health or well-being

The measurement of various indicators will be discussed later in this chapter.

Status changes involve a movement from one life situation to another. Rapp and Poertner (1992) argue that measures of status changes need to meet four criteria: (1) The list of possible statuses needs to be exhaustive, (2) the statuses need to be mutually exclusive, (3) the statuses should be hierarchically ordered from least desirable to most desirable, and (4) the measures need to be sensitive to change. They provide an example of a list of living arrangement statuses for clients with chronic mental illness (1992, pp. 118–119):

1. Psychiatric hospital ward
2. General hospital psychiatric ward

3. Nursing home or IC-MH
4. Emergency shelter
5. Adult foster care
6. Lives with relatives, is largely dependent
7. Group home
8. Halfway house
9. Boarding house
10. Lives with relatives, is largely independent
11. Supervised apartment program
12. Shares apartment, is capable of self-care
13. Lives alone or with spouse, is capable of self-care

In a partnership approach, *clients* would construct the list, based upon their desires and priorities.

One method for demonstrating program success based on status changes derived from service plan activities is *goal attainment scaling* (Pietrzak, Ramler, Renner, Ford, & Gilbert, 1990). An example of an outcome value scale would be the following:

- Most unfavorable outcome thought likely (–2)
- Less than expected success (-1)
- Expected level of success (0)
- Better than expected success (+1)
- Best anticipated success (+2).

Each plan outcome would be scored in this way, and a total score would be obtained for each client. Increases in the sum of total scores for all clients in a program would suggest program success.

One case example in Chapter 9 involved Michael King, a young man who needed a part-time job, and Michael's plan included actions to help him locate employment. (see p. 233) Using the scale above, possible actual outcomes could be scored as follows:

- Michael does not learn of any appropriate jobs. (–2)
- Michael has some job interviews but is not hired. (–1)
- Michael gets a job with limited hours and no possibility of advancement. (0)
- Michael gets a job that allows him to work as many hours as he wants but offers no possibility for advancement. (+1)
- Michael gets a job that allows him to work as many hours as he wants and provides training for career advancement. (+2)

A detailed discussion of score calculations and weighted scales can be found in Pietrzak et al. (1990).

Client- versus Agency-Level Outcomes

In a program evaluation study, outcomes need to be assessed for the program as a whole and not just for individual clients. Thus, evaluators will want to know what percentage of program clients are satisfied with the services they have received and what percentage of clients have experienced status changes and at what level. Changes in these percentages over time may be indicators of program improvement.

Agency-level evaluations also might look at whether the principles of a partnership approach are being incorporated into service provision. Records can be reviewed and clients and staff members can be observed and questioned to learn whether service plans are based on the clients' definitions of the situation rather than the professionals'. In addition, evaluators can explore the relationship between service plan activities and clients' stated concerns and between service outcomes and changes in clients' opportunity structures.

Such measures address whether microlevel interventions by agency personnel have been successful in expanding clients' opportunity structures and in promoting positive definitions of the situation. In the case of mesolevel activities such as grant writing and political action, the population in question may be larger than the clients currently being served by a particular agency. One way to assess the impact of such activities is by conducting a series of community needs assessments (see Chapter 10). If the needs in a community decrease after the establishment of a new service or the expansion of an old one, evaluators may be able to conclude that this mesolevel intervention has resulted in a communitywide status change. Many needs assessment instruments also address satisfaction with available services. An increase in satisfaction after the implementation of a new or expanded program also may be an indicator of success. The methods discussed below relate to both micro- and mesolevel evaluation studies.

Methods

As in the case of identifying client resources and concerns, the process of service evaluation can be conducted through either quantitative or qualitative methods. All the methods used in the identification process are also appropriate for use in service evaluation. As noted in earlier chapters, quantitative methods such as surveys tend to be more efficient and easier to administer. However, such methods are not as good at capturing meanings and contexts as more qualitative methods, such as participant observation and depth interviewing. Rodwell (1995) writes, "[In qualitative evaluation] maximum power remains with the participants, who shape not only the appropriate evaluation questions, but the evaluation results. The participants, particularly the families, remain in charge of the evaluation process" (p. 192).

Similarly, Wells and Freer (1994) suggest that service users may conceptualize outcomes very differently from providers and that qualitative methods are best suited to eliciting their conceptualizations. Further, they note that qualitative approaches can be valuable in explaining intervention failures. Even when evaluations indicate the overall success of programs, practitioners should be interested in understanding why services have not worked for some clients or for certain categories of clients.

Qualitative methods also are better suited to discovering unintended consequences of service provision. As Bruhn and Rebach (1996) suggest, interventions may have both intended and unintended outcomes. Evaluators need to be especially alert to negative "side effects" that program participation may entail. For example, a program that successfully empowers some family members may have the effect of "disempowering" other family members.

Guba and Lincoln (1989) also argue that various stakeholders are likely to have different definitions or constructions of program success. They suggest the method of "hermeneutic dialectic circles" as a means of understanding stakeholders' "claims, concerns, and issues." This method will be discussed shortly. Sluyter (1998) suggests that accepting the definitions of nonclient stakeholders can jeopardize positive outcomes for clients. He offers the example of a state legislator who supports an abusive staff member because he does not believe that his own corporal punishment as a child had a detrimental effect on his well-being. Because evaluators are typically paid by stakeholders other than clients, they may find themselves in situations in which acceptance of the clients' perspectives creates a conflict for them. Sometimes an appeal to the principles of total quality management discussed earlier can be helpful in convincing funders that quality in human services is "defined by the customer" (Martin, 1993).

Regardless of the method used, clients should be consulted in the process of designing evaluation instruments. They can be asked to suggest questions for interviews or satisfaction surveys; in addition, they may have preferences about the types of methods to be used. The discussion of method choice at the beginning of Chapter 9 is also relevant here. The following sections will review various qualitative and quantitative methods, including those discussed earlier in the volume, in terms of their value in judging program success.

Observation

Chapter 6 described observation techniques that could be used to identify clients' resources, concerns, and priorities for the purpose of service plan development. These techniques can be used in service evaluation as well. As noted in Chapter 6, the partner observer observes ongoing social processes without disrupting or imposing an outside point of view. Observations can occur in settings familiar to the service user, such as a home or workplace, or at a human service agency.

Who Should Observe?

Sometimes objectivity is enhanced if the observer is not the staff member who has been providing services to a client or family. However, an unknown observer may not be as welcome in a client's home or other setting, and the people being observed may be more guarded and may not act naturally in the presence of a stranger, especially a stranger in a judgment role. If outside observers are used, they should take the time to get to know the staff and clients before attempting to observe. Time also is important in understanding context and meaning.

What Should Be Observed?

In service evaluation, observations can focus on either of the outcomes discussed in the last section: satisfaction with services or client status changes based on the accomplishment of service plan activities.

SATISFACTION WITH SERVICES. The best situation for observing satisfaction with services is within the program setting. The observer can watch interactions between clients and staff in an attempt to answer the following questions:

- Do clients seem to be at ease, enthusiastic, and involved when interacting with program staff, or do they seem cautious, reticent, or hostile?
- Do clients keep service appointments and arrive on time?
- Do clients mention increases in resources or decreases in concerns as a result of service efforts?
- Do clients seem to like and respect the staff?

ACCOMPLISHMENT OF SERVICE PLAN ACTIVITIES. In addition to observing interactions, observers can, with permission from staff and clients, look at written agency records, including service plans. One method for record review is *content analysis*. In this method, categories or themes are elicited from the data and their frequency of occurrence is noted. For example, in one study of an early intervention program, an analysis of service plans revealed five major categories of concern: (1) information about the child's condition or disability, (2) information about the child's progress and development, (3) information about available services, (4) information regarding likely life-stage transitions, and (5) information about parent resources (Darling & Baxter, 1996, p. 266). Following this evaluation, the program expanded its resource library to better address these categories. Patton (1987) notes that a content analysis should be conducted by more than one person to assure uniformity of categories or themes. More quantitative methods, such as goal attainment scaling (described earlier in this chapter) also could be used in conjunction with observation of written records.

In general, in evaluating partnership-based programs, record reviewers should look for terms that suggest that services are client-driven rather than professional-driven. Some terms and phrases that suggest partnership include:

- Strengths
- Resources
- Concerns
- [The client] wants . . .
- [The client] is interested in . . .
- [The client] hopes . . .

On the other hand, phrases like "[The client] denies . . . ," "[The client] should . . . ," and "[The client] must . . . ," among others may suggest a status inequality approach.

Observation of service plans of course also can provide simple evidence about whether plan activities are being accomplished. Most plans provide (or should provide) space next to each action statement to indicate whether or not it has been accomplished. Sometimes the notation will be the date of accomplishment; other times, just the client's initials will appear. Thus, the evaluator can simply count the number of actions that have been completed and calculate the percentage of completed actions based on the total number written.

STATUS CHANGES. Just as a first home observation can provide information about the nature of a family's resources and concerns, a second observation can provide information about changes in resources and concerns. For example, at program entry, a home visit might reveal that a family has little furniture or other material resources. A follow-up visit that reveals a well-furnished home would suggest that the family's situation had improved. Many of the indicators noted earlier in this chapter in the areas of material support and informal support can be observed during both initial and follow-up home visits. Certainly, a family's situation can change for reasons other than program participation, but apparent improvement might be attributable to services received, especially when supported by other data (such as corresponding plan activities that have been noted as having been accomplished).

Interviewing

As indicated in Chapter 7, depth interviewing can provide a good understanding of a client's situation and definition of the situation. When used in service evaluation, depth interviewing can provide an equally good understanding of the impact of the program on the lives of clients and can suggest ways to improve service delivery. The following excerpt from an evaluation interview provides an indication of program success:

> Family B
>
> The main thing is having more help from my mother. [Interviewer says "How is that?"] She always used to avoid any contact with Allie, but Brenda (program worker) suggested that she be invited to come on one of the program days, and as soon as she saw what Brenda got her to do, there was no stopping her. She (mother) asked a lot of questions, and Brenda gave me a leaflet to give to her. It's been much better since then, and last week she even volunteered to have Allie for a weekend later in the month so that Bob and I can have a bit of a rest. I didn't want to, but Bob said we should and we should go to a movie like we used to. Mom says she will even pay for the movie. [Mother smiles broadly.] [Interviewer says, "So things are better with your mother now?"] Yes, we've always been a close family, but my mother was afraid to handle Allie; that's definitely changed. (Darling & Baxter, 1996, p. 274)

Interviews can be used to elicit information about both program satisfaction and changes in client status as a result of program participation. The nature of interviewing provides a basis for greater certainty about the link between service efforts and client outcomes than that provided by either observation or questionnaires.

Interviewing can be used either with individual clients, as in the example above, or with groups of clients. Just as focus group interviews can be useful in needs assessment (see Chapter 10), interviews with groups of service users can be useful in program evaluation. Evaluators can bring small groups together and ask questions like, "What do you like best about the services provided here?" or "What do you think we could do to make the services better?" Group interviews are less time-consuming than individual interviews, although some group members may be reluctant to speak openly and honestly in the presence of others.

Guba and Lincoln (1989) describe a group interview method they call hermeneutic dialectic circles to elicit the opinions of clients and other stakeholders. The method begins with individual interviews and progresses to a group interview in an attempt to obtain a consensual construction of reality. The first step in the process involves interviewing one member of a stakeholder group, in this case, a client. At the close of the interview, this client is asked to name another client "who feels very different from the way you do." At the close of this second interview, this client is asked to comment on the views that were stated by the first client and to nominate a third respondent. This last respondent presents his or her views and is then asked to react to the views of the first two respondents, and so on. The process continues until the comments become redundant or until two or more distinct and irreconcilable constructions emerge. The interviewer may then bring together all respondents and ask them to discuss their differences in an attempt to achieve consensus.

Such a process would probably work best in a program where clients were known to one another, such as a group home or a support group. In more individualized service situations, principles of confidentiality and the nature of service delivery would limit the ability of clients to suggest other respondents. The process could still be used in those situations, but respondents would have to be suggested by staff members, possibly biasing the results to suggest higher client satisfaction than actually exists.

Questionnaires

Measuring Status Changes

The survey methods described in Chapter 8 also can be used in service evaluation. Questionnaires commonly have been used in evaluation research from both the status inequality and partnership perspectives. Questionnaires based on a status inequality model have tended to be used to assess status changes in clients. Standardized instruments have been designed to measure changes in family functioning, child abuse potential, parenting skills, and other client characteristics. Questionnaires also have been used in partnership-based evaluations to measure changes in social support networks and other environmental resources. Many such instruments are described in Pecora et al. (1995).

In addition, partnership-based programs could assess status changes by asking clients to design instruments to measure changes in their level of functioning. Such instruments could be based on client-identified concerns and priorities discovered through the methods discussed in Chapters 6, 7, and 8. For example, the professionally defined purpose of a program might be to enhance child development through the improvement of parenting skills. However, a number of the program's clients may have priorities that relate to improvements in their access to material resources such as housing or transportation. A partnership-based evaluation instrument in this case would include items about access to these resources in addition to or instead of items about parenting skills.

Instruments designed for the identification of client concerns such as the Parent Needs Survey (see Chapter 8) also can be used in service evaluation. For example, in the program I administered, the Parent Needs Survey was used at intake and again at 6-month intervals until a client left the program. A comparison of these pre- and postservice administrations could be used to document changes in the number and intensity of parent concerns. Presumably, a successful program will result in a decrease in concerns. Thus, a sum of concerns at intake for all parents in the program can be obtained, and this sum can be compared with the comparable sum at various service intervals. The instrument also allows for weighted concern scores, because respondents choose from among three scaled alternatives that address the intensity of their concerns.

Measuring Client Satisfaction

Questionnaires also are the most commonly used method of assessing client satisfaction with program services. Satisfaction surveys are relatively easy to administer and analyze and can be distributed to large numbers of clients within a short period of time. However, as noted in Chapter 8, survey methods have some limitations, including client illiteracy and lack of contextual information, among others. In addition, questionnaires typically ask only about clients' satisfaction with existing services, which may be a poor indication of service quality or the need for additional or different services. Thus, evaluators might want to combine satisfaction surveys with other methods, including needs assessment techniques discussed in Chapter 10.

Some of the topics to be covered in a satisfaction survey were suggested earlier in this chapter and include communication, competency, and empathy, among others. Simeonsson (1988) also suggests the dimension of appropriateness. Services not only must be delivered well, they also must address the concerns of individual clients.

The principles of questionnaire design presented in Chapter 8 also apply to client satisfaction surveys. Rapp and Poertner (1992) suggest some additional principles that are especially applicable to surveys of this type:

- Avoid double negatives. (Do not use a question like "Did the counselor seem to dislike you?")
- Avoid response choices that inflate satisfaction. (People are more likely to choose "satisfied" than "dissatisfied" on a scale using those dimensions. "Agree/disagree" or "Never/all of the time" scales may be preferable.)
- Include both open-ended questions and space to explain answers to closed-ended questions.
- Pretest the scale.

Some of the dimensions of client satisfaction were suggested earlier in this chapter. Simeonsson (1988) argues that measures of satisfaction should at a minimum evaluate the following aspects:

- Communication
- Perceived competence of staff
- Quality and appropriateness of services
- Perceived empathy and sensitivity of staff

King, Morris, and Fitz-Gibbon (1987) make some good general suggestions for evaluating client satisfaction. They also suggest ways of determining whether clients believe that a program is based on partnership. Figure 11.1 shows a scale adapted from their suggestions for use in an early intervention program (Darling & Baxter, 1996, p. 279).

Rather than "reinventing the wheel," practitioners generally should look first for existing satisfaction surveys. Some instruments have been widely validated and can be adapted for a variety of programs. For example, Coulter (1997)

Family Consultation Questionnaire
IFSP/IEP Procedures Evaluation

The following are statements about whether families have been asked for their views and always consulted during the IFSP/IEP procedures. We are interested in knowing which statements you agree with and which you disagree with. For this reason we ask you to indicate, using the 1-to-4 scale after each statement, whether it was always true, generally true, seldom true, or never true. Please circle your answer and use the lines below the statement to make your own comments.

	ALWAYS TRUE 1	GENERALLY TRUE 2	SELDOM TRUE 3	NEVER TRUE 4
We were consulted about where the interviews would be held Comment:	1	2	3	4
We were consulted about who would be present at the family interview. Comment:	1	2	3	4
We were consulted about everything in the IFSP. Comment:	1	2	3	4
We were consulted about the program for our child. Comment:	1	2	3	4

Figure 11.1. Example of a scale to measure family satisfaction with a program. From Darling & Baxter (1996, p. 279), with permission.

describes the Patient Satisfaction Questionnaire (PSQ), which measures seven dimensions of care: (1) interpersonal manner of the provider, (2) technical quality, (3) accessibility and convenience, (4) finances, (5) efficacy and outcomes, (6) continuity of care, and (7) overall satisfaction.

Some surveys are designed to measure satisfaction with different services provided by the same agency. Figures 11.2 and 11.3 are examples of surveys of this type.

Quality Performance Measure

A Information and Referral

1. Overall, how satisfied are you with the information and referral program?

Very Dissatisfied				Very Satisfied
1	2	3	4	5

2. Do your contacts with the information and referral program result in referrals to agencies whose services you are eligible for?

Almost Never				Almost Always
1	2	3	4	5

3. When you call the information and referral program, do you usually get connected on the first attempt?

Almost Never				Almost Always
1	2	3	4	5

B. Home-Delivered Meals

1. Overall, how satisfied are you with the home-delivered meals program?

Very Dissatisfied				Very Satisfied
1	2	3	4	5

2. Do your home-delivered meals arrive hot?

Almost Never				Almost Always
1	2	3	4	5

3. Do your home-delivered meals arrive on time (within 10 minutes of scheduled delivery times)?

Almost Never				Almost Always
1	2	3	4	5

C. Counseling

1. Overall, how satisfied are you with the counseling program?

Very Dissatisfied				Very Satisfied
1	2	3	4	5

2. Do you see the same counselor each time you visit the agency?

Almost Never				Almost Always
1	2	3	4	5

3. Do your counseling sessions start on time (within 10 minutes of the scheduled time)?

Almost Never				Almost Always
1	2	3	4	5

Figure 11.2. Client Satisfaction Survey Questionnaire. From Martin & Kettner (1996, p. 49), with permission.

After checking all of the services received, say, "Now I'd like to ask you how satisfied you were with each service you received in the past year. After I read the service, please tell me if you were 'very satisfied', 'satisfied,' 'somewhat dissatisfied,' 'very dissatisfied,' or you had 'no particular feelings one way or the other.'" Now read the services the client reported using in the past year, marking the satisfaction rating with a '1' in the appropriate column.

Services	Ever received as a parent	Received in last year	Very satisfied	Satisfied	Somewhat dissatisfied	Very dissatisfied	No feelings
Family counseling							
Group counseling							
Individual counseling for you							
Individual counseling for one of your children							
Crisis center or "hot line"							
Day treatment							
Alcohol counseling							
Drug abuse counseling							
Psychiatric hospitalization							
School/social work counseling							
Homemaker service							
Youth club							
Big Brothers/Big Sisters							
Parent education class							
Support group, like AA							

Visiting nurse, public health nurse							
Free breakfast—lunch program at school							
Assistance in finding housing							
Emergency housing							
Job training							
Job finding through employment office							
Day care							
Health care at hospital or clinic							
Planned Parenthood/family planning							
Legal aid							
Food pantry/food giveaway							
Battered women's shelter							
Transportation							

From P. J. Peccra, M. W. Fraser, K. E. Nelson, J. McCroskey, & W. Meezan, Evaluating Family-Based Services. New York: Aldine DeGruyter, 1995, pp. 82–83, with permission.

Figure 11.3. Example of instrument to measure client satisfaction with services.

Some general questions that may be useful in client satisfaction surveys include the following:

- Would you recommend this program to a friend who had concerns like yours? Why or why not?
- In what way(s) do you think the program could be made better?
- What do you like best about the program?
- What do you like least about the program?

Although most satisfaction surveys are designed to be administered to clients, instruments designed to be completed by staff also can be used to address program quality. For example, staff can be questioned about their attitudes toward clients and service provision in order to determine whether they favor partnership or status inequality intervention styles. Some dimensions that could be addressed in such a questionnaire might include respect for the client's (vs. the professional's) definition of the situation (e.g., the statement, "Clients usually know what is best for themselves and their families," with an agree/disagree scale) or focus on system (vs. client) change (e.g., the statement, "Most of the time in human services clients are responsible for causing their own problems," with an agree/disagree scale).

Some Methodological Issues

The design of a program evaluation involves certain considerations about the process to be used. These considerations include decisions about the number of people to be studied, whether or not to use an experimental design, the method or method combination to use, and the reliability and validity of the results.

Group versus Single-Subject Designs and the Issue of Sampling

Single-subject designs derive from an assumption that each client is unique and should be studied separately (Rutman & Mowbray, 1993). The method of goal attainment scaling discussed earlier is sometimes used in single-subject designs to monitor the progress of individual clients. Such methods avoid some of the pitfalls of using standardized tests based on status inequality models. Scores of individual clients can still be totaled to indicate whether or not the program in general is succeeding in producing desired outcomes.

On the other hand, measuring the progress of every client is a time-consuming process that is probably most valuable in formative studies. In summative evaluations, researchers often are able to look at a smaller sample of clients, who are believed to be representative of the client population as a whole. A further consideration in single-subject designs involves potential difficulties with reliability and validity. Goal attainment scales and similar measures tend to be subjective, and what one client might define as the "best outcome expected," another might define merely as the "expected outcome." Although subjectivity is less of an issue in partnership than in status inequality-based programs, obtaining data that are consistent enough to be compared over time is always important.

All the methods discussed in this chapter—observation, interviewing, and questionnaires—can be used with samples of clients as well as with the entire client population. When selecting samples, evaluators need to be careful that those selected to be studied are representative of the population as a whole. In addition, they need to be sure that the sample size is sufficient to allow for statistical testing of group differences. Most standard textbooks in research methods provide guidance on randomly selecting a sample from a larger population and also may contain tables of required sample sizes needed to conduct various statistical tests.

Experimental Evaluation and Control Group Designs

Many texts in evaluation research advocate the use of experimental or quasi-experimental designs. In the simplest of these designs, one group of clients receives the services of the program being evaluated while another receives no services at all. The two groups are usually matched on important characteristics, such as socioeconomic status and problem severity. Typically pre- and postservice tests are administered to both groups to measure change over time. Presumably, if the service is working, treated subjects (the experimental group) will show greater improvement than those who are not treated (the control group).

In human services, such a rigorous approach may be desirable but impractical to implement for the following reasons:

- Funding for experimental research usually is not readily available, especially in the case of smaller agencies.
- When services are believed to be effective, permitting a group of clients in need to receive no services at all may be unethical.
- Service providers usually spend almost all their time serving clients and are likely to have little or no time for research that is not a direct part of the service delivery process.
- Experimental methods usually require specialized training at a level beyond that of most service providers.
- Less rigorous available methods, although inferior in some ways, usually can be used to satisfy funders and other stakeholders about program efficacy.

Some human service situations provide a simple and ethical alternative to control group designs. Unfortunately, because of limited resources, many programs today have waiting lists. Unless a triage system is in use, these lists typically include clients whose concerns are comparable in most ways to those of clients who are being served. A simple checklist such as the Parent Needs Survey (see Chapter 8) can be administered to waiting list clients at the same time it is administered to those receiving services and again at regular intervals. If the program is effective, the number and magnitude of the concerns of program participants will diminish, while these dimensions will remain unchanged (or increase) among those on the waiting list. Ideally, such a method would still require some consideration of matching characteristics in the two groups.

Selecting Methods

Some of the strengths and weaknesses of the methods of observation, interviewing, and questionnaire administration were discussed in previous chapters. In addition, some characteristics of these methods have special implications for service evaluation.

One consideration in observation studies involves the presence of the evaluator. If evaluation is not normally an ongoing aspect of service delivery, the natural situation will be altered to some extent by the evaluation process itself. The pros and cons of using an outside evaluator were discussed earlier in this chapter. Furthermore, any evaluator, whether internal or external to the organization, introduces a new element into the service situation. People do not do or say the same things they might normally do or say when they know they are being judged (cf the discussion of self-presentation in Chapter 4). The effect of the evaluator can be lessened to some extent by allowing enough time to develop familiarity. However, evaluation results always should be read with an awareness of the potential for evaluator-induced bias.

Another kind of bias in evaluation studies involving interviews or questionnaires is possible deliberate distortion of responses by clients who have seemingly unrelated concerns or requirements. Rossi (1997), for example, cites the case of a study of births to mothers receiving Aid to Families with Dependent Children (AFDC) in New Jersey after the imposition of a "family cap." Although the birthrate appeared to decline after the imposition of the cap, Rossi suggests that mothers may have stopped reporting births, because they would no longer receive additional income for doing so. The "decline," then, may have been the result of reporting error. In a human service situation, clients who are about to be discharged from a program may have less incentive than those who expect to continue receiving services to respond accurately to a satisfaction survey.

Ware (1997) cites another potential bias in survey research that can result from the lack of standardization in scale construction. For example, the scale, *excellent, average, fair, poor, very poor*, will produce more "excellent" responses than the scale, *excellent, very good, good, fair, poor*. Such differences can be problematic in cross-agency comparisons or in the same agency if scale categories are changed from one survey administration to the next.

An awareness of potential biases may influence the choice of methods in some cases. In all cases, this awareness should at least affect the interpretation of evaluation results. In designing any evaluation, then, the practitioner will need to consider the likely validity of the instruments and methods that are being considered.

Validity and Reliability

Validity indicates the degree to which an instrument or method produces the data it was intended to produce. *Reliability* concerns the extent to which an instrument or method will produce the same results in the same conditions on different occasions. In the context of service evaluation, the evaluator must consider whether observed changes are the result of the program being evaluated or whether they can be explained by some alternative process. Thus, problems in validity and reliability can result from the design of the instruments themselves (internal validity) or from factors extraneous to the evaluation process (external validity).

Some of the threats to internal validity were discussed in the last section. Scales always should be validated in smaller pilot studies before they are used with large numbers of clients in a full-scale evaluation. Earlier chapters suggested methods such as comparing interview and questionnaire data for the same clients to assess the validity of questionnaire responses. Standard textbooks on research methods provide additional suggestions for developing valid questionnaires. In the case of qualitative methods, Darling and Baxter (1996, pp. 291–292) suggest the following techniques for increasing both validity and reliability:

- Make use of multiple data collection procedures.
- Document in detail the data collection procedures used.
- Record extensive descriptive information and verbatim accounts that can be checked by other observers.
- If it can be done unobtrusively, use recording devices such as tape recorders or video cameras; then, with permission, allow other staff and clients to view or listen to the tapes independently.
- Always explore disagreements among participants and provide an opportunity for resolution.
- Spend as much time as possible with participants.
- Do observations in natural settings.

The primary threat to external validity may be factors other than program participation that may affect clients. Dunst (1986) reviewed 57 studies designed to assess the impact of early intervention programs and concluded that these programs were only one of many factors affecting families. Rossi and Freeman (1993) have documented a number of factors that compete with program interventions:

- *Endogenous changes:* Change occurs naturally in any social situation.
- *Exogenous changes:* Change also occurs continually in the larger society. Changes in the economy, in social policy, and in other areas can affect human service clients.
- *Interfering events:* Short-term events affecting clients can enhance or mask other changes. Such events include births, deaths, marriages, and relocations, among others.
- *Maturational trends:* Individuals experience developmental changes with aging and movement from one life cycle stage to another.
- *Uncontrolled selection:* Evaluators may not be able to influence who will participate in a study, and study volunteers may not be representative of the population as a whole.

To counteract as many of these factors as possible, evaluators should try to use entire populations or representative samples and should try to combine quantitative measures with more qualitative techniques that explore the nature of other changes that may be occurring.

Reporting and Using Evaluation Results

Communicating Findings

Most evaluation reports contain narrative descriptions of both qualitative and quantitative results as well as tabular presentations of quantitative findings. Direct quotes from depth interviews and from responses to open-ended survey questions also are helpful in illustrating outcomes.

Both tables and bar graphs (histograms) provide graphic representations of quantitative data. Table 11.1 illustrates the tabular presentation of client satisfaction among groups receiving different interventions. Figure 11.4 illustrates a change in client satisfaction over time for groups receiving different interventions. Such graphs also can be used to illustrate changes in the accomplishment of service plan activities over time, changes in client resources and concerns over time, or changes in the magnitude of concerns over time.

Formative evaluation reports usually provide information to assist in the identification, development, and improvement of alternative plans for the use of strategies and resources to achieve the stated goals of the program (Irwin, 1989). A formative report on a new program might contain:

- Background information about the program and its clients
- Characteristics of the program, including funding sources and a description of intervention techniques

Table 11.1. Parents' Responses to the Question "How Satisfied Are You with the Early Intervention Program?" by Type of Program[a]

Parent-Perceived Satisfaction with EI	Home-Based %[b]	Home-Based N	Combined Home and Center %	Combined Home and Center N	Center-Based %	Center-Based N
Not at all satisfied with the program	22.6	7	5.3	1	20.0	4
Not completely satisfied with the program	19.4	6	26.3	5	20.0	4
Satisfied with the program	16.1	5	5.3	1	10.0	2
Very satisfied with the program	41.9	13	63.2	12	50.0	10
Total	100.0	31	100.0	19	100.0	20

[a] From Darling & Baxter (1996, p. 294), with permission. [b] Percentages are rounded to the nearest tenth.

- Evaluation measures, including information about sample selection and methods being used
- Description of results
- Discussion of results
- Recommendations

A summative evaluation report would contain similar sections but might be based on more rigorous methods and a larger sample. Summative reports also usually address specific program objectives that were included in proposals for funding. For example, if the grant proposal promised that the program would achieve high satisfaction in at least 75% of program clients, the evaluation report

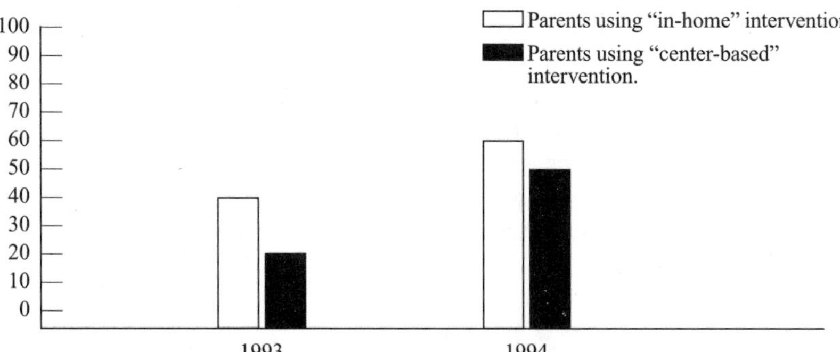

Figure 11.4. Example of a graph showing change in client satisfaction over time. Darling & Baxter (1996, p. 295), with permission.

might include a bar graph showing percentages of clients indicating high satisfaction at several points in time. Summative reports generally should follow these guidelines:

- Begin with an executive summary of major findings.
- Gear the report to the interests of the audience.
- Focus on program goals and resist the temptation to include extraneous information.
- Use tables and graphics such as graphs and diagrams whenever possible.
- Include some quotes or anecdotal descriptions to illustrate findings.
- Provide recommendations that will result in program improvement.

Linking Evaluation and Planning

Although evaluation reports of course must address the expectations of those who fund a program, they also should be useful to practitioners who want to improve the delivery of services to clients. As Mullen and Magnabosco (1997, p. 317) have written, "Although organizational and professional survival and learning are important reasons for developing outcomes measurement systems, quality human services must eventually meet the test of benefiting citizens."

A related consideration involves which citizens are benefiting from the services. If, for example, a program chooses to serve the least needy clients in order to produce better outcomes, a glowing evaluation report may not be an indication of success. In today's environment of managed care and for-profit services, the poorest and sickest clients are sometimes excluded from needed services. As a result, programs that appear to be successful should be carefully scrutinized for inclusiveness.

Good administrators will make use of evaluation results as part of an ongoing planning process. Just as action statements are written for client service plans, organizational plans can contain such statements as well. An evaluation finding that clients are not satisfied with the services they are receiving or that service plan activities are not being carried out might be an indication that additional staff training is needed. Figure 11.5 illustrates an organizational plan that might be based on such a finding. Other organizational action statements might include the reorganization of service delivery practices or the adoption of new intervention strategies.

Chapter Summary

This chapter discussed the final component of the partnership-based model of practice: service evaluation. Some basic principles of evaluation research were presented. The importance of outcomes in evaluation research was discussed, along with the relationship between outcomes, outputs, and service activities. The most important outcomes in partnership-based practice—client satisfaction and status changes—were presented and discussed, and methods for measuring these outcomes were explored. Finally, the presentation of evaluation results was addressed, along with the relevance of evaluation results to program planning.

Suggested Exercises

1. Figure 9.3 (Chapter 9) is a service plan for the Jones family. Review the action statements listed in the plan. Then, for each action statement, write at least

Northwest Rehabilitation Center Strategic Plan

Key Strategic Issue #1: Employees of Northwest Rehabilitation Center (NWRC) do not have knowledge and skills necessary to consistently meet the needs of clients, families, and the community.

Key Outcome #1: NWRC will have a staff education program that helps employees continuously develop the knowledge and skills needed to consistently meet the needs of clients, families, and the community.

Strategies

1. NWRC will establish a staff development improvement team that will provide guidance and oversight for the agency's staff education program. The team will be made up of a cross section of employees from both the clinical and support sides of the house and will be established by September 1, 19xx.
2. The staff development team will conduct an analysis of training needs of all agency employees and provide a report to the Staff Development Team by January 15, 19xx.
3. Based on the results of the survey and analysis, the staff development team will propose a comprehensive, competency-based core curriculum for all agency employees by June 30, 19xx.
4. The staff development unit of the agency will pilot test the competency-based curriculum between July 1 and August 31, 19xx, and will propose revisions for implementation on October 1, 19xx.
5. Agency employees will complete the required core curriculum by July 31 of the following year.

Outcome Measures

1. Milestones in the development of the core curriculum
2. Number of employees completing the required training
3. Skill test scores of employees completing curriculum
4. Improved performance of employees on job tasks as measured by supervisors or assessments
5. Evaluation of the curriculum by participants
6. Percentage of compliance with external accreditation standards regarding staff training requirements.

From G. V. Sluyer (1998). *Improving Organizational Performance: A Practical Guidebook for the Human Services Field*. Thousand Oaks, CA: Sage, p. 45.

Figure 11.5. An example of an organizational plan linked to evaluation. From Sluyter (1998, p. 45), with permission.

one projected output. Use these outputs to determine the outcomes for the Jones family that this plan is designed to achieve.

2. Design an evaluation study for a fictitious human service agency. This agency serves clients with a history of drug abuse. The program being evaluated is a home visiting program for mothers of infants and toddlers. During the 3-year period being evaluated, 45 clients are served. The goal of the program is to promote optimal child development while supporting the mothers and preventing relapse. Your design should include the following elements:

- A plan for identifying agency clients to serve as subjects for this evaluation (either all clients served or a representative sample). You may want to use different sets of respondents for the interview and questionnaire sections below.
- A description of a plan for a structured observation of some aspect of the agency's operation.
- A list of topics that you would include in depth interviews with agency professionals and/or clients. Explain why you have chosen these topics.
- A survey instrument (based on the principles of good questionnaire design covered in Chapter 8) to determine client satisfaction with the home visiting program.
- A description of a possible controlled study comparing clients served by this agency with people in a similar situation who are not receiving these services. You should discuss how you would obtain the respondents in your comparison group and indicate which methods you would use (any combination of observation, interviewing, and/or questionnaires). How might the results of this study be used by this agency?

Suggestions for Further Reading

Martin, L.L., & Kettner, P.M. (1996). *Measuring the performance of human service programs*. Thousand Oaks, CA: Sage.

Mullen, E.J., & Magnabosco, J.L. (1997). *Outcomes measurement in human services*. Washington, DC: NASW Press.

Pecora, P.J., Fraser, M.W., Nelson, K.E., McCroskey, J., & Meezan, W. (1995). *Evaluating family-based services*. New York: Aldine deGruyter.

Rapp, C.A., & Poertner, J. (1992). *Social administration: A client-centered approach*. White Plains, NY: Longman.

Rossi, P.H., & Freeman, H.E. (1993). *Evaluation: A systematic approach*. Newbury Park, CA: Sage.

Review of the Process of Partnership-Based Practice

Figure 1.1 presented a model of the process of partnership-based practice. The process begins with the client's opportunity structure. Opportunity structures consist of the resources available to individuals in society and are shaped by their socioeconomic status, gender, race, ethnicity, community of residence, family ties, access to services, and other variables. Some opportunities are determined by the values and structures of the larger society, including factors such as racism and the status of the national economy, whereas others result from conditions within the individual's family and community. Opportunity structures place constraints on some courses of action while promoting other courses of action.

Individuals become aware of their opportunity structures through a process of symbolic interaction. Through their interactions with the significant others in their environment, people learn to define their situations in society. Thus, definitions of the situation typically vary among members of different social classes and racial and ethnic groups. The definition of the situation includes an awareness of the availability of resources or opportunities, as well as concerns about resources that are perceived to be lacking or unavailable. In addition, concerns tend to be prioritized, that is, some concerns are defined as more important or pressing than others.

When individuals experience concerns that they believe they are unable to address with available resources, they sometimes seek help from human service agencies. Just as individuals experience constraints relating to their opportunity structures, help from agencies may be limited by socially structured barriers inherent in agency organization. In particular, bureaucracy sometimes creates obstacles to service access. In addition, professionals themselves may create barriers by playing their roles in unhelpful ways.

In order to successfully address their clients' concerns, professionals need to engage in a process of identifying clients' definitions of their resources, concerns, and priorities. The primary identification methods are observation, interviewing, and questionnaire development and administration. Each of these methods has both advantages and disadvantages, and the use of several methods in combination is usually preferable to the use of any one method alone. In addition, professionals need to be guided by differing subcultural expectations and client preferences.

After the identification process has been completed, the professional works with the client to develop a service plan. This plan contains action statements designed to produce client-desired outcomes. These statements specify the ways in which the professional will act to expand the client's opportunity structure. In order to increase available opportunities, professionals need to maintain a high level of awareness of resources available in the community, along with a repertory of techniques for obtaining resources that do not currently exist.

Intervention in human services may take place at two levels: micro and meso. At the microlevel, the professional expands the client's opportunity structure by making the client aware of existing resources and enabling the client to gain access to those resources. Sometimes, advocacy is necessary to link clients with resources that are not immediately available. When needed resources do not exist at all in the community, the professional will need to engage in mesolevel intervention in the form of grant writing, political action, or other activities. These activities are designed to expand the opportunities available to larger populations of clients rather than to individuals.

Because some client concerns are the result of socially structured conditions at a macrolevel, traditional forms of human service intervention may not be able to address them adequately. Overcoming barriers such as racism and economic depressions requires social change on a broad scale. Although professionals can, as individuals, become involved in social movements designed to bring about societal-level changes, they need to understand that they may not be able to address all of their clients' concerns within the structure of the human service system.

The final step in the service process is evaluation. Professionals need to be sure that the services they are providing are in fact producing the outcomes that their clients desire. Outcomes to be assessed include client satisfaction and status changes. Status changes reflect the expansion of opportunity structures. Thus, the process is circular and ends where it began—with the opportunity structure of the client.

The human service system has been undergoing significant changes in recent years. Older status inequality models are being replaced by partnership approaches that respect the client's definition of the situation. Much of the change that has occurred has been atheoretical. Professionals in fields as diverse as health care, social work, and education have been working to listen more closely to their clients, in some cases because their clients have demanded that they be taken seriously, and in other cases because consumerism has become valued on ethical or practical grounds. This volume has suggested that sociological theory provides the missing foundation for a partnership approach. Sociological theory and methods are valuable, then, in establishing a framework for human service practice.

Clinical sociology encompasses intervention at various levels. At the micro- and mesolevels, much of the intervention that takes place occurs within the realm of the human service system. Thus, the model described in this volume is an important contribution to the clinical sociological literature. In addition to sociological practitioners, human service professionals from a variety of disciplines should find the model valuable in the implementation of newer partnership approaches. All professionals, regardless of discipline, will need to work together in the new millennium if they wish to expand opportunities for as many people as possible.

References

Abidin, R.R. (1983). *Parenting stress index.* Charlottesville, VA: Pediatric Psychology Press.

Adams, P., & Krauth, K. (1995). Working with families and communities: The patch approach. In P. Adams & K Nelson (Eds.), *Reinventing human services; Community- and family-centered practice.* (pp. 8–108). New York: Aldine de Gruyter.

Adams, P., & Nelson, K. (Eds.). (1995). *Reinventing human services: Community- and family-centered practice.* New York: Aldine de Gruyter.

Adapting research to cultures and countries. (1995/96, Fall/Winter). *Impact World Institute on Disability Semi Annual Report, 3*(1), 5.

Alvirez, D., & Bean, T.D. (1976). The Mexican-American family. In C. H. Mindel & R.W. Habenstein (Eds.), *Ethnic families in America: Patterns and variations* (pp. 271–292). New York: Elsevier.

Anderson, P. (1988, June). *Serving culturally diverse populations of infants and toddlers with disabilities.* Paper presented at the meeting of the Society for Disability Studies, Washington, DC.

Aneshensel, C.D., Pearlin, L.I., Mullan, J.T., Zaiet, S.H., & Whitlatch, C.J. (1995). *Profiles in caregiving: The unexpected career.* San Diego: Academic Press.

Anspach, R.R. (1993). *Fateful choices in the intensive-care nursery.* Berkeley: University of California Press.

Antonucci, T.C., & Depner, C.E. (1982). Social support and informal helping relationships. In T.A. Wills (Ed.), *Basic processes in helping relationships* (pp. 233–254). New York: Academic Press.

Attneave, C. (1982). American Indians and Alaska native families: Emigrants in their own homeland. In M. McGoldrick (Ed.), *Ethnicity and family therapy* (pp. 55–83). New York: Guilford.

Axtell, R.E. (1991). *Gestures: The do's and taboos of body language around the world.* New York: John Wiley & Sons.

Ayer, S. (1984). Community care: The failure of professionals to meet family needs. *Child: Health and Development, 10,* 127–140.

Azziz, R. (1981, July). The Hispanic patient. *Pennsylvania Medicine,* 22–25.

Bailey, D.B., Jr., Simionsson, R.J., Winton, P.J., Huntington, G., Comfort, M., Isbell, P., O'Donnell, K., & Helm, J.M. (1986). Family focused intervention: A functional model for planning, implementing, and evaluating individualized family services in early intervention. *Journal of the Division for Early Childhood, 12* (3), 195–207.

Barnes, H.E. (1948). Lester Frank Ward: The reconstruction of society by social science. In H.E. Barnes (Ed.), *An Introduction to the history of sociology* (pp. 126–143). Chicago: The University of Chicago Press.

Bartz, K.W., & Levine, E.S. (1978). Childbearing by black parents: A description and comparison to Anglo and Chicano parents. *Journal of Marriage and the Family, 40,* 709–719.

Bateman, N. (1995). *Advocacy skills: A handbook for human service professionals.* Brookfield, VT: Ashgate Publishing Company.

Batson, C.D., O'Quin, K., & Pych, V. (1982). An attribution theory analysis of trained helpers' inferences about clients' needs. In T.A. Wills (Ed.), *Basic processes in helping relationships* (pp. 59–80). New York: Academic Press.

Baxter, C. (1987). Professional services as support: Perceptions of parents. *Australia and New Zealand Journal of Developmental Disabilities, 13,* 243–253.

Becker, H. (1963). *Outsiders: Studies in the sociology of deviance.* New York: The Free Press.

Becker, H.S., & Geer, B. (1967). Participant observation and interviewing: A comparison. In J.G. Manis & B.N. Meltzer (Eds.), *Symbolic interaction: A reader in social psychology* (pp. 109–119). Boston: Allyn & Bacon.

Beinart, P. (1997, August 9). Jews, Latinos and the US political landscape. *The Globe and Mail,* p. 21.

Bell, R.R. (1965). Lower class negro mothers' aspirations for their children. *Social Forces, 43,* 493–500.

Berg, B.L. (1995). *Qualitative research methods for the social sciences.* Boston: Allyn & Bacon.

Bergmann, B.R. (1996). *Saving our children from poverty: What the United States can learn from France.* New York: Russell Sage Foundation.

Berkowitz, S. (1996). Using qualitative and mixed-method approaches. In R. Reviere, S. Berkowitz, C.C. Carter, & C.G. Ferguson (Eds.), *Needs assessment: A creative and practical guide for social scientists* (pp. 53–70). Washington, DC: Taylor & Francis.

Bernstein, N. (1996, September 15). Giant companies entering race to run state welfare programs. *The New York Times*, p.1.

Berrick, J.D. (1995). *Faces of poverty: Portraits of women and children on welfare.* New York: Oxford University Press.

Biklen, D. (1974). *Let our children go: An organizing manual for advocates and parents*. Syracuse, NY: Human Policy Press.

Bonilla-Santiago, G. (1996). Latino battered women: Barriers to service delivery and cultural considerations. In A.R. Roberts (Ed.), *Helping battered women: New perspectives and remedies* (pp. 229–234). New York: Oxford University Press.

Bowman, B. (1992) Who is at risk for what and why. *Journal of Early Intervention, 16*(2), 101–200.

Boykin, A.W. (1983). The academic performance of Afro-American children. In J. Spence (Ed.), *Achievement and achievement motives*. San Francisco: Freeman.

Bradburn, N.M., & Sudman, S. (1979). *Improving interview method and questionnaire design.* San Francisco: Jossey-Bass.

Brewer, E.J., Jr., McPherson, M., Magrab, P.R., & Hutchins, V.L. (1989). Family-centered, community-based, coordinated care for children with special health care needs. *Pediatrics, 83,* 1055–1060.

Briggs, C.L. (1986). *Learning how to ask: A sociological appraisal of the interview in social science research*. Cambridge, England: Cambridge University Press.

Brody, R. (1991). Preparing effective proposals. In R.L. Edwards & J.A. Yankey (Eds.), *Skills for effective human service management* (pp. 44–61). Silver Spring, MD: NASW Press.

Bromley, M. (1989). New beginnings for Cambodian refugees—or further disruptions? *Social Work, 32,* 236–239.

Bronfenbrenner, U. (1979). *The ecology of human development*. Cambridge, MA: Harvard University Press.

Browner, C.H., Preloran, H.M., & Cox, S.J. (1999). Ethnicity, bioethics, and prenatal diagnosis: The amniocentesis decisions of Mexican-origin women and their partners. *American Journal of Public Health, 89,* 1658–1666.

Bruhn, J.G., & Rebach, H.M. (1996). *Clinical sociology: An agenda for action.* New York: Plenum Press.

Cameron, G. & Vanderwoerd, J. (1997). *Protecting children and supporting families: Promising programs and organizational realities.* New York: Aldine de Gruyter.

Capossela, C., & Warnock, S. (1997). *Share the care: How to organize a group to care for someone who is seriously ill.* New York: Fireside.

Carter, C.C. (1996). Using and communicating findings. In R. Reviere, S. Berkowitz, C.C. Carter, & C.G. Ferguson (Eds.), *Needs assessment: A creative and practical guide for social scientists* (pp. 185–201). Washington, DC: Taylor & Francis.

Cavalieri, W., Clarke, D., & Bolych, C. (1997, August). *Using research as an emancipatory tool: Injection drug users reclaim their voice and power.* Paper presented at the meeting of the Society for the Study of Social Problems, Toronto, ON.

Chafel, J.A. (1993). Child poverty: Overview and outlook. In J.A. Chafel (Ed.), *Child poverty and public policy* (pp. 1–8). Washington, DC: The Urban Institute Press.

Chan, S. (1990). Early intervention with culturally diverse families of infants and toddlers with disabilities. *Infants and Young Children, 3,* 78–87.

Charmaz, K. (1991). *Good days, bad days: The self in chronic illness and time.* New Brunswick, NJ: Rutgers University Press.

Clark, R.E., & LaBeff, E.E. (1982). Death telling: Managing the delivering of bad news. *Journal of Health and Social Behavior, 23,* 366–380.

Cloward, R.A., & Ohlin, L.E. (1960). *Delinquency and opportunity: A theory of delinquent gangs.* New York: The Free Press.

Cohen, R., & Lavach, C. (1995). Strengthening partnerships between families and service providers. In P. Adams & K. Nelson (Eds.), *Reinventing human services: Community-and family-centered practice* (pp. 261–277). New York: Aldine de Gruyter.

Colon, E. (1980). The family life cycle of the multiproblem poor family. In E.A. Carter & M. McGoldrick (Eds.), *The family life cycle: A framework for family therapy* (pp. 343–381). New York: Gardner.

Coltrane, S. (1998). Changing patterns of family work: Chicano men and housework. In S.J. Ferguson (Ed.), *Shifting the center: Understanding contemporary families* (pp. 547–562). Mountainview, CA: Mayfield.

Conrad, P., & Schneider, J.W. (1980). *Deviance and medicalization: From badness to sickness.* St. Louis: C.V. Mosly.

Cook, D.A., & Fine, M. (1995). "Motherrwit": Childrearing lessons from African American mothers of low income. In B.B. Swadener & S. Lubeck (Eds.), *Children and families "at promise": Deconstructing the discourse of risk* (pp. 118–142). Albany: State University of New York Press.

Cooley, C.H. (1964). *Human nature and the social order.* New York: Schocken.

Cooley, W.C. (1994). Graduate medical education in pediatrics: Preparing reliable allies for parents of children with special health care needs. In R.B. Darling & M.J. Peter (Eds.), *Families, physicians, and children with special health needs: Collaborative medical education models* (pp. 109–120). Westport, CT: Greenwood.

Coopersmith, S. (1967). *The antecedents of self-esteem.* San Francisco: W.H. Freeman.

Core principles of family-centered health care. (1998, Summer). *Advances, 4(1),* 2–3.

Coulter, I.D. (1997). The development of health-related quality-of-life measures at RAND. In E.J. Mulen & J.L. Magnabosco (Eds.), *Outcomes measurement in human services* (pp. 209–217). Washington, DC: NASW Press.

Crandall, R., & Allen, R.D. (1982). The organizational context of helping relationships. In T.A. Wills (Ed.), *Basic processes in helping relationships* (pp. 431–452). New York: Academic Press.

Crnic, K.A., Friedrich, W.N., & Greenburg, M.T. (1983). Adaptation of families with mentally retarded children: A model of stress, coping, and family ecology. *American Journal of Mental Deficiency,* 125–138.

Daniels, A.K. (1978). The social construction of military psychiatric diagnosis. In J.G. Manis & B.N. Meltzer (Eds.), *Symbolic interaction: A reader in social psychology* (3rd edition) (pp. 380–391). Boston: Allyn & Bacon.

Darling, J. (1977). Bachelorhood and late marriage: An interactionist interpretation. *Symbolic Interaction, 1,* 44–45.

Darling, R.B. (1979). *Families against society: A study of reactions to children with birth defects.* Beverly Hills, CA: Sage.

Darling, R.B. (1988). Parental entrepreneurship: A consumerist response to professional dominance. *Journal of Social Issues, 44,* 141–158.

Darling, R.B. (1994). Overcoming obstacles to early intervention referral: The development of a video-based training model for community physicians. In R.B. Darling & M.J. Peter (Eds.), *Families, physicians, and children with special health needs: Collaborative medical education models* (pp. 135–148). Westport, CT: Greenwood.

Darling, R.B., & Baxter, C. (1996). *Families in focus: Sociological methods in early interventions.* Austin, TX: Pro-Ed.

Darling, R.B., & Darling, J. (1982). *Children who are different: Meeting the challenges of birth defects in society.* St. Louis: Mosby.

Darling, R.B., & Darling, J. (1992). Early intervention: A field moving toward a sociological perspective. *Sociological Studies of Child Development, 5,* 9–22.

Darling, R.B., & Peter, M.I. (Eds.). (1994). *Families, physicians, and children with special health needs: Collaborative medical education models.* Westport, CT: Greenwood.

Davis, A.Y. (1997). Race and criminalization: Black Americans and the punishment industry. In W. Lubiano (Ed.), *The house that race built: Black Americans, US Terrain* (pp. 264–279). New York: Pantheon.

Davis, F. (1960). Uncertainty in medical prognosis: Clinical and functional. *American Journal of Sociology, 66,* 41–47.

Davis, F. (1961). Deviance disavowal: The management of strained interaction by the visibly handicapped. *Social Problems, 9,* 120–132.

DePaulo, B.M. (1982). Social–psychological processes in informal help seeking. In T.A. Wills (Ed.), *Basic processes in helping relationships* (pp. 255–279). New York: Academic Press.

Developing systems of support with American Indian families of youth with disabilities. (1998, Summer). *Health Issues, 6,* 9–10.

Dickman, I., & Gordan, S. (1985). *One miracle at a time: How to get help for your disabled child—From the experience of other parents.* New York: Simon & Schuster.

Dillard, J.L. (1972). *Black English: Its history and usage in the United States.* New York: Random House.

Dilsworth-Anderson, P., Burton, L., & Turner, W.I. (1993). The importance of values in the study of culturally diverse families. *Family Relations, 42,* 238–242.

Dodson, J. (1981). Conceptualization of black families. In H.P. McAdoo (Ed.), *Black families* (pp. 23–36). Beverly Hills: Sage.

Doherty, W.J. (1985). Family intervention in health care. *Family Relations, 34,* 129–137.

Douglas, J.D. (1985). *Creative interviewing.* Beverly Hills, CA: Sage.

Dunst, C.J. (1986). Overview of the efficacy of early intervention programs. In L. Bickman & D.L. Weatherford (Eds.), *Evaluating early intervention programs for severely handicapped children and their families* (pp. 79–148). Austin, TX: Pro-Ed.

Dunst, C.J., Trivette, C.M., & Cross, A.H. (1988). Social support networks of Appalachian and non-Appalachian families with handicapped children: Relationship to personal and family well-being. In S. Keefe (Ed.), *Mental health in Appalachia.* Lexington: University of Kentucky Press.

Dunst, C.J., Trivette, C.M., & Deal, A.G. (1987). *Enabling and empowering families: Principles and guidelines for practice.* Cambridge, MA: Brookline.

Edelman, M.W. (1985). The sea is so wide and my boat is so small: Problems facing black children today. In H.P. McAdoo & J.L. McAdoo (Eds.), *Black children: Social, educational, and parental environments* (pp. 72–82). Beverly Hills, CA: Sage.

Edgerton, R.B. (1993). *The clock of competence: Stigma in the lives of the mentally retarded.* Berkeley: University of California Press.

Edin, K., & Harris, K.M. (1997, August). *Getting off and staying off: Race differences in the work route off welfare.* Paper presented at the meeting of the American Sociological Association, Toronto, ON.
Elden, M., & Chisholm, R.F. (1993). Emerging varieties of action research: Introduction to special issues. *Human Relations, 45,* 121–142.
Ellis, M. (1995, July). Grandmother raising five children finds lifeline in family support. *The Family Support Reader, 1,* 6.
Elman, N.S. (1991). Family therapy. In M. Seligman (Ed.), *The family with a handicapped child* (2nd ed., pp. 369–406). Boston: Allyn & Bacon.
Erlich, J.L., Rothman, J., & Teresa, J.G. (1999). *Taking action in organizations and communities.* Dubuque, IA: Eddie Bowers Publishing.
Falicov, C.J. (1982). Mexican families. In M. McGoldrick, J.K. Pearce, & J. Giordano (Eds.), *Ethinicity and family therapy* (pp. 134–163). New York: Guilford.
Falicov, C.J., & Karrer, B.M. (1980). Cultural variations in the family life cycle: The Mexican-American family. In E.A. Carter & M. McGoldrick (Eds.), *The family life cycle: A framework for family therapy* (pp. 383–426). New York: Gardner.
Families as advisors: A checklist for attitudes. (1992, September). *Advances in Family-Centered Care,* 5.
Family-centered service delivery. (1997, Summer). *Families and Disability Newsletter,* 1.
Family support center opened the door to independence. (1995, January). *The Family Support Reader, 1,* 6–7.
Featherstone, H. (1980). *A difference in the family.* New York: Basic Books.
Fein, E.B. (1997, November 23). Language barriers are hindering health care. *The New York Times,* pp. 1, 20.
Foddy, W. (1993). *Constructing questions for interviews and questionnaires: Theory and practice in social research.* Cambridge, England: Cambridge University Press.
Fong, R. (1994). Family preservation: Making it work for Asians. *Child Welfare, LXXIII,* 331–341.
Fracasso, M.P. (1994). Studying the social and emotional development of Hispanic children in the United States: Addressing research challenges. *Zero to Three, 15,* 24–27.
Franklin, A.J., & Boyd-Franklin, N. (1985). A psycho-educational perspective on black parenting. In H.P. McAdoo (Ed.), *Black families* (pp. 194–210). Beverly Hills: Sage.
Fraser, M.W., Pecora, P.J., & Haapala, D.A. (1991). *Families in crisis: The impact of intensive family preservation services.* Hawthorne, NY: Aldine de Gruyter.
Freidson, E. (1970a). *Profession of medicine: A study of the sociology of applied knowledge.* New York: Dodd, Mead & Company.
Freidson, E. (1970b). *Professional dominance.* Chicago: Aldine.
Gans, H.J. (1995). *The war against the poor: The underclass and antipoverty policy.* New York: Basic Books.
García-Preto, N. (1982). Puerto Rican families. In M. McGoldrick, J.K. Pearce, & J. Giordano (Eds.), *Ethnicity and family therapy* (pp. 164–186). New York: Guilford.
Garfinkel, H. (1956). Conditions of successful degradation ceremonies. *American Journal of Sociology, 61,* 420–424.
Garson, B. (1988). *The electronic sweatshop: How computers are transforming the office of the future into the factory of the past.* New York: Penguin.
Gelles, R.J. (1996). *The book of David: How preserving families can cost children's lives.* New York: Basic Books.
George, S.M., & Dickerson, B.J. (1995). The role of the grandmother in poor single-mother families and households. In B.J. Dickerson (Ed.)., *African-American single mothers: Understanding their lives and families* (pp. 146–163). Thousand Oaks, CA: Sage.
Glaser, B.G., & Strauss, A.L. (1965). *Awareness of dying.* Chicago: Aldine.
Glaser, B.G., & Strauss, A.L. (1967). *The discovery of grounded theory: Strategies for qualitative research.* New York: Aldine De Gruyter.

Gliedman, J., & Roth, W. (1980). *The unexpected minority: Handicapped children in America.* New York: Harcourt Brace Jovanovich.

Goffman, E. (1958). *The presentation of self in everyday life.* Edinburgh: University of Edinburgh Social Sciences Research Centre.

Goffman, E. (1961). *Asylums: Essays on the social situation of mental patients and other inmates.* Garden City, NY: Doubelday Anchor.

Goffman, E. (1963). *Stigma: Notes on the management of spoiled identity.* Englewood Cliffs, NJ: Prentice-Hall.

Golfus, B. (1994). The do-gooder. In B. Shaw (Ed.), *The ragged edge: The disability experience from the pages of the first fifteen years of The Disability Rag* (pp. 165–172). Louisville, KY: The Advocado Press.

Goodman, J.F. (1994). "Empowerment" versus "best interests": Client–professional relationships. *Infants and Young Children, 6,* vi–x.

Gorden, R.L. (1992). *Basic interviewing skills.* Prospect Heights, IL: The Waveland Press.

Guba, E.G., & Lincoln, Y.S. (1989). *Fourth generation evaluation.* Newbury Park, CA: Sage.

Guide to Citizen Education. (March, 1995). *The Nation's Health,* p. 20.

Guttmacher, S., & Elinson, J. (1971). Ethno-religious variation in perception of illness. *Social Science and Medicine, 5,* 117–125.

Hagedorn, J.M. (1995). *Forsaking our children: Bureaucracy and reform in the child welfare system.* Chicago: Lake View Press.

Halley, A.A., Kopp, J., & Austin, M.J. (1992). *Delivering human services: A learning approach to practice.* New York: Longman.

Hanson, M.J. (1981). A model for early intervention with culturally diverse single and multiparent families. *Topics in Early Childhood Special Education, 1,* 37–44.

Harrison, A., Serafica, F., & McAdoo, H. (1984). Ethnic families of color. In R.D. Parke (Ed.), *Review of child development research* (vol. 7, pp. 329–371). Chicago: University of Chicago Press.

Harry, B. (1992a). *Cultural diversity, families, and the special education system: Communication and empowerment.* New York: Teachers College Press.

Harry, B. (1992b). Making sense of disability: Low-income Puerto Rican parents' theories of the problem. *Exceptional Children, 59,* 27–40.

Harry, B., & Kalyanpur, M. (1994). Cultural understandings of special education: Implications for professional interactions with culturally diverse families. *Disability and Society, 9,* 145–165.

Harry, B., Torguson, C., Katkavich, J., & Guerrero, M. (1993). Crossing social class and cultural barriers in working with families: Implications for teacher training. *Teaching Exceptional Children, 25*(1), 48–51.

Hartman, A. (1978, October). Diagrammatic assessment of family relationships. *Social Casework,* 465–476.

Haug, M., & Lavin, B. (1983). *Consumerism in medicine: Challenging physician authority.* Beverly Hilss, CA: Sage.

Harris & D.C. Maloney (Eds.), *Human services: Contemporary issues and trends* (pp. 335–340). Boston: Allyn & Bacon.

Hedges, A. (1985). Group interviewing. In R. Walker (Ed.), *Applied qualitative research* (pp. 71–91). London: Gower.

Hendrickson, J.M., & Omer, D. (1995). School-based comprehensive services: An example of interagency collaboration. In P. Adams & K. Nelson (Eds.), *Reinventing human services: Community- and family-centered practice* (pp. 145–162). New York: Aldine de Gruyter.

Herz, R.M., & Rosen, E.J. (1982). Jewish families. In M. McGoldrick, J.K. Pearce, & J. Giordano (Eds.), *Ethnicity and family therapy* (pp. 364–392). New York: Guilford.

Hewitt, J.P. (1998). *The myth of self-esteem: Finding happiness and solving problems in America.* New York: St. Martin's Press.

Hines, P.M., & Boyd-Franklin, N. (1982). Black families. In M. McGoldrick, J.K. Pearce, & J. Giordano (Eds.), *Ethnicity and family therapy* (pp. 84–107). New York: Guilford.

Hinkle, R.C., Jr., & Hinkle, G.J. (1954). *The development of modern sociology.* New York: Random House.

Hockenberry, J. (1995). *Moving violations: War zones, wheelchairs, and declarations of independence.* New York: Hyperion.

Hostler, S.L. (1991). Family-centered care. *Pediatric Clinics of North America, 38,* 1545–1560.

Huang, L.J. (1976). The Chinese-American family. In C.H. Mindel & R.W. Habenstein (Eds.), *Ethnic families in America: Patterns and variations* (pp. 124–147). New York: Elsevier.

Ireys, H.T., & Nelson, R.P. (1992). New federal policy for children with special health care needs: Implications for pediatricians. *Pediatrics, 90,* 321–327.

Irwin, L.K. (1989). Evaluating family support programs. In G.H.S. Singer & L.K. Irwin (Eds.), *Support for caregiving families* (pp. 329–334). Baltimore: Paul H. Brookes.

JFK Child Development Center. (1981). *HOME Screening Questionnaire.* Denver: LADOCA Publishing.

Jennings, M. (1994, December). A mother talks to Mrs. Clinton. *Children's Health Issues, 2,* 2–3.

Johnson, B., McGonigel, M., & Kaufmann, R. (1989). *Guidelines and recommended practices for the individualized family service plan.* Washington, DC: Association for the Care of Children's Health.

Judd, C.M., Smith, E.R., & Kidder, L.H. (1991). *Research methods n social relations.* Orlando, FL: Holt, Rinehart & Winston.

Kadushin, A., & Kadushin, G. (1997). *The social work interview: A guide for human service professionals.* New York: Columbia University Press.

Kahn, S. (1982). *Organizing: A guide for grassroots leaders.* New York: McGraw-Hill.

Karuza, J., Jr., Zevon, M.A., Rabinowitz, V.C.,, & Brickman, P. (1982). Attribution of responsibility by helpers and recipients. In T.A. Wills (Ed.), *Basic processes in helping relationships* (pp. 107–129). New York: Academic Press.

Kavanagh, K.H., & Kennedy, P.H. (1992). *Promoting cultural diversity: Strategies for health care professionals.* Newbury Park, CA: Sage.

Kaysen, S. (1993). *Girl, interrupted.* New York: Random House.

Kazak, A.E., & Marvin, R.S. (1984). Differences, difficulties, and adaption: Stress and social networks in families with a handicapped child. *Family Relations, 33,* 67–77.

Kazak, A.E., & Wilcox, B.L. (1984). The structure and function of social support networks in families with handicapped children. *American Journal of Community Psychology, 12,*645–661.

Keefe, S.E., Padilla, A.M., & Carlos, M.L. (1979). The Mexican-American extended family as an emotional support system. *Human Organization, 38,* 144–152.

Kilty, K.M., & Joseph, A. (1997, August). *Institutional racism and sentencing disparities for cocaine possession.* Paper presented at the meeting of the Society for the Study of Social Problems, Toronto, ON.

Kinch, J.W. (1968). Experiments in factors related to self-concept change. *Journal of Social Psychology, 74,* 251–258.

King, J.A., Morris, T., & Fitz-Gibbon, C. (1987). *How to assess program implementation.* Newbury Park, CA: Sage.

Kirk, J., & Miller, M.L. (1986). *Reliability and validity in qualitative research.* Beverly Hills, CA: Sage.

Kirk, S.A., & Kutchins, H. (1992). *The selling of DSM: The rhetoric of science in psychiatry.* New York: Aldine de Gruyter.

Kitano, H.M.L., & Kikumura, A. (1976). The Japanese American family. In C.H. Mindel & R.W. Habenstein (Eds.), *Ethnic families in America: Patterns and variations* (pp. 41–60). New York: Elsevier.

Kline, E., Acosta, F.X., Austin, W., & Johnson, R.G., Jr. (1980). The misunderstood Spanish-speaking patient. *American Journal of Psychiatry, 137* (12), 1530–1533.

Kluegel, J.R., & Smith, E.R. (1982). Whites' beliefs about blacks' opportunity. *American Sociological Review, 47,* 518–532.

Kozol, J. (1988). *Rachel and her children: Homeless families in America.* New York: Fawcett Columbine.

Kozol, J. (1991). *Savage inequalities: Children in America's schools.* New York: Crown.

Kozol, J. (1995). *Amazing grace: The lives of children and the conscience of a nation.* New York: Crown.

Kuhn, M., & McParland, T.S. (1954). An empirical investigation of self-attitudes. *American Sociological Review, 19,* 68–76.

Laosa, L.M. (1974). Child care and the culturally different child. *Child Care Quarterly, 3,* 214–224.

Laosa, L.M. (1978). Maternal teaching strategies in Chicano families of varied educational and socioeconomic levels. *Child Development, 49,* 1129–1135.

Lauffer, A. (1997). *Grants, etc.* Thousand Oaks, CA: Sage.

Lee, E. (1982). A social systems approach to assessment and treatment for Chinese American families. In M. McGoldrick, J.K. Pearce, & J. Giordano (Eds.), *Ethnicity and family therapy* (pp. 527–551). New York: Guilford.

Lee, J.A.B. (1994). *The empowerment approach to social work practice.* New York: Columbia University Press.

Leifeld, L., & Murray, T. (1995). Advocating for Aric: Strategies for full inclusion. In B.B. Swadener & S. Lubeck (Eds.), *Children and families "at promise": Deconstructing the discourse of risk* (pp. 238–261). Albany: State University of New York Press.

Lemert, E.M. (1967). *Human deviance, social problems, and social control.* Englewood Cliffs, NJ: Prentice-Hall.

Lewis, J., & Greenstein, R.M. (1994). A first year medical student curriculum about family views of chronic and disabling conditions. In R.B. Darling & M.J. Peter (Eds.), *Families, physicians, and children with special health needs: Collaborative medical education models* (pp. 77–100). Westport, CT: Greenwood.

Lewis, J.A., Lewis, M.D., & Souflee, F., Jr. (1993). *Management of human service programs* (2nd ed.). Belmont, CA: Wadsworth.

Lewis, O. (1959). *Five families: An intimate and objective revelation of family life in Mexico today: A dramatic study of the culture of poverty.* New York: Basic Books.

Lieberman, A.F. (1990). Infant–parent intervention with recent immigrants: Reflections on a study with Latino families. *Zero to Three, 10,* 8–11.

Liebow, E. (1993). *Tell them who I am: The lives of homeless women.* New York: Penguin.

Likert, R.A. (1932). Technique for the measurement of attitudes. *Archives of Psychology, 21.*

Link, B.G., Struening, E.L., Rahav, M., Phelan, J.C., & Nuttbrock, L. (1997). On stigma and its consequences: Evidence from a longitudinal study of men with dual diagnoses of mental illness and substance abuse. *Journal of Health and Social Behavior, 38,* 177–190.

Locust, C. (1988, June). *Integration of American Indian and scientific concepts of disability: Cross-cultural perspectives.* Paper presented at the meeting of the Society for Disability Studies, Washington, DC.

Lofland, J., & Lofland, L.H. (1995). *Analyzing social settings: A guide to qualitative observation and analysis.* Belmont, CA: Wadsworth.

Lynch, E.W., & Hanson, M.J. (Eds.). (1992). *Developing cross-cultural competence: A guide for working with young children and their families.* Baltimore: Paul Brookes.

Mairs, N. (1996). *Waist-high in the world: A life among the nondisabled.* Boston: Beacon Press.

Mandlebaum, A., & Wheeler, M.E. (1960). The meaning of a defective child to parents. *Social Casework, 41,* 360–367.

Manns, W. (1981). Support system of significant others in black families. In H.P. McAdoo (Ed.), *Black families* (pp. 238–251). Beverly Hills: Sage.

Marcos, L.R. (1979). Effects of interpreters on the evaluation of psychopathology in non-English-speaking patients. *American Journal of Psychiatry, 136,* 171–174.

Martin, L.L. (1993). *Total quality management in human service organizations.* Newbury Park, CA: Sage.

Martin, L.L., & Kettner, P.M. (1996). *Measuring the performance of human service programs.* Thousand Oaks, CA: Sage.

Massey, D.S., Zambrana, R.E., & Alonzo Bell, S. (1995). Contemporary issues in Latino families: Future directions for research, policy, and practice. In R.E. Zambrana (Ed.), *Understanding Latino families: Scholarship, policy, and practice* (pp. 190–204). Thousand Oaks, CA: Sage.

McAdoo, J.L. (1981). Involvement of fathers in the socialization of black children. In H.P. McAdoo (Ed.), *Black families.* Beverly Hills: Sage.

McGoldrick, M. (1982). Ethnicity and family therapy: An overview. In M. McGoldrick, J.K. Pearce, & J. Giordano (Eds.), *Ethnicity and family therapy* (pp. 3–30). New York: Guilford.

McHugh, P. (1968). *Defining the situation: The organization of meaning in social interaction.* Indianapolis: Boobs-Merrill.

McNeal, N., & Leach, P. (1997a, Winter). Health care strategies for working with the Amish community. *Pennsylvania Rural Health News, 7,* 3.

McNeal, N., & Leach, P. (1997b, Spring). Health care strategies for working with the Amish community. *Pennsylvania Rural Health News, 7,* 3.

Mercer, J.R. (1965). Social systems perspective and clinical perspective: Frames of reference for understanding career patterns of persons labeled as mentally retarded. *Social Problems, 13,* 18–34.

Mills, C.W. (1959). *The sociological imagination.* New York: Oxford University Press.

Minichiello, V., Aroni, R., Timewell, E., & Alexander, L. (1990). *In-depth interviewing: Researching people.* Melbourne: Longman Cheshire.

Minuchin, S. (1974). *Families and family therapy.* Cambridge, MA: Harvard University Press.

Minuchin, S. (1995). Foreword: Simple fable for a complex problem. In P. Adams & K. Nelson (Eds.), *Reinventing human services: Community- and family-centered practice* (pp. vii–ix). New York: Aldine de Gruyter.

Moeller, C.J. (1986). The effect of professionals on the family of a handicapped child. In R.R. Fewell & P.F. Vadasy (Eds.), *Families of handicapped children* (pp. 149–166). Austin, TX: Pro-Ed.

Moffett, D. (1997, February 16). Center to give families a hand. *The (Johnstown, PA) Tribune-Democrat,* p. 1.

Monette, D.R., Sullivan, T.J., & DeJong, C.R. (1994). *Applied social research: Tool for the human services.* Fort Worth: Harcourt Brace.

Monette, D.R., Sullivan, T.J., & DeJong, C.R. (1998). *Applied social research: Tool for the human services.* Fort Worth: Harcourt Brace.

Moore, E.D. (1991). Influencing legislation for the human services. In R.L. Edwards & J.A. Yankey (Eds.), *Skills for effective human service management* (pp. 76–89). Silver Spring, MD: NASW Press.

Moore, E.K. (1981). Policies affecting the status of black children and families. In H.P. McAdoo (Ed.), *Black families* (pp. 278–290). Beverly Hills: Sage.

Mullen, E.J., & Magnabosco, J.L. (1997). *Outcomes measurement in human services.* Washington, DC: NASW Press.

National Community Mental Healthcare Council. (1997). *Principles for behavioral healthcare delivery.* Rockville, MD: Author.

Nelson, K., & Allen, M. (1995). Family-centered social services: Moving toward system change. In P. Adams & K. Nelson (Eds.), *Reinventing human services: Community- and family-centered practice* (pp. 109–125). New York: Aldine de Gruyter.

Neuman, L.W. (1991). *Social research methods.* Needham Heights, MA: Allyn & Bacon.

O'Looney, J. (1996). *Redesigning the work of human services.* Westport, CT: Quorum.

Ortiz, V. (1995). Diversity of Latino families. In R.E. Zambrana (Ed.), *Understanding Latino families: Scholarship, policy, and practice* (pp. 18–39). Thousand Oaks, CA: Sage.

Osgood, C.E., Suci, G.J., & Tannenbaum, P.H. (1957). *The measurement of meaning.* Urbana: University of Illinois Press.

Parsons, T (Ed.). (1947). *Max Weber: The theory of social and economic organization.* New York: Oxford University Press.

Parsons, T. (1951). *The social system.* New York: The Free Press.

Past harassments still a cause of pain. (1995, November 6). *Johnstown Tribune-Democrat,* p. B2.

Patton, M.Q. (1987). *How to use qualitative methods in evaluation.* Newbury Park, CA: Sage.

Patton, M.Q. (1997). *Utilization-focused evaluation: The new century text.* Thousand Oaks, CA: Sage.

Pecora, P.J., Fraser, M.W., Nelson, K.E., McCroskey, J., & Meezan, W. (1995). *Evaluating family-based services.* New York: Aldine DeGruyter.

Pennsylvania Partnerships for Children. (1997). *Practical pointers on lobbying.*

Perske, R. (1972). The dignity of risk. In W. Wolfensberger (Ed.), *Normalization: The principle of normalization in human services* (pp. 194–200). Toronto: National Institute on Mental Retardation.

Peter, D. (1999). The client role: A help or a hindrance? *Disability and Society, 14,* 805–818.

Peter, M.I., & Sia, C.C.J. (1994). Preparing physicians through continuing medical education. In R.B. Darling & M.J. Peter (Eds.), *Families, physicians, and children with special health needs: Collaborative medical education models* (pp. 124–134). Westport, CT: Greenwood.

Pietrzak, J., Ramler, M., Renner, T., Ford, L., & Gilbert, N. (1990). *Practical program evaluation: Examples from child abuse prevention.* Newbury Park, CA: Sage.

Pizzo, P. (1983). *Parent to parent: Working together for ourselves and our children.* Boston: Beacon Press.

Polk, C. (1994). Therapeutic work with African-American families. *Zero to Three, 15,* 9–11.

Porteous, D. (1996). Methodologies for needs assessment. In J. Percy-Smith (Ed.), *Needs assessments in public policy* (pp. 32–46). Buckingham, England: Open University Press.

Powell, D.R. (1995). Including Latino fathers in parent education and support programs: Development of a program model. In R.E. Zambrana (Ed.), *Understanding Latino families: Scholarship, policy, and practice* (pp. 85–106). Thousand Oaks, CA: Sage.

Prattes, O. (1973). Section A: Beliefs of the Mexican-American family. In D. Hymovich & M. Barnard (Eds.), *Family health care* (pp. 128–137). New York: McGraw-Hill.

Quesada, G.M. (1976). Language and communication barriers for health delivery to a minority group. *Social Science and Medicine, 10,* 323–327.

Quine, L., & Pahl, J. (1986). First diagnosis of severe mental handicap: Characteristics of unsatisfactory encounters between doctors and parents. *Social Science and Medicine,* 22, 53–62.

Quint, J.C. (1965). Institutionalized practices of information control. *Psychiatry, 28,* 119–132.

Rapp, C.A., & Poertner, J. (1992). *Social administration: A client-centered approach.* White Plans, NY: Longman.

Ray, M.B. (1961). The cycle of abstinence and relapse among heroin addicts. *Social Problems, 9,* 132–140.

Reskin, B. (1993). Sex segregation in the workplace. *Annual Review of Sociology, 19,* 241–270.

Richan, W.C. (1991). *Lobbying for social change.* New York: Haworth Press.

Rodwell, M.K. (1995). Constructivist research: A qualitative approach. In P.J. Pecora et al. (Eds.), *Evaluating family-based services* (pp. 191–214). New York: Aldine DeGruyter.

Romaine, M.E. (1982). Clinical management of the Spanish-speaking patient: Pleasures and pitfalls. *Clinical Management in Physical Therapy, 2,* 9–10.

Roschelle, A.R. (1997). *No more kin: Exploring race, class, and gender in family networks.* Thousand Oaks, CA: Sage.

Rosenberg, M. (1965). *Society and the adolescent self-image.* Princeton, NJ: Princeton University Press.

Rossi, P.H. (1997). Program outcomes: Conceptual and measurement issues. In E.J. Mullen & J.L. Magnabosco (Eds.), *Outcomes measurements in human services* (pp. 20–34). Washington, DC: NASW Press.

Rossi, P.H., & Freeman, H.E. (1993). *Evaluation: A systematic approach.* Newbury Park, CA: Sage.

Rotunno, M., & McGoldrick, M. (1982). Italian families. In M. McGoldrick, J.K. Pearce, & J. Giordano (Eds.), *Ethnicity and family therapy* (pp. 340–363). New York: Guilford.

Rubin, H.J., & Rubin, I.S. (1995). *Qualitative interviewing: The art of hearing data.* Thousand Oaks, CA: Sage.

Rutman, L., & Mowbray, G. (1983). *Understanding program evaluation.* Beverly Hills, CA: Sage.

Sadker, M., & Sadker, D. (1994). *Failing at fairness.* New York: Scribner.

Samantrai, K. (1996). *Interviewing in health and human services.* Chicago: Nelson-Hall.

Schatzman, L., & Strauss, A.L. (1973). *Field research: Strategies for a natural sociology.* Englewood Cliffs, NJ: Prentice-Hall.

Scheff, T. (1966). *Being mentally ill: A sociological theory.* Chicago: Aldine.

Schonell, F.J. & Rorke, M. (1960). A second survey of the effects of a subnormal child on the family unit. *American Journal of Mental Deficiency, 64,*862–868.

Schonell, F.J. & Watts, B.H. (1956). A first survey of the effects of a subnormal child on the family unit. *American Journal of Mental Deficiency, 61,* 210–219.

Schorr, L. (1995). *The case for shifting to results-based accountability.* Washington, DC: Center for the Study of Social Policy.

Schorr, L.B. (1997). *Common purpose: Strengthening families and neighborhoods to rebuild America.* New York: Doubleday.

Schreiber, J.M., & Homiak, J.P. (1981). Mexican Americans. In A. Harwood (Ed.), *Ethnicity and medical care* (pp. 264–336). Cambridge, MA: Harvard University Press.

Schwartz, D.B. (1987). *Who cares? Rediscovering community.* Boulder, CO: Westview Press.

Seligman, M., & Darling, R.B. (1997). *Ordinary families, special children: A systems approach to childhood disability* (2nd ed.). New York: Guilford.

Shadish, W.R., Jr., Cook, T.D., & Leviton, L.C. (1991). *Foundations of program evaluation: Theories of practice.* Newbury Park, CA: Sage.

Shapiro, J. & Tittle, K. (1986). Psychosocial adjustment of poor Mexican mothers of disabled and nondisabled children. *American Journal of Orthopsychiatry, 56,* 289–302.

Shibutani, T. (1961). *Society and personality: An interactionist approach to social psychology.* Englewood Cliffs, NJ: Prentice Hall.

Shon, S.P., & Ja, D.Y. (1982). Asian families: In M. McGoldrick, J.K. Pearce, & J. Giordano (Eds.), *Ethnicity and family therapy* (pp. 208–228). New York: Guilford.

Simeonsson, R. (1988). Evaluating the effects of family-focused intervention. In D. Bailey & R. Simeonsson (Eds.), *Family assessment and early intervention* (p. 257). Columbus, OH: Merrill.

Simon, B.L. (1994). *The empowerment tradition in American social work: A history.* New York: Columbia University Press.

Sluyter, G.V. (1998). *Improving organizational performance: A practical guidebook for the human services field.* Thousand Oaks, CA: Sage.

Smith, E.R., & Kluegel, J.R. (1984). Beliefs and attitudes about women's opportunity. *Social Psychology Quarterly, 47,* 81–95.

Snow, D.A., & Anderson, L. (1993). *Down on their luck: A study of homeless street people.* Berkeley: University of California Press.

Solnit, A., & Stark, M.H. (1961). Mourning and the birth of a defective child. *The Psychoanalytic Study of the Child, 16,* 523–537.

Sontag, J.C., & Schacht, R. (1994). An ethnic comparison of parent participation and information needs in early intervention. *Exceptional Children, 60,* 422–433.

Spano, S.L. (1994). The miracle of Michael. In R.B. Darling & M.I. Peter (Eds.), *Families, physicians, and children with special health needs: Collaborative medical education models* (pp. 29–50). Westport, CT: Auburn House.

Specht, H. & Courtney, M.E. (1994). *Unfaithful angels: How social work has abandoned its mission.* New York: The Free Press.

Spector, R.E. *Cultural diversity in health and illness.* New York: Appleton-Century-Crofts.

Stack, C. (1974). *All our kin.* New York: Basic Books.

Staples, R. (1976). The black American family. In C.H. Mindel & R.W. Habenstein (Eds.), *Ethnic families in America: Patterns and variations* (pp. 221–247). New York: Elsevier.

Stecher, B.M., & Davis, W.A. (1987). *How to focus an evaluation.* Newbury Park, CA: Sage.

Stein, R.C. (1983). Hispanic parent perspectives and participation in the children's special education program: Comparisons by program and race. *Learning Disability Quarterly, 6,* 432–439.

Stewart, D.W., & Shamdasani, P.N. (1998). Focus group research: Exploration and discovery. In L. Bickman & D.J. Rog (Eds.), *Handbook of applied social research methods* (pp. 505–526). Thousand Oaks, CA: Sage.

Stoneham, Z. (1985). Family involvement in early childhood special education programs. In N.H. Fallen & W. Umansky (Eds.), *Young children with special needs* (2nd ed., pp. 442–469). Columbus, OH: Charles E. Merrill.

Stotland, J. (1984, February). Relationship of parents to professionals: A challenge to professionals. *Journal of Visual Impairment and Blindness,* 69–74.

Strauss, A. (1962). Transformations of identity. In A.M. Rose (Ed.), *Human behavior and social processes* (pp. 63–85). Boston: Houghton Mifflin.

Sudarkasa, N. (1981). Interpreting the African heritage in Afro-American family organization. In H.P. McAdoo (Ed.), *Black families* (pp. 37–53). Beverly Hills: Sage.

Sullivan, H.S. (1947). The human organism and its necessary environment. In *Conceptions of modern psychiatry* (pp. 14–27). Washington, DC: William Alanson White Psychiatric Foundation.

Sussman, G.I. (1983). Action research: A sociotechnical systems perspective. In G. Morgan (Ed.), *Beyond method: Strategies for social research* (pp. 95–114). Beverly Hills, CA: Sage.

Svarstad, B.L., & Lipton, H.E. (1977). Informing parents about mental retardation: A study of professional communication and parent acceptance. *Social Science and Medicine, 11,* 645–651.

Swadener, B.B., & Lubeck, S. (1995). *Children and families "at promise": Deconstructing the discourse of risk.* Albany: State University of New York Press.

Tannen, D. (1994). *Talking from 9 to 5—Women and men in the workplace: Language, sex and power.* New York: Avon books.

Taylor, S.J., & Bogdan, R. (1984). *Introduction to qualitative research methods: The search for meanings.* New York: John Wiley & Sons.

Thomas, W.I. (1928). *The child in America: Behavior problems and programs.* New York: Alfred A. Knopf.

Thurman, Q.C. (1995). Community policing: The police as a community resource. In P. Adams & K. Nelson (Eds.), *Reinventing human services: Community- and family-centered practice* (pp. 175–187). New York: Aldine de Gruyter.

Timberlake, E., & Cook, K. (1984). Social work and the Vietnamese refugee. *Social Work, 29,* 108–114.

Toch, H., & Grant, J.D. (1982). *Reforming human services: Change through participation.* Newbury Park, CA: Sage.

Tolson, T.F.J., & Wilson, M.N. (1990). The impact of two-and three-generational black family structure on perceived family climate. *Child Development, 61,* 416–428.

Topics in Early Childhood Special Education. (1986). *6*(2).

Topics in Early Childhood Special Education. (1990). *10*(1).

Turnbull, A.P. & Turnbull, H.R., III. (1990). *Families, professionals, and exceptionality: A special partnership.* Columbus, OH: Merrill.

University of Pittsburgh Office of Child Development. (1991). Black families: An inquiry into the issues. *Developments, 5*(1), 5–8.

VanDenBerg, J., & Grealish, E.M. (1997). Finding family strengths: A multiple-choice test. *Reaching Today's Youth, The Community Circle of Caring Journal, 1* (http://www.air.org/cecp/wraparound/articles.html).

Vega, W.A. (1995). The study of Latino families: A point of departure. In R.E. Zambrana (Ed.), *Understanding Latino families: Scholarship, policy, and practice* (pp. 3–17).; Thousand Oaks, CA: Sage.

Ware, J.E., Jr. (1997). Health care outcomes from the patient's point of view. In E.J. Mullen & J.L. Magnabosco (Eds.), *Outcomes measurement in human services* (pp. 44–67). Washington, DC: NASW Press.

Wasow, M. (1997). Outcomes measurement and the mental health consumer advocacy movement. In E.J. Mullen & J.L. Magnabosco (Eds.), *Outcomes measurement in human services* (pp. 160–169). Washington, DC: NASW Press.

Wayman, K.I., Lynch, E.W., & Hanson, M.J. (1991). Home-based early intervention services: Cultural sensitivity in a family systems approach. *Topics in Early Childhood Special Education, 10,* 56–75.

Weber, M. (1949). *Theory of social and economic organization.* New York: The Free Press.

Weiss, C. (1986). Validity of mother's interview responses. *Public Opinion Quarterly, 32,* 622–633.

Wells, A.S. (1998, April 5). For baby boomers, a 90s kind of sit-in. *New York Times, Education Life,* pp. 22–23, 33–34.

Wells, K. & Biegel, D.E. (Eds.). (1991). *Family preservation services: Research and evaluation.* Newbury Park, CA: Sage.

Wells, K., & Freer, R. (1994). Reading between the lines: The case for qualitative research in intensive family preservation services. *Children and Youth Services Review, 16,* 399–415.

Wendeborn, J.D. (1982). Administrative considerations in treating the Hispanic patient. *Clinical Management in Physical Therapy, 2,* 6–7.

White, C.J. (1995). Native Americans at promise: Travel in borderlands. In B.B. Swadener & S. Lubeck (Eds.), *Children and families "at promise": Deconstructing the discourse of risk* (pp. 163–184). Albany: State University of New York Press.

Whittaker, J.K., Kenney, J., Tracy, E.M., & Booth, C. (Eds.). (1990). *Reaching high risk families: Intensive family preservation in human services.* Hawthorne, NY: Aldine de Gruyter.

Wice, B., & Fernandez, H. (1984, October). Meeting the bureaucracy face to face: Parent power in the Philadelphia schools. *Exceptional Parent,* 36–41.

Wilensky, H.L., & Lebeaux, C.N. (1965), *Industrial society and social welfare.* New York: The Free Press.

Williams, H.B., & Williams, E. (1979). Some aspects of childrearing practices in three minority subcultures in the United States. *Journal of Negro Education, 48,* 408–418.

Winton, P.J., & Bailey, D.B., Jr. (1988). The family-focused interview: A collaborative mechanism for family assessment and goal setting. *Journal of the Division for Early Childhood, 12*(3), 195–207.

Wolfensberger, W. (1972). *Normalization: The principle of normalization in human services.* Toronto: National Institute on Mental Retardation.

Wood, G.G., & Middleman, R.R. (1989). *The structural approach to direct practice in social work: A textbook for students and front-line practitioners.* New York: Columbia University Press.

Yee, L.Y. (1988). Asian children. *Teaching Exceptional Children, 20*(4), 49–50.

Zambrana, R.E., Dorrington, C., & Hayes-Bautista, D. (1995). Family and child health: A neglected vision. In R.E. Zambrnana (Ed.), *Understanding Latino families: Scholarship, policy, and practice* (pp. 157–176). Thousand Oaks, CA: Sage.

Zigler, E., & Black, K.B. (1989). America's family support movement: Strengths and limitations. *American Journal of Orthopsychiatry, 59,* 6–19.

Zinn, M.B., & Eitzen, D.S. (1993). *Diversity in families.* New York: Harper Collins.

About the Author

Rosalyn Benjamin Darling is Associate Professor of Sociology and Coordinator of the doctoral program in Administration and Leadership Studies at Indiana University of Pennsylvania, where she also teaches courses in human services theory and administration, disability and society, and at-risk children. Prior to accepting a full-time university appointment six years ago, Dr. Darling served for 15 years as a program supervisor and as the Executive Director of Beginnings, an agency serving young children and their families. In that capacity, she also served as President of the Early Intervention Providers Association of Pennsylvania and as a member of various state-level policy advisory committees. She currently serves on the National Commission on Applied and Clinical Sociology. Dr. Darling is the author of six other books, as well as numerous articles and book chapters.

Index